2004 EDITION

INJURY FACTS®

NATIONAL SAFETY COUNCIL

FORMERLY ACCIDENT FACTS®

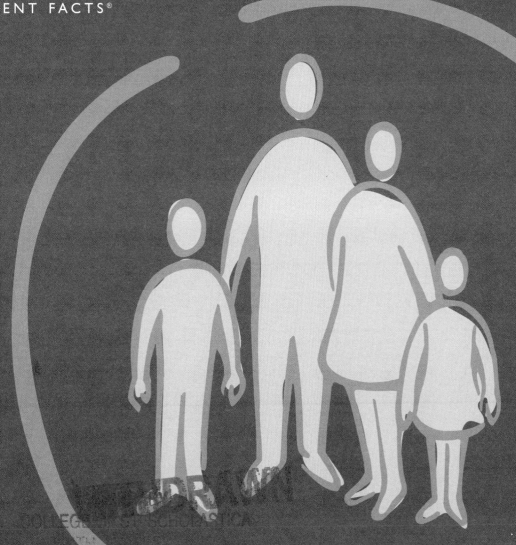

The National Safety Council, chartered by an act of Congress, is a nongovernmental, not-for-profit, public service organization devoted solely to educating and influencing society to adopt safety, health, and environmental policies, practices, and procedures that prevent and mitigate human suffering and economic losses arising from preventable causes.

Injury Facts®, the Council's annual statistical report on unintentional injuries and their characteristics and costs, was prepared by:

Research and Statistical Services Group
Mei-Li Lin, Executive Director
Alan F. Hoskin, Manager, Statistics Department
Kevin T. Fearn, Sr. Statistical Associate
Kathleen T. Porretta, Production Manager
Sergey Sinelnikov, Research Associate

Questions or comments about the content of *Injury Facts*® should be directed to the Research and Statistics Department, National Safety Council, 1121 Spring Lake Drive, Itasca, IL 60143, or telephone 630-775-2322, or fax 630-285-0242, or E-mail rssdept@nsc.org.

For price and ordering information, write Customer Relations, National Safety Council, 1121 Spring Lake Drive, Itasca, IL 60143, or telephone 800-621-7619, or fax 630-285-0797.

Acknowledgments
The information presented in *Injury Facts*® was made possible by the cooperation of many organizations and individuals, including state vital and health statistics authorities, state traffic authorities, state workers' compensation authorities, trade associations, Bureau of the Census, Bureau of Labor Statistics, Consumer Product Safety Commission, Federal Highway Administration, Federal Railroad Administration, International Labour Office, International Road Federation, National Center for Health Statistics, National Fire Protection Association, National Highway Traffic Safety Administration, National Transportation Safety Board, National Weather Service, Mine Safety and Health Administration, and the World Health Organization. Specific contributions are acknowledged in footnotes and source notes throughout the book.

Visit the National Safety Council's website:

http://www.nsc.org

Suggested citation: National Safety Council. (2004). *Injury Facts*®, *2004 Edition*. Itasca, IL: Author.

Library of Congress Catalog Card Number: 99–74142

Printed in U.S.A.   ISBN 0–87912–258–7   NSC Press Product No. 02304–0000

FOREWORD

Unintentional-injury deaths were down 2% in 2003 compared to the revised 2002 total. Unintentional-injury deaths were estimated to total 101,500 in 2003 and 103,500 in 2002.

The resident population of the United States was 290,810,000 in 2003, an increase of 1% from 2002. The death rate in 2003 was 34.9 per 100,000 population — 3% lower than the rate in 2002 and 3% greater than the lowest rate on record, which was 34.0 in 1992.

The graph on page v shows the overall trends in the number of unintentional-injury deaths, the population, and the death rate per 100,000 population. A more complete summary of the situation in 2003 and recent trends is given on page 2.

Changes in the 2004 Edition

Once again, some important changes have been made to improve *Injury Facts*®. A new chapter on International Data has been added beginning on page 165. It includes data on all unintentional-injury deaths, motor-vehicle deaths, and work-related deaths by country. The chapter on Home and Community has been reorganized to keep the overall estimates together at the beginning of the chapter with the special subjects following.

Look for *new* data on …

• Relative risk of work injury by age and sex

• Comprehensive estimates of work injuries

• Mining injury data from MSHA

• High-visibility enforcement of safety belt laws

• Senior safety and mobility

• War and terrorism deaths

• Ozone

• Childhood asthma

• Drowning

• Electrocutions

• Falls and hip fractures

• And more

and *updated* or *expanded* data on …

• General mortality

• Industry division profiles

• Occupational injury and illness incidence rates by industry

• Workers' compensation claims and costs

• Comparing safety of transportation modes

• Highway work zones

• Sports injuries

• Consumer product-related injuries

• State-level data

• And more

We welcome your comments and suggestions to improve *Injury Facts*®. Information on how to contact us is given on page ii.

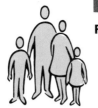

UNINTENTIONAL-INJURY DEATHS, DEATH RATES, AND POPULATION, UNITED STATES, 1903–2003

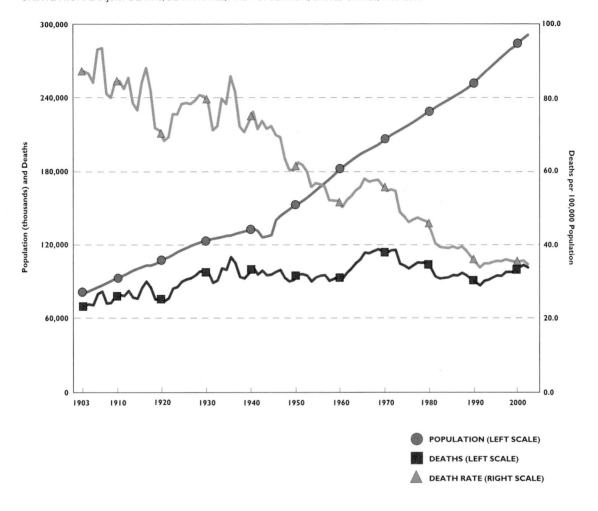

POPULATION (LEFT SCALE)

DEATHS (LEFT SCALE)

DEATH RATE (RIGHT SCALE)

INJURY FACTS®

NATIONAL SAFETY COUNCIL

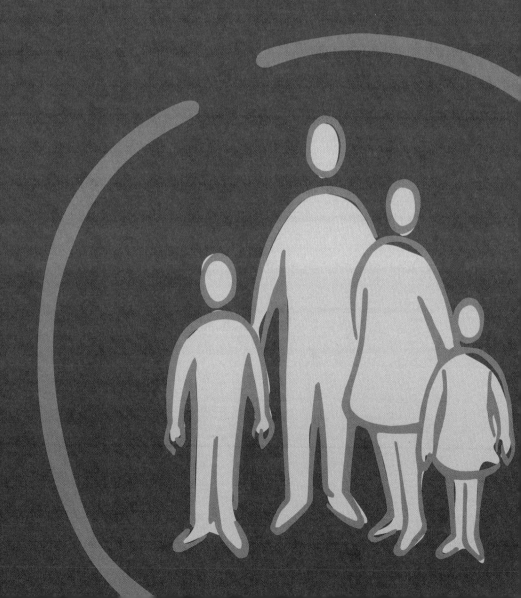

2

Unintentional-injury deaths were down 2% in 2003 compared to the revised 2002 total. Unintentional-injury deaths were estimated to total 101,500 in 2003 and 103,500 in 2002. The 2003 estimate is virtually unchanged from the 2001 final count of 101,537. The 2003 figure is 17% greater than the 1992 total of 86,777 (the lowest annual total since 1924) and 13% below the 1969 peak of 116,385 deaths.

The death rate in 2003 was 34.9 per 100,000 population — 3% greater than the lowest rate on record, which was 34.0 in 1992. The 2003 death rate was 3% lower than the 2002 revised rate of 35.9.

Comparing 2003 to 2002, public, home, and work deaths decreased while motor-vehicle deaths increased. The population death rates in the public, home, and work classes also declined and the rate increased in the motor-vehicle class.

The motor-vehicle death total was up 2% in 2003. The motor-vehicle death rate per 100,000,000 vehicle-miles was 1.56 in 2003, up 1.3% from the revised 2002 rate (1.54) and down 0.6% from the revised 2001 rate of 1.57.

According to the latest final data (2001), unintentional injuries continued to be the fifth leading cause of death, exceeded only by heart disease, cancer, stroke, and chronic lower respiratory diseases. Preliminary death certificate data for 2002 indicate that unintentional injuries will remain in fifth place.

Nonfatal injuries also affect millions of Americans. In 2002, about 23.7 million people — about 1 out of 12 — sought medical attention for an injury. About 2.7 million people were hospitalized for injuries and about 39.2 million were treated in hospital emergency departments in 2002. In 2001, about 11.1 million visits to outpatient departments and about 99.8 million visits to physicians' offices were due to injuries.

The economic impact of these fatal and nonfatal unintentional injuries amounted to $607.7 billion in 2003. This is equivalent to about $2,100 per capita, or about $5,700 per household. These are costs that every individual and household pays whether directly out of pocket, through higher prices for goods and services, or through higher taxes.

Between 1912 and 2003, unintentional-injury deaths per 100,000 population were reduced 55% (after adjusting for the classification change in 1948) from 82.4 to 34.9. The reduction in the overall rate during a period when the nation's population tripled has resulted in 4,800,000 fewer people being killed due to unintentional injuries than there would have been if the rate had not been reduced.

ALL UNINTENTIONAL INJURIES, 2003

Class	2003 Deaths	Change from 2002	Deaths per 100,000 Persons	Disabling Injuries[a]
All Classes[b]	101,500	–2%	34.9	20,700,000
Motor-vehicle	44,800	+2%	15.4	2,400,000
Public nonwork	42,600			2,300,000
Work	2,000			100,000
Home	200			([c])
Work	4,500	–5%	1.5	3,400,000
Nonmotor-vehicle	2,500			3,300,000
Motor-vehicle	2,000			100,000
Home	33,100	–6%	11.4	7,900,000
Nonmotor-vehicle	32,900			7,900,000
Motor-vehicle	200			([c])
Public	21,300	–1%	7.3	7,100,000

Source: National Safety Council estimates (rounded) based on data from the National Center for Health Statistics, Bureau of Labor Statistics, state departments of health, state traffic authorities, and state industrial commissions. The National Safety Council adopted the Bureau of Labor Statistics' Census of Fatal Occupational Injuries count for work-related unintentional injuries retroactive to 1992 data. See the Glossary for definitions and the Technical Appendix for revised estimating procedures. Beginning with 1999 data, which became available in September 2001, deaths are now classified according to the 10th revision of the International Classification of Diseases. Overall, about 3% more deaths are classified as due to "unintentional injuries" under the new classification system than under the 9th revision. The difference varies across causes of death. See the Technical Appendix for more information on comparability. Caution should be used in comparing data classified under the two systems.
[a]Disabling beyond the day of injury. Disabling injuries are not reported on a national basis, so the totals shown are approximations based on ratios of disabling injuries to deaths developed by the National Safety Council. The totals are the best estimates for the current year. They should not, however, be compared with totals shown in previous editions of this book to indicate year-to-year changes or trends. See the Glossary for definitions and the Technical Appendix for estimating procedures.
[b]Deaths and injuries above for the four separate classes add to more than the All Classes figures due to rounding and because some deaths and injuries are included in more than one class. For example, 2,000 work deaths involved motor vehicles in transport and are in both the Work and Motor-vehicle totals and 200 motor-vehicle deaths occurred on home premises and are in both Home and Motor-vehicle. The total of such duplication amounted to about 2,200 deaths and 100,000 injuries in 2003.
[c]Less than 10,000.

UNINTENTIONAL-INJURY DEATHS BY CLASS, UNITED STATES, 2003

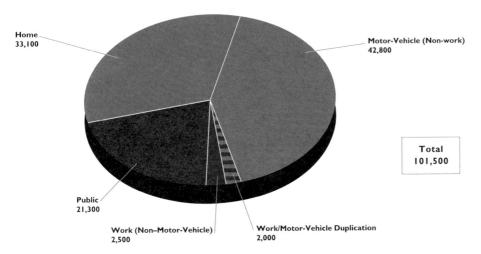

Home
33,100

Motor-Vehicle (Non-work)
42,800

Total
101,500

Public
21,300

Work (Non–Motor-Vehicle)
2,500

Work/Motor-Vehicle Duplication
2,000

UNINTENTIONAL DISABLING INJURIES BY CLASS, UNITED STATES, 2003

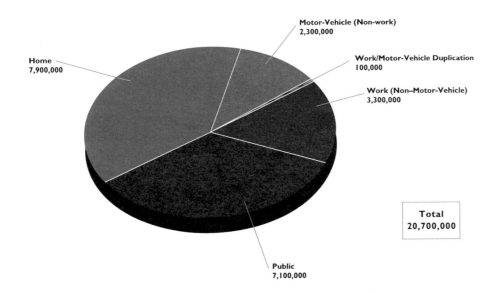

Motor-Vehicle (Non-work)
2,300,000

Work/Motor-Vehicle Duplication
100,000

Work (Non–Motor-Vehicle)
3,300,000

Home
7,900,000

Total
20,700,000

Public
7,100,000

COSTS OF UNINTENTIONAL INJURIES BY CLASS, 2003

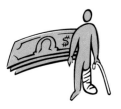

The total cost of unintentional injuries in 2003, $607.7 billion, includes estimates of economic costs of fatal and nonfatal unintentional injuries together with uninsured employer costs, vehicle damage costs, and fire losses. Wage and productivity losses, medical expenses, administrative expenses, and uninsured employer costs are included in all four classes of injuries. Cost components unique to each class are identified below.

Motor-vehicle costs include property damage from motor-vehicle accidents. Work costs include the value of property damage in on-the-job motor-vehicle accidents and fires. Home and public costs include estimated fire losses, but do not include other property damage costs.

Besides the estimated $607.7 billion in economic losses from unintentional injuries in 2003, lost quality of life from those injuries is valued at an additional $1,366.6 billion, making the comprehensive cost $1,974.3 billion in 2003.

Cost estimating procedures were revised extensively for the 1993 edition of *Accident Facts®*. New components were added, new benchmarks adopted, and a new discount rate assumed (see the Technical Appendix). In general, cost estimates are not comparable from year to year. As additional or more precise data become available, they are used from that point forward. Previously estimated figures are not revised.

CERTAIN COSTS OF UNINTENTIONAL INJURIES BY CLASS, 2003 ($ BILLIONS)

Cost	Total[a]	Motor-Vehicle	Work	Home	Public Nonmotor-Vehicle
Total	**$607.7**	**$240.7**	**$156.2**	**$135.1**	**$95.4**
Wage and productivity losses	301.5	82.4	78.3	84.3	60.5
Medical expenses	118.7	31.5	30.9	33.5	24.4
Administrative expenses[b]	103.7	75.8	28.7	6.0	4.9
Motor-vehicle damage	48.8	48.8	2.0	(c)	(c)
Uninsured employer cost	24.5	2.2	13.7	5.0	4.0
Fire loss	10.5	(c)	2.6	6.3	1.6

Source: National Safety Council estimates. See the Technical Appendix.
[a]Duplication between work and motor-vehicle, which amounted to $19.7 billion, was eliminated from the total.
[b]Home and public insurance administration costs may include costs of administering medical treatment claims for some motor-vehicle injuries filed through health insurance plans.
[c]Not included; see comments above.

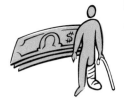

COSTS OF UNINTENTIONAL INJURIES BY CLASS, 2003

TOTAL COST $607.7 BILLION

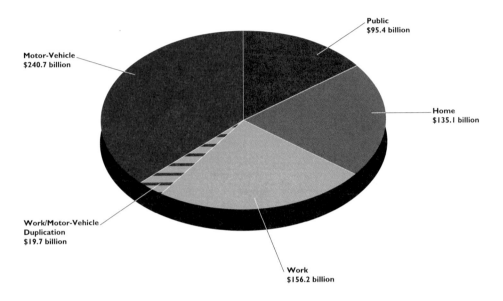

Public
$95.4 billion

Motor-Vehicle
$240.7 billion

Home
$135.1 billion

Work/Motor-Vehicle
Duplication
$19.7 billion

Work
$156.2 billion

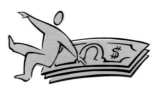

Wage and Productivity Losses

A person's contribution to the wealth of the nation usually is measured in terms of wages and household production. The total of wages and fringe benefits together with an estimate of the replacement-cost value of household services provides an estimate of this lost productivity. Also included is travel delay for motor-vehicle accidents.

Medical Expenses

Doctor fees, hospital charges, the cost of medicines, future medical costs, and ambulance, helicopter, and other emergency medical services are included.

Administrative Expenses

Include the administrative cost of public and private insurance, and police and legal costs. Private insurance administrative costs are the difference between premiums paid to insurance companies and claims paid out by them. It is their cost of doing business and is a part of the cost total. Claims paid by insurance companies are not identified separately, as every claim is compensation for losses such as wages, medical expenses, property damage, etc.

Motor-Vehicle Damage

Includes the value of damage to vehicles from motor-vehicle crashes. The cost of normal wear and tear to vehicles is not included.

Uninsured Employer Costs

This is an estimate of the uninsured costs incurred by employers, representing the dollar value of time lost by uninjured workers. It includes time spent investigating and reporting injuries, giving first aid, hiring and training of replacement workers, and the extra cost of overtime for uninjured workers.

Fire Loss

Includes losses from both structure fires and nonstructure fires such as vehicles, outside storage, crops, and timber.

Work–Motor-Vehicle Duplication

The cost of motor-vehicle crashes that involve persons in the course of their work is included in both classes, but the duplication is eliminated from the total. The duplication in 2003 amounted to $19.7 billion and was made up of $4.0 billion in wage and productivity losses, $1.6 billion in medical expenses, $11.7 billion in administrative expenses, $2.0 billion in vehicle damage, and $0.4 billion in uninsured employer costs.

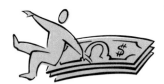

COSTS OF UNINTENTIONAL INJURIES BY COMPONENT, 2003

TOTAL COST $607.7 BILLION

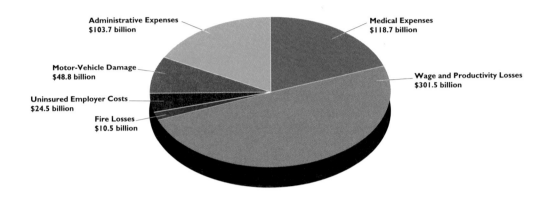

Administrative Expenses
$103.7 billion

Medical Expenses
$118.7 billion

Motor-Vehicle Damage
$48.8 billion

Wage and Productivity Losses
$301.5 billion

Uninsured Employer Costs
$24.5 billion

Fire Losses
$10.5 billion

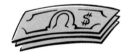

COST EQUIVALENTS

The costs of unintentional injuries are immense — billions of dollars. Since figures this large can be difficult to comprehend, it is sometimes useful to reduce the numbers to a more understandable scale by relating them to quantities encountered in daily life. The table below shows how the costs of unintentional injuries compare to common quantities such as taxes, corporate profits, or stock dividends.

COST EQUIVALENTS, 2003

The Cost of ...	Is Equivalent to ...
... All Injuries ($607.7 billion)	...80 cents of every dollar paid in federal personal income taxes, **or** ...57 cents of every dollar spent on food in the U.S.
... Motor-Vehicle Crashes ($240.7 billion)	...purchasing 630 gallons of gasoline for each registered vehicle in the U.S., **or** ...more than $1,200 per licensed driver.
... Work Injuries ($156.2 billion)	...36 cents of every dollar of corporate dividends to stockholders, **or** ...18 cents of every dollar of pre-tax corporate profits, **or** ...exceeds the combined profits reported by the top 25 Fortune 500 companies.
... Home Injuries ($135.1 billion)	...a $97,500 rebate on each new single-family home built, **or** ...44 cents of every dollar of property taxes paid.
... Public Injuries ($95.4 billion)	...a $10.5 million grant to each public library in the U.S., **or** ...a $97,100 bonus for each police officer and firefighter.

Source: National Safety Council estimates.

DEATHS DUE TO UNINTENTIONAL INJURIES, 2003

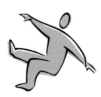

TYPE OF EVENT AND AGE OF VICTIM

All Unintentional Injuries

The term "unintentional" covers most deaths from injury and poisoning. Excluded are homicides (including legal intervention), suicides, deaths for which none of these categories can be determined, and war deaths.

	Total	Change from 2002	Death Rate[a]
Deaths	101,500	−2%	34.9

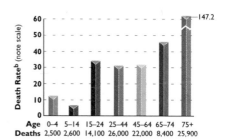

Motor-Vehicle Accidents

Includes deaths involving mechanically or electrically powered highway-transport vehicles in motion (except those on rails), both on and off the highway or street.

	Total	Change from 2002	Death Rate[a]
Deaths	44,800	+2%	15.4

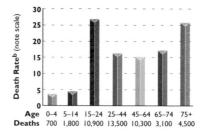

Falls

Includes deaths from falls from one level to another or on the same level. Excludes falls in or from transport vehicles, or while boarding or alighting from them.

	Total	Change from 2002	Death Rate[a]
Deaths	16,200	+6%	5.6

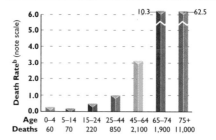

Poisoning

Includes deaths from drugs, medicines, other solid and liquid substances, and gases and vapors. Excludes poisonings from spoiled foods, salmonella, etc., which are classified as disease deaths.

	Total	Change from 2002	Death Rate[a]
Deaths	13,900	−14%	4.8

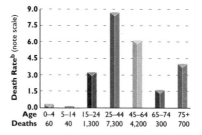

Choking

Includes deaths from unintentional ingestion or inhalation of food or other objects, resulting in the obstruction of respiratory passages.

	Total	Change from 2002	Death Rate[a]
Deaths	4,300	−2%	1.5

See footnotes on page 9.

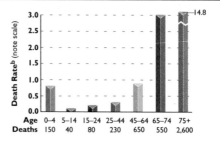

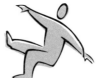

Drowning

Includes nontransport-related drownings such as those resulting from swimming, playing in the water, or falling in. Excludes drownings in floods and other cataclysms, which are classified to the cataclysm, and boating-related drownings.

	Total	Change from 2002	Death Rate[a]
Deaths	2,900	−3%	1.0

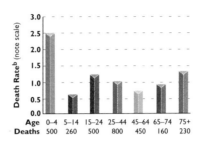

Age	0–4	5–14	15–24	25–44	45–64	65–74	75+
Deaths	500	260	500	800	450	160	230

Fires, Flames, and Smoke

Includes deaths from exposure to fires, flames, and smoke, and from injuries in fires — such as falls and being struck by falling objects. Excludes burns from hot objects or liquids.

	Total	Change from 2002	Death Rate[a]
Deaths	2,600	−7%	0.9

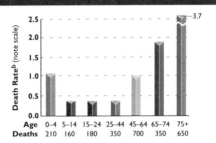

Age	0–4	5–14	15–24	25–44	45–64	65–74	75+
Deaths	210	160	180	350	700	350	650

Mechanical Suffocation

Includes deaths from hanging and strangulation, and suffocation in enclosed or confined spaces, cave-ins, or by bed clothes, plastic bags, or similar materials.

	Total	Change from 2002	Death Rate[a]
Deaths	1,200	−20%	0.4

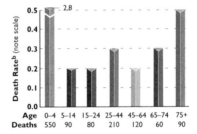

Age	0–4	5–14	15–24	25–44	45–64	65–74	75+
Deaths	550	90	80	210	120	60	90

Natural Heat or Cold

Includes deaths resulting from exposure to excessive natural heat and cold (e.g., extreme weather conditions).

	Total	Change from 2002	Death Rate[a]
Deaths	800	0%	0.3

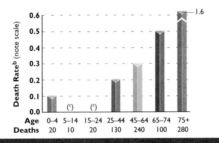

Age	0–4	5–14	15–24	25–44	45–64	65–74	75+
Deaths	20	10	20	130	240	100	280

All Other Types

Most important types included are: firearms, struck by or against object, machinery, electric current, and air, water, and rail transport.

	Total	Change from 2002	Death Rate[a]
Deaths	14,800	−5%	5.1

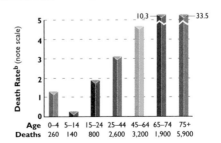

Age	0–4	5–14	15–24	25–44	45–64	65–74	75+
Deaths	260	140	800	2,600	3,200	1,900	5,900

Note: Category descriptions have changed due to adoption of ICD-10. See Technical Appendix for comparablity.
[a]Deaths per 100,000 population.
[b]Deaths per 100,000 population in each age group.
[c]Death rate less than 0.05.

LEADING CAUSES OF DEATH

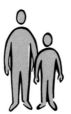

Unintentional injuries are the fifth leading cause of death overall and first among persons in age groups from 1 to 34. By single years of age, unintentional injuries are the leading cause from 1 to 39.

Causes are ranked for both sexes combined. Some leading causes for males and females separately may not

be shown. Beginning with 1999 data, deaths are classified according to the 10th revision of the *International Classification of Diseases*. See the Technical Appendix for comparability.

DEATHS AND DEATH RATES BY AGE AND SEX, 2001

Cause	Number of Deaths			Death Rates[a]		
	Total	Male	Female	Total	Male	Female
All Ages[b]						
All Causes	2,416,425	1,183,421	1,233,004	847.6	845.5	849.6
Heart disease	700,142	339,095	361,047	245.6	242.3	248.8
Cancer (malignant neoplasms)	553,768	287,075	266,693	194.2	205.1	183.8
Stroke (cerebrovascular disease)	163,538	63,177	100,361	57.4	45.1	69.2
Chronic lower respiratory diseases	123,013	59,697	63,316	43.1	42.7	43.6
Unintentional injuries	**101,537**	**66,060**	**35,477**	**35.6**	**47.2**	**24.4**
Motor-vehicle	43,788	30,064	13,724	15.4	21.5	9.5
Falls	15,019	8,089	6,930	5.3	5.8	4.8
Poisoning	14,078	9,885	4,193	4.9	7.1	2.9
Choking[c]	4,185	2,113	2,072	1.5	1.5	1.4
Drowning	3,281	2,560	721	1.2	1.8	0.5
All other unintentional injuries	21,186	13,349	7,837	7.4	9.5	5.4
Diabetes mellitus	71,372	32,841	38,531	25.0	23.5	26.5
Influenza and pneumonia	62,034	27,342	34,692	21.8	19.5	23.9
Alzheimer's disease	53,852	15,762	38,090	18.9	11.3	26.2
Nephritis and nephrosis	39,480	18,852	20,628	13.8	13.5	14.2
Septicemia	32,238	14,307	17,931	11.3	10.2	12.4
Under 1 Year						
All Causes	**27,568**	**15,477**	**12,091**	**684.5**	**752.3**	**613.7**
Congenital anomalies	5,513	2,954	2,559	136.9	143.6	129.9
Short gestation, low birth weight, n.e.c.	4,410	2,426	1,984	109.5	117.9	100.7
Sudden infant death syndrome	2,234	1,317	917	55.5	64.0	46.5
Maternal complications of pregnancy	1,499	847	652	37.2	41.2	33.1
Complications of placenta, cord, membranes	1,018	582	436	25.3	28.3	22.1
Respiratory distress	1,011	574	437	25.1	27.9	22.2
Unintentional injuries	**976**	**541**	**435**	**24.2**	**26.3**	**22.1**
Mechanical suffocation	552	316	236	13.7	15.4	12.0
Motor-vehicle	144	66	78	3.6	3.2	4.0
Drowning	68	30	38	1.7	1.5	1.9
Choking[c]	62	42	20	1.5	2.0	1.0
Fires and flames	50	30	20	1.2	1.5	1.0
All other unintentional injuries	100	57	43	2.5	2.8	2.2
Bacterial sepsis	696	404	292	17.3	19.6	14.8
Diseases of the circulatory system	622	326	296	15.4	15.8	15.0
Intrauterine hypoxia and birth asphyxia	534	295	239	13.3	14.3	12.1
1 to 4 Years						
All Causes	**5,107**	**2,899**	**2,208**	**33.3**	**37.0**	**29.5**
Unintentional injuries	**1,714**	**1,045**	**669**	**11.2**	**13.3**	**8.9**
Motor-vehicle	626	356	270	4.1	4.5	3.6
Drowning	458	291	167	3.0	3.7	2.2
Fires and flames	225	142	83	1.5	1.8	1.1
Choking[c]	74	45	29	0.5	0.6	0.4
Mechanical suffocation	64	38	26	0.4	0.5	0.3
All other unintentional injuries	267	173	94	1.7	2.2	1.3
Congenital anomalies	557	282	275	3.6	3.6	3.7
Cancer (malignant neoplasms)	420	229	191	2.7	2.9	2.6
Homicide	415	238	177	2.7	3.0	2.4
Heart disease	225	121	104	1.5	1.5	1.4
Influenza and pneumonia	112	57	55	0.7	0.7	0.7
Septicemia	108	60	48	0.7	0.8	0.6
Certain conditions originating in the perinatal period	72	44	28	0.5	0.6	0.4
Benign neoplasms	58	30	28	0.4	0.4	0.4
Stroke (cerebrovascular disease)	54	25	29	0.4	0.3	0.4

See source and footnotes on page 12.

DEATHS AND DEATH RATES BY AGE AND SEX, 2001, Cont.

Cause	Number of Deaths			Death Rates[a]		
	Total	Male	Female	Total	Male	Female
5 to 14 Years						
All Causes	**7,095**	**4,168**	**2,927**	**17.3**	**19.8**	**14.6**
Unintentional injuries	**2,836**	**1,803**	**1,033**	**6.9**	**8.6**	**5.2**
Motor-vehicle	1,686	1,029	657	4.1	4.9	3.3
Drowning	333	237	96	0.8	1.1	0.5
Fires and flames	252	152	100	0.6	0.7	0.5
Mechanical suffocation	79	63	16	0.2	0.3	0.1
Falls	66	46	20	0.2	0.2	0.1
All other unintentional injuries	420	276	144	1.0	1.3	0.7
Cancer (malignant neoplasms)	1,008	533	475	2.5	2.5	2.4
Congenital anomalies	376	210	166	0.9	1.0	0.8
Homicide	326	193	133	0.8	0.9	0.7
Suicide	279	214	65	0.7	1.0	0.3
Heart disease	272	138	134	0.7	0.7	0.7
Benign neoplasms	105	52	53	0.3	0.2	0.3
Chronic lower respiratory diseases	104	61	43	0.3	0.3	0.2
Influenza and pneumonia	92	47	45	0.2	0.2	0.2
Stroke (cerebrovascular disease)	80	42	38	0.2	0.2	0.2
15 to 24 Years						
All Causes	**32,252**	**23,963**	**8,289**	**80.7**	**117.0**	**42.6**
Unintentional injuries	**14,411**	**10,832**	**3,579**	**36.1**	**52.9**	**18.4**
Motor-vehicle	10,725	7,778	2,947	26.8	38.0	15.1
Poisoning	1,362	1,080	282	3.4	5.3	1.4
Drowning	596	544	52	1.5	2.7	0.3
Falls	256	232	24	0.6	1.1	0.1
Fires and flames	209	137	72	0.5	0.7	0.4
All other unintentional injuries	1,263	1,061	202	3.2	5.2	1.0
Homicide	5,297	4,541	756	13.3	22.2	3.9
Suicide	3,971	3,409	562	9.9	16.6	2.9
Cancer	1,704	1,024	680	4.3	5.0	3.5
Heart disease	999	647	352	2.5	3.2	1.8
Congenital anomalies	505	306	199	1.3	1.5	1.0
Human immunodeficiency virus infection	225	105	120	0.6	0.5	0.6
Stroke (cerebrovascular disease)	196	103	93	0.5	0.5	0.5
Influenza and pneumonia	181	106	75	0.5	0.5	0.4
Chronic lower respiratory diseases	173	100	73	0.4	0.5	0.4
25 to 34 Years						
All Causes	**41,683**	**28,757**	**12,926**	**104.8**	**143.1**	**65.7**
Unintentional injuries	**11,839**	**9,092**	**2,747**	**29.8**	**45.2**	**14.0**
Motor-vehicle	6,937	5,236	1,701	17.4	26.0	8.6
Poisoning	2,507	1,862	645	6.3	9.3	3.3
Drowning	374	328	46	0.9	1.6	0.2
Falls	340	295	45	0.9	1.5	0.2
Fires and flames	247	161	86	0.6	0.8	0.4
All other unintentional injuries	1,434	1,210	224	3.6	6.0	1.1
Homicide	5,204	4,157	1,047	13.1	20.7	5.3
Suicide	5,070	4,199	871	12.7	20.9	4.4
Cancer	3,994	1,860	2,134	10.0	9.3	10.8
Heart disease	3,160	2,068	1,092	7.9	10.3	5.5
Human immunodeficiency virus infection	2,101	1,421	680	5.3	7.1	3.5
Stroke (cerebrovascular disease)	601	311	290	1.5	1.5	1.5
Diabetes mellitus	595	341	254	1.5	1.7	1.3
Congenital anomalies	458	249	209	1.2	1.2	1.1
Chronic liver disease and cirrhosis	387	259	128	1.0	1.3	0.7
35 to 44 Years						
All Causes	**91,674**	**58,164**	**33,510**	**203.2**	**259.1**	**147.9**
Cancer	16,569	7,297	9,272	36.7	32.5	40.9
Unintentional injuries	**15,945**	**11,612**	**4,333**	**35.4**	**51.7**	**19.1**
Motor-vehicle	7,083	5,016	2,067	15.7	22.3	9.1
Poisoning	5,036	3,522	1,514	11.2	15.7	6.7
Falls	647	544	103	1.4	2.4	0.5
Drowning	462	376	86	1.0	1.7	0.4
Fires and flames	441	308	133	1.0	1.4	0.6
All other unintentional injuries	2,276	1,846	430	5.0	8.2	1.9
Heart disease	13,326	9,346	3,980	29.5	41.6	17.6
Suicide	6,635	5,180	1,455	14.7	23.1	6.4
Human immunodeficiency virus infection	5,867	4,360	1,507	13.0	19.4	6.7
Homicide	4,268	3,122	1,146	9.5	13.9	5.1
Chronic liver disease and cirrhosis	3,336	2,206	1,130	7.4	9.8	5.0
Stroke (cerebrovascular disease)	2,491	1,267	1,224	5.5	5.6	5.4
Diabetes mellitus	1,958	1,181	777	4.3	5.3	3.4
Influenza and pneumonia	983	556	427	2.2	2.5	1.9

See source and footnotes on page 12.

LEADING CAUSES OF DEATH (CONT.)

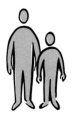

DEATHS AND DEATH RATES BY AGE AND SEX, 2001, Cont.

Cause	Number of Deaths			Death Rates[a]		
	Total	Male	Female	Total	Male	Female
45 to 54 Years						
All Causes	168,065	104,848	63,217	428.8	544.9	316.8
Cancer	49,562	25,071	24,491	126.4	130.3	122.7
Heart disease	36,399	26,280	10,119	92.9	136.6	50.7
Unintentional injuries	13,344	9,743	3,601	34.0	50.6	18.0
Motor-vehicle	5,564	3,938	1,626	14.2	20.5	8.1
Poisoning	3,547	2,503	1,044	9.0	13.0	5.2
Falls	1,024	821	203	2.6	4.3	1.0
Fires and flames	419	288	131	1.1	1.5	0.7
Drowning	359	299	60	0.9	1.6	0.3
All other unintentional injuries	2,431	1,894	537	6.2	9.8	2.7
Chronic liver disease and cirrhosis	7,259	5,295	1,964	18.5	27.5	9.8
Suicide	5,942	4,504	1,438	15.2	23.4	7.2
Stroke (cerebrovascular disease)	5,910	3,205	2,705	15.1	16.7	13.6
Diabetes mellitus	5,343	3,154	2,189	13.6	16.4	11.0
Human immunodeficiency virus infection	4,120	3,241	879	10.5	16.8	4.4
Chronic lower respiratory diseases	3,324	1,702	1,622	8.5	8.8	8.1
Homicide	2,467	1,832	635	6.3	9.5	3.2
55 to 64 Years						
All Causes	244,139	144,958	99,181	965.1	1,193.4	754.2
Cancer	90,223	49,244	40,979	356.7	405.4	311.6
Heart disease	62,486	42,519	19,967	247.0	350.1	151.8
Chronic lower respiratory diseases	11,166	5,702	5,464	44.1	46.9	41.6
Stroke (cerebrovascular disease)	9,608	5,277	4,331	38.0	43.4	32.9
Diabetes mellitus	9,570	5,241	4,329	37.8	43.1	32.9
Unintentional injuries	7,658	5,228	2,430	30.3	43.0	18.5
Motor-vehicle	3,465	2,309	1,156	13.7	19.0	8.8
Falls	1,004	718	286	4.0	5.9	2.2
Poisoning	798	500	298	3.2	4.1	2.3
Fires and flames	378	236	142	1.5	1.9	1.1
Choking[c]	330	194	136	1.3	1.6	1.0
All other unintentional injuries	1,683	1,271	412	6.7	10.5	3.1
Chronic liver disease and cirrhosis	5,750	4,028	1,722	22.7	33.2	13.1
Suicide	3,317	2,563	754	13.1	21.1	5.7
Nephritis and nephrosis	3,284	1,714	1,570	13.0	14.1	11.9
Septicemia	3,111	1,606	1,505	12.3	13.2	11.4
65 to 74 Years						
All Causes	430,960	241,581	189,379	2,353.9	2,912.2	1,891.4
Cancer	147,018	81,699	65,319	803.0	984.9	652.4
Heart disease	116,299	70,637	45,662	635.2	851.5	456.0
Chronic lower respiratory diseases	30,751	15,877	14,874	168.0	191.4	148.6
Stroke (cerebrovascular disease)	22,598	11,649	10,949	123.4	140.4	109.4
Diabetes mellitus	16,731	8,437	8,294	91.4	101.7	82.8
Unintentional injuries	7,835	4,751	3,084	42.8	57.3	30.8
Motor-vehicle	2,990	1,786	1,204	16.3	21.5	12.0
Falls	1,833	1,090	743	10.0	13.1	7.4
Choking[c]	539	294	245	2.9	3.5	2.4
Fires and flames	411	229	182	2.2	2.8	1.8
Poisoning	291	170	121	1.6	2.0	1.2
All other unintentional injuries	1,771	1,182	589	9.7	14.2	5.9
Nephritis and nephrosis	7,356	3,826	3,530	40.2	46.1	35.3
Influenza and pneumonia	6,650	3,732	2,918	36.3	45.0	29.1
Septicemia	5,998	3,044	2,954	32.8	36.7	29.5
Chronic liver disease and cirrhosis	5,486	3,335	2,151	30.0	40.2	21.5
75 Years and Older[b]						
All Causes	1,367,882	558,606	809,276	8,038.1	8,849.6	7,559.6
Heart disease	466,497	187,096	279,401	2,741.3	2,964.0	2,609.9
Cancer	243,204	120,087	123,117	1,429.1	1,902.5	1,150.1
Stroke (cerebrovascular disease)	121,892	41,235	80,657	716.3	653.3	753.4
Chronic lower respiratory diseases	76,154	35,604	40,550	447.5	564.1	378.8
Alzheimer's disease	49,823	14,019	35,804	292.8	222.1	334.5
Influenza and pneumonia	48,873	19,800	29,073	287.2	313.7	271.6
Diabetes mellitus	36,977	14,376	22,601	217.3	227.8	211.1
Nephritis and nephrosis	25,766	11,599	14,167	151.4	183.8	132.3
Unintentional injuries	24,979	11,413	13,566	146.8	180.8	126.7
Falls	9,794	4,303	5,491	57.6	68.2	51.3
Motor-vehicle	4,568	2,550	2,018	26.8	40.4	18.9
Choking[c]	2,516	1,135	1,381	14.8	18.0	12.9
Fires and flames	677	315	362	4.0	5.0	3.4
Poisoning	441	196	245	2.6	3.1	2.3
All other unintentional injuries	6,983	2,914	4,069	41.0	46.2	38.0
Septicemia	19,420	7,676	11,744	114.1	121.6	109.7

Source: Adapted from Anderson, R.N., & Smith, B.L. (2003). Deaths: Leading Causes for 2001. National Vital Statistics Reports, 52(9), 13–19, 69; with additional National Safety Council tabulations of NCHS mortality data.
[a] Deaths per 100,000 population in each age group.
[b] Includes 431 deaths where the age is unknown.
[c] Inhalation or ingestion of food or other objects.

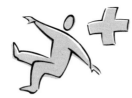

LEADING CAUSES OF NONFATAL INJURIES

LEADING CAUSES OF NONFATAL UNINTENTIONAL INJURIES TREATED IN HOSPITAL EMERGENCY DEPARTMENTS BY AGE GROUP, UNITED STATES, 2002

Rank	All Ages	<1	1–4	5–9	10–14	15–24	25–34	35–44	45–54	55–64	65+
						Age Group					
1	Falls 7,410,159	Falls 126,459	Falls 870,950	Falls 676,444	Falls 659,923	Struck by/against 951,581	Falls 702,946	Falls 765,275	Falls 684,042	Falls 490,737	Falls 1,638,883
2	Struck by/against 4,490,051	Struck by/against 33,023	Struck by/against 390,945	Struck by/against 449,222	Struck by/against 622,615	Motor-vehicle occupant 902,186	Overexertion 701,783	Overexertion 656,122	Overexertion 393,539	Struck by/against 185,922	Motor-vehicle occupant 193,068
3	Overexertion 3,286,856	Fire/burn 13,193	Other bite/sting[a] 126,710	Cut/pierce 135,098	Overexertion 288,074	Falls 794,288	Struck by/against 671,811	Struck by/against 609,021	Struck by/against 385,139	Motor-vehicle occupant 179,527	Struck by/against 190,501
4	Motor-vehicle occupant 2,988,064	Other bite/sting[a] 10,926	Foreign body 106,331	Pedalcyclist 118,046	Cut/pierce 170,062	Overexertion 758,312	Motor-vehicle occupant 609,636	Motor-vehicle occupant 515,768	Motor-vehicle occupant 332,260	Overexertion 175,009	Overexertion 156,231
5	Cut/Pierce 2,278,105	Motor-vehicle occupant 9,336	Cut/pierce 87,836	Other bite/sting[a] 96,330	Pedalcyclist 142,085	Cut/pierce 492,172	Cut/pierce 461,058	Cut/pierce 394,133	Cut/pierce 272,953	Cut/pierce 142,911	Cut/pierce 115,708
6	Other bite/sting[a] 880,910	Poisoning 8,814	Poisoning 78,828	Motor-vehicle occupant 79,531	Unknown/unspecified 129,388	Unknown/unspecified 174,572	Other bite/sting[a] 121,398	Other specified[c] 129,831	Other bite/sting[a] 94,895	Other bite/sting[a] 57,805	Other bite/sting[a] 70,093
7	Unknown/unspecified 742,188	Foreign body 8,776	Overexertion 74,530	Overexertion 76,811	Motor-vehicle occupant 115,920	Other bite/sting[a] 126,498	Other specified[c] 110,163	Other bite/sting[a] 115,409	Other specified[c] 93,356	Other specified[c] 37,399	Unknown/unspecified 47,825
8	Other transport[b] 594,127	Unknown/unspecified 6,916	Fire/burn 62,073	Foreign body 54,164	Other transport[b] 65,375	Other transport[b] 125,085	Unknown/unspecified 109,749	Poisoning 97,480	Poisoning 74,802	Other transport[b] 34,315	Other transport[b] 44,759
9	Foreign body 577,622	Inhalation/suffocation 6,452	Motor-vehicle occupant 50,331	Dog bite 51,882	Other bite/sting[a] 60,780	Other specified[c] 111,000	Other transport[b] 95,680	Unknown/unspecified 92,403	Foreign body 57,803	Unknown/unspecified 28,358	Poisoning 31,073
10	Other specified[c] 558,206	Overexertion 6,336	Unknown/unspecified 48,293	Unknown/unspecified 48,079	Dog bite 41,516	Fire/burn 91,571	Foreign body 95,478	Other transport[b] 89,150	Other transport[b] 57,758	Foreign body 26,901	Foreign body 28,723
All Causes											
Number	26,359,496	2,276,376		1,904,190	2,433,723	4,989,157	4,067,291	3,849,832	2,703,396	1,489,669	2,645,863[d]
Per 1,000 population	91.4	116.1		95.7	115.1	122.9	101.9	84.7	67.4	56.0	74.3[d]

Source: NEISS All Injury Program, Office of Statistics and Programming, National Center for Injury Prevention and Control, CDC, and Consumer Product Safety Commission.
[a] Other than dog bite.
[b] Includes occupant of any transport vehicle other than a motor vehicle or motor cycle (e.g., airplane, rail car, boat, ATV, animal rider).
[c] Includes electric current, explosions, fireworks, radiation, animal scratch, etc. Excludes all causes listed in the table and bb/pellet gunshot, drowning and near drowning, firearm gunshot, suffocation, machinery, natural and environmental conditions, pedestrians, and motorcyclists.
[d] Includes 2,507 cases with age unknown.

Falls are the leading cause of nonfatal injuries that are treated in hospital emergency departments (ED), according to data from the All Injury Program, a cooperative program involving the National Center for Injury Prevention and Control, CDC, and the Consumer Product Safety Commission. About seven and one half million people were treated in an ED for fall-related injuries in 2002. Falls were the leading cause of nonfatal injuries for all age groups except those 15–24 years old, for which struck by or against an object or person was the leading cause. Struck by or against, overexertion, and motor-vehicle crashes involving vehicle occupants were also leading causes for most age groups.

LEADING CAUSES OF UNINTENTIONAL-INJURY DEATH BY AGE, 2001

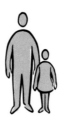

LEADING CAUSES OF UNINTENTIONAL-INJURY DEATH BY AGE, UNITED STATES, 2001

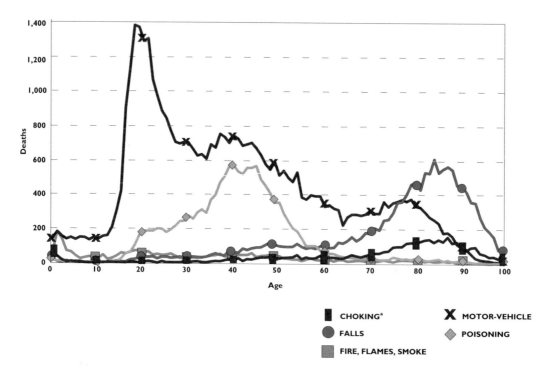

Motor-vehicle crashes, falls, poisonings, choking (suffocation by inhalation or ingestion of food or other object), fires and flames, drownings, and mechanical suffocation were the seven leading causes of unintentional-injury death in the United States in 2001. The graph above depicts the number of deaths attributed to the top five causes by single years of age through age 99.

In 2001, motor-vehicle crashes were the leading cause of unintentional-injury death for all ages combined and the leading cause of unintentional-injury deaths for each single year of age from 2 to 77. Furthermore, for those aged 6 through 33, motor-vehicle crashes caused more deaths than any other injury or illness, combining to account for 25% of the total.

The distribution of 2001 motor-vehicle fatalities shows a sharp increase for persons aged 15 to 19, rising from 420 for 15-year-olds to 1,371 for 19-year-olds. The greatest number of motor-vehicle fatalities occurred to persons aged 18 and 19 in 2001.

The second leading cause of unintentional-injury death overall in 2001 was falls. Falls were the leading cause of unintentional-injury death of persons aged 78 and older and the second leading cause from ages 59 through 77 for each year of age; deaths resulting from falls peaked

at 608 for individuals age 84. Poisoning was the third leading cause of unintentional-injury death in the United States in 2001. Poisoning fatalities reached a high of 567 for 40-year-old individuals and were the second leading cause of unintentional-injury death for persons aged 18 to 58.

Choking was the fourth leading cause of unintentional-injury death in 2001. Choking deaths peaked at age 87 with 155 deaths. It was the second leading cause of unintentional-injury deaths for each year of age over 85. Fires and flames were the fifth leading cause of unintentional-injury death in 2001. Fatalities due to fires and flames reached a high of 68 for 41-year-olds (the third leading cause for that age) and were the second leading cause of unintentional-injury death for children aged 5 to 8.

The sixth leading cause of unintentional-injury death was drownings, which peaked at 182 for 1-year-olds. Drownings were the second leading cause of injury death for children and adolescents between ages 1 and 18. Mechanical suffocation was the seventh leading cause overall and the leading cause for infants under 1 year old with 552 deaths.

Source: National Safety Council tabulations of National Center for Health Statistics data. See the Technical Appendix for ICD-10 codes for the leading causes and comparability with prior years.
a Inhalation or ingestion of food or other objects.

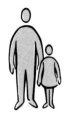

UNINTENTIONAL-INJURY DEATH RATES BY AGE, 2001

UNINTENTIONAL-INJURY DEATH RATES BY AGE, UNITED STATES, 2001

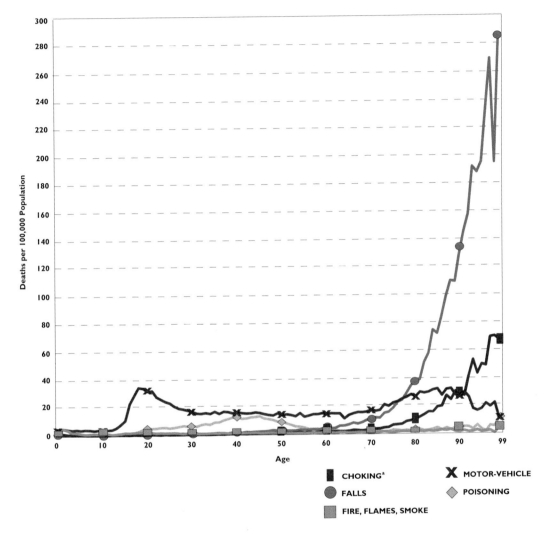

On a rate basis, motor-vehicle deaths by single year of age in 2001 rose to a high of 34.1 per 100,000 population for persons 18 years of age. This rate declined to an average of about 14.7 for those aged 30 to 69, then increased to another high at 32.1 for those 88 years of age.

While motor-vehicle crashes are a significant problem for all ages, deaths resulting from falls for certain older ages have even higher death rates. Beginning at about age 70, the death rate from falls increases dramatically. At age 78 the falls death rate surpasses that for motor-vehicle, with the death rate continuing to rise with increasing age.

The poisoning death rate remains low until about age 14, where it starts to increase up to its peak rate of 13.0 at 45 years of age then falls again.

Death rates due to choking on inhaled or ingested food or other objects are quite low for most ages. Rates are slightly elevated for infants and toddlers and rise rapidly beginning at about age 70. The death rates for drownings show peaks at very young ages and again at some very old ages.

The graph above depicts death rates per 100,000 population for the five leading causes of unintentional-injury deaths in 2001 for single years of age through age 99.

Source: National Safety Council tabulations of National Center for Health Statistics data. See the Technical Appendix for ICD-10 codes for the leading causes and comparability with prior years.
a Inhalation or ingestion of food or other objects.

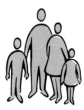

UNINTENTIONAL-INJURY DEATHS BY SEX AND AGE, UNITED STATES, 2001

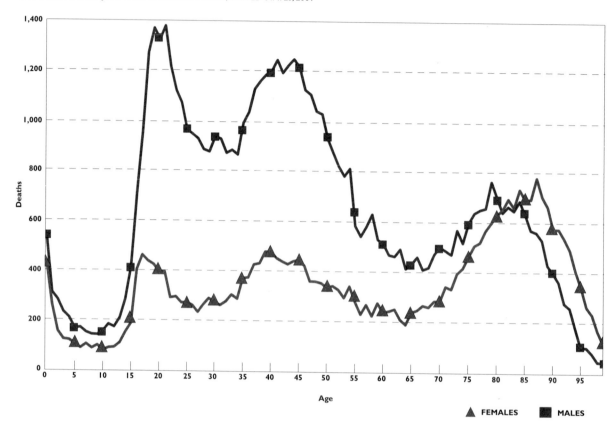

Males incur more deaths due to unintentional injuries than females at all ages from birth to age 80. During those years the difference between the unintentional-injury death totals by gender ranges from 42 at age 9 to 982 at age 21. The excess number of deaths for males compared to females is most evident from the late teenage years to the late forties where the gap begins to narrow. Beginning at age 81, deaths of females exceed those of males by as little as 12 deaths to as much as 257 at age 92.

Unintentional-injury deaths during the first 95 years are at their lowest level for both sexes from about age 4 to about age 13. For males the highest number of deaths (1,378) occurs at age 21 and the totals remain high until the late forties to early fifties. For females, however, the highest totals occur among the elderly from about age 75 and older. The greatest number of female deaths (780) occurs at age 87.

The graph above shows the number of unintentional-injury deaths for each sex by single years of age from under 1 year old through age 99. It is based on death certificate data from the National Center for Health Statistics.

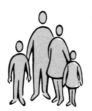

UNINTENTIONAL-INJURY DEATH RATES BY SEX AND AGE, UNITED STATES, 2001

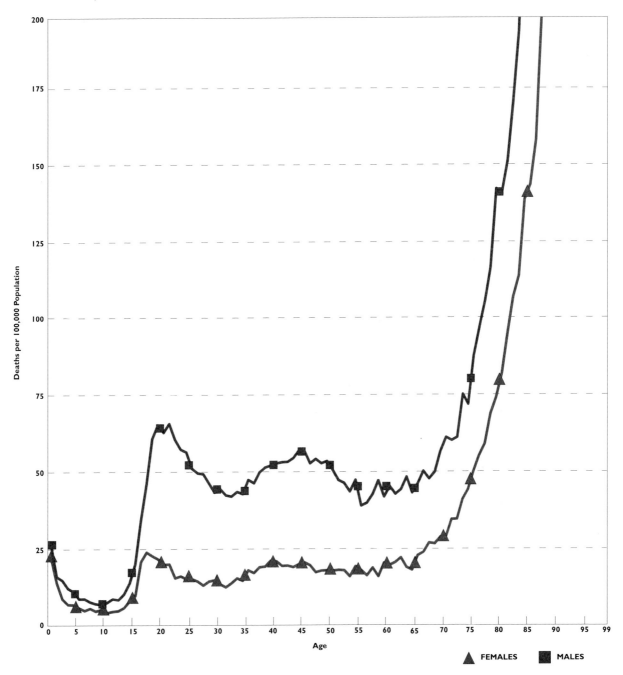

Throughout the lifespan, males have greater unintentional-injury death rates for each year of age compared to females.

The graph above shows the unintentional-injury death rates for males and females by single years of age from under 1 year old to about age 85. It is based on National Center for Health Statistics mortality data and U.S. Census Bureau population data.

Death rates for both sexes are lowest from birth until the mid-teenage years where rates rise rapidly. Rates then remain fairly constant until the late sixties where they again rise steadily with increasing age. Rates for males in their late nineties are generally between 406 and 846 per 100,000 population. Rates for females in their late nineties average around 393. For comparison, the overall unintentional-injury death rate for all ages and both sexes is 35.6.

ALL DEATHS DUE TO INJURY

MORTALITY BY SELECTED EXTERNAL CAUSES, UNITED STATES, 1999–2001

Type of Accident or Manner of Injury	2001[a]	2000	1999
All External Causes of Mortality, V01–Y98[b]	**160,099**	**151,268**	**151,109**
Deaths Due to Unintentional (Accidental) Injuries, V01–X59,Y85–Y86	**101,537**	**97,900**	**97,860**
Transport Accidents, V01–V99, Y85	**47,288**	**46,749**	**46,423**
Pedestrian, V01–V09	6,071	5,870	6,047
Pedalcyclist, V10–V19	792	740	800
Motorcycle rider, V20–V29	3,042	2,765	2,316
Occupant of three-wheeled motor vehicle, V30–V39	11	23	33
Car occupant, V40–V49	14,946	14,813	14,549
Occupant of pick-up truck or van, V50–V59	3,739	3,268	3,133
Occupant of heavy transport vehicle, V60–V69	374	369	422
Bus occupant, V70–V79	37	20	62
Animal rider or occupant of animal-drawn vehicle, V80	116	97	110
Occupant of railway train or railway vehicle, V81	26	30	54
Occupant of streetcar, V82	3	1	1
Other and unspecified land transport accidents, V83–V89	16,036	16,850	16,992
Occupant of special industrial vehicle, V83	*10*	*15*	*18*
Occupant of special agricultural vehicle, V84	*239*	*273*	*348*
Occupant of special construction vehicle, V85	*18*	*37*	*38*
Occupant of all-terrain or other off-road motor vehicle, V86	*751*	*717*	*603*
Other and unspecified person, V87–V89	*15,018*	*15,808*	*15,985*
Water transport accidents, V90–V94	591	630	679
Drowning, V90, V92	*413*	*466*	*501*
Other and unspecified injuries, V91, V93–V94	*178*	*164*	*178*
Air and space transport accidents, V95–V97	918	777	715
Other and unspecified transport accidents and sequelae, V98–V99, Y85	586	496	51
Other specified transport accidents, V98	*1*	*2*	*8*
Unspecified transport accident, V99	*3*	*4*	*6*
Nontransport Unintentional (Accidental) Injuries, W00–X59, Y86	**54,249**	**51,151**	**51,437**
Falls, W00–W19	15,019	13,322	13,162
Fall on same level from slipping, tripping, and stumbling, W01	*564*	*565*	*611*
Other fall on same level, W00, W02–W03, W18	*2,570*	*1,885*	*820*
Fall involving bed, chair, other furniture, W06–W08	*734*	*650*	*624*
Fall on and from stairs and steps, W10	*1,462*	*1,307*	*1,421*
Fall on and from ladder or scaffolding, W11–W12	*439*	*412*	*375*
Fall from out of or through building or structure, W13	*580*	*506*	*550*
Other fall from one level to another, W09, W14–W17	*840*	*687*	*772*
Other and unspecified fall, W04–W05, W19	*7,830*	*7,310*	*7,989*
Exposure to inanimate mechanical forces, W20–W49	2,752	2,768	2,739
Struck by or striking against object, W20–W22	*853*	*877*	*842*
Caught between objects, W23	*116*	*84*	*93*
Contact with machinery, W24, W30–W31	*648*	*676*	*622*
Contact with sharp objects, W25–W29	*81*	*80*	*68*
Firearms discharge, W32–W34	*802*	*776*	*824*
Explosion and rupture of pressurized devices, W35–W38	*38*	*30*	*33*
Fireworks discharge, W39	*6*	*5*	*7*
Explosion of other materials, W40	*138*	*167*	*166*
Foreign body entering through skin or natural orifice, W44–W45	*33*	*36*	*38*
Other and unspecified inanimate mechanical forces, W41–W43, W49	*37*	*37*	*46*
Exposure to animate mechanical forces, W50–W64	160	204	214
Struck by or against another person, W50–W52	*45*	*61*	*52*
Bitten or struck by dog, W54	*25*	*26*	*25*
Bitten or struck by other mammals, W53, W55	*65*	*65*	*69*
Bitten or stung by nonvenomous insect and other arthropods, W57	*9*	*9*	*10*
Bitten or crushed by other reptiles, W59	*0*	*31*	*45*
Other and unspecified animate mechanical forces, W56, W58, W60, W64	*16*	*12*	*13*
Accidental drowning and submersion, W65–W74	3,281	3,482	3,529
Drowning and submersion while in or falling into bathtub, W65–W66	*322*	*341*	*320*
Drowning and submersion while in or falling into swimming pool, W67–W68	*596*	*567*	*530*
Drowning and submersion while in or falling into natural water, W69–W70	*1,054*	*1,135*	*1,212*
Other and unspecified drowning and submersion, W73–W74	*1,309*	*1,439*	*1,467*
Other accidental threats to breathing, W75–W84	5,555	5,648	5,503
Accidental suffocation and strangulation in bed, W75	*456*	*327*	*330*
Other accidental hanging and strangulation, W76	*279*	*333*	*307*
Threat to breathing due to cave-in, falling earth, and other substances, W77	*56*	*64*	*47*
Inhalation of gastric contents, W78	*422*	*382*	*417*
Inhalation and ingestion of food causing obstruction of respiratory tract, W79	*742*	*744*	*640*
Inhalation and ingestion of other objects causing obstruction of respiratory tract, W80	*3,021*	*3,187*	*2,828*
Confined to or trapped in a low-oxygen environment, W81	*20*	*15*	*16*
Other and unspecified threats to breathing, W83–W84	*559*	*596*	*918*

See source and footnotes on page 19.

MORTALITY BY SELECTED EXTERNAL CAUSES, UNITED STATES, 1999–2001, Cont.

Type of Accident or Manner of Injury	2001[a]	2000	1999
Exposure to electric current, radiation, temperature, and pressure, W85–W99	431	419	479
Electric transmission lines, W85	83	99	127
Other and unspecified electric current, W86–W87	326	296	310
Radiation, W88–W91	0	0	0
Excessive heat or cold of man-made origin, W92–W93	8	12	18
High and low air pressure and changes in air pressure, W94	13	12	22
Other and unspecified man-made environmental factors, W99	1	0	2
Exposure to smoke, fire, and flames, X00–X09	3,309	3,377	3,348
Uncontrolled fire in building or structure, X00	2,673	2,776	2,676
Uncontrolled fire not in building or structure, X01	61	68	78
Controlled fire in building or structure, X02	44	50	56
Controlled fire not in building or structure, X03	41	29	32
Ignition of highly flammable material, X04	53	65	73
Ignition or melting of nightwear, X05	5	9	6
Ignition or melting of other clothing and apparel, X06	125	116	112
Other and unspecified smoke, fire, and flames, X08–X09	307	264	315
Contact with heat and hot substances, X10–X19	114	110	123
Contact with hot tap-water, X11	57	55	51
Other and unspecified heat and hot substances, X10, X12–X19	57	55	72
Contact with venomous animals and plants, X20–X29	61	80	61
Contact with venomous snakes and lizards, X20	7	12	7
Contact with venomous spiders, X21	5	5	6
Contact with hornets, wasps, and bees, X23	43	54	43
Contact with other and unspecified venomous animal or plant, X22, X24–X29	6	9	5
Exposure to forces of nature, X30–X39	1,100	1,223	1,488
Exposure to excessive natural heat, X30	300	301	594
Exposure to excessive natural cold, X31	599	742	598
Lightning, X33	44	50	64
Earthquake and other earth movements, X34–X36	28	35	46
Cataclysmic storm, X37	54	49	129
Flood, X38	35	5	15
Exposure to other and unspecified forces of nature, X32, X39	40	41	42
Accidental poisoning by and exposure to noxious substances, X40–X49	14,078	12,757	12,186
Nonopioid analgesics, antipyretics, and antirheumatics, X40	208	176	168
Antiepileptic, sedative-hypnotic, antiparkinsonism, and psychotropic drugs n.e.c., X41	763	704	671
Narcotics and psychodysleptics [hallucinogens] n.e.c., X42	6,509	6,139	6,009
Other and unspecified drugs, medicaments, and biologicals, X43–X44	5,544	4,693	4,307
Alcohol, X45	303	302	320
Gases and vapors, X46–X47	656	631	597
Other and unspecified chemicals and noxious substances, X48–X49	95	112	114
Overexertion, travel and privation, X50–X57	137	185	191
Accidental exposure to other and unspecified factors and sequelae, X58–X59, Y86	8,252	7,576	8,414
Intentional self-harm, X60–X84, Y87.0, *U03	**30,622**	**29,350**	**29,199**
Intentional self-poisoning, X60–X69	5,191	4,859	4,893
Intentional self-harm by hanging, strangulation, and suffocation, X70	6,198	5,688	5,427
Intentional self-harm by firearm, X72–X74	16,869	16,586	16,599
Other and unspecified means and sequelae, X71, X75–X84, Y87.0	2,360	2,217	2,280
Terrorism, *U03	4	—	—
Assault, X85–Y09, Y87.1, *U01	**20,308**	**16,765**	**16,889**
Assault by firearm, X93–X95	11,348	10,801	10,828
Assault by sharp object, X99	1,971	1,805	1,879
Other and unspecified means and sequelae, X85–X92, X96–X98, Y00–Y09, Y87.1	4,067	4,159	4,182
Terrorism, *U01	2,922	—	—
Event of undetermined intent, Y10–Y34, Y87.2, Y89.9	**4,198**	**3,819**	**3,917**
Poisoning, Y10–Y19	2,909	2,557	2,595
Hanging, strangulation, and suffocation, Y20	131	104	110
Drowning and submersion, Y21	235	231	243
Firearm discharge, Y22–Y24	231	230	324
Exposure to smoke, fire, and flames, Y26	76	76	70
Falling, jumping, or pushed from a high place, Y30	77	55	59
Other and unspecified means and sequelae, Y25, Y27–Y29, Y31–Y34, Y87.2, Y89.9	539	566	516
Legal intervention, Y35, Y89.0	**396**	**359**	**398**
Legal intervention involving firearm discharge, Y35.0	323	270	299
Legal execution, Y35.5	63	80	88
Other and unspecified means and sequelae, Y35.1–Y35.4, Y35.6–Y35.7, Y89.0	10	9	11
Operations of war and sequelae, Y36, Y89.1	**17**	**16**	**23**
Complications of medical and surgical care and sequelae, Y40–Y84, Y88.0–Y88.3	**3,021**	**3,059**	**2,823**

Source: National Center for Health Statistics. Deaths are classified on the basis of the tenth revision of The International Classification of Diseases (ICD-10), which became effective in 1999.
Note: n.e.c. = not elsewhere classified.
[a] Latest official figures.
[b] Numbers following titles refer to external cause of injury and poisoning classifications in ICD-10.

DEATHS BY AGE, SEX, AND TYPE

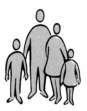

UNINTENTIONAL-INJURY DEATHS BY AGE, SEX, AND TYPE, UNITED STATES, 2001[a]

Age & Sex	Total[b]	Motor-vehicle	Falls	Poisoning	Choking[c]	Fires/Flames	Drowning[d]	Mechanical Suffocation	Natural Heat/Cold	All Types Males	All Types Females
All Ages	101,537	43,788	15,019	14,078	4,185	3,309	3,281	1,370	899	66,060	35,477
0–4	2,690	770	55	46	136	275	526	616	33	1,586	1,104
5–14	2,836	1,686	66	50	33	252	333	79	6	1,803	1,033
15–24	14,411	10,725	256	1,362	55	209	596	90	24	10,832	3,579
25–44	27,784	14,020	987	7,543	233	688	836	267	141	20,704	7,080
45–64	21,002	9,029	2,028	4,345	673	797	565	169	262	14,971	6,031
65–74	7,835	2,990	1,833	291	539	411	159	56	119	4,751	3,084
75+	24,979	4,568	9,794	441	2,516	677	266	93	314	11,413	13,566
Males	66,060	30,064	8,089	9,885	2,113	1,998	2,560	929	603		
Females	35,477	13,724	6,930	4,193	2,072	1,311	721	441	296		

Source: National Safety Council tabulations of National Center for Health Statistics mortality data.
[a]Latest official figures.
[b]Includes types not shown separately.
[c]Inhalation or ingestion of food or other objects.
[d]Excludes transport drownings.

Of the 101,537 unintentional-injury deaths in 2001, men accounted for 65% of all deaths. Women had the greatest share of deaths in the 75 and over age group (54% women). By type of accident, men accounted for 78% of all drowning deaths, but only 50% of deaths due to choking (inhalation or ingestion of food or other object obstructing breathing).

UNINTENTIONAL-INJURY DEATH RATES BY AGE, SEX, AND TYPE, UNITED STATES, 2001[a]

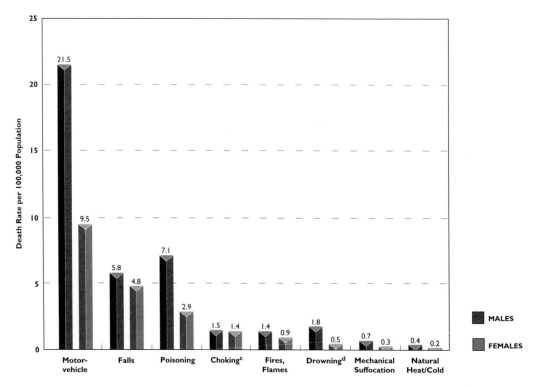

See footnotes in table above.

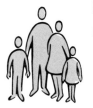

UNINTENTIONAL-INJURY DEATHS BY MONTH AND TYPE, UNITED STATES, 2001[a]

Month	All Types	Motor-vehicle	Falls	Poisoning	Choking[b]	Fires/Flames	Drowning[c]	Mechanical Suffocation	Natural Heat/Cold	Struck By/Against	All Other Types
Total	**101,537**	**43,788**	**15,019**	**14,078**	**4,185**	**3,309**	**3,281**	**1,370**	**899**	**853**	**14,755**
January	8,079	3,083	1,324	1,132	378	485	112	110	172	72	1,211
February	7,330	2,878	1,158	985	350	400	118	121	121	66	1,133
March	7,935	3,262	1,233	1,114	377	340	159	111	68	74	1,197
April	8,161	3,428	1,176	1,229	342	268	259	115	35	72	1,237
May	8,574	3,810	1,215	1,180	352	199	380	134	29	76	1,199
June	8,605	3,728	1,175	1,196	305	199	533	112	48	70	1,239
July	9,354	4,059	1,309	1,257	326	187	620	102	100	89	1,305
August	9,230	4,047	1,266	1,316	360	164	490	126	129	69	1,263
September	8,222	3,752	1,217	1,113	344	203	214	98	26	76	1,179
October	8,807	4,055	1,375	1,183	344	257	150	113	29	81	1,220
November	8,535	3,833	1,234	1,122	324	245	128	114	43	62	1,430
December	8,705	3,853	1,337	1,251	383	362	118	114	99	46	1,142
Average	**8,461**	**3,649**	**1,252**	**1,173**	**349**	**276**	**273**	**114**	**75**	**71**	**1,230**

Source: National Safety Council tabulations of National Center for Health Statistics mortality data.
[a]Latest official figures.
[b]Inhalation or ingestion of food or other objects.
[c]Excludes water transport drownings.

UNINTENTIONAL-INJURY DEATHS BY MONTH, UNITED STATES, 2001

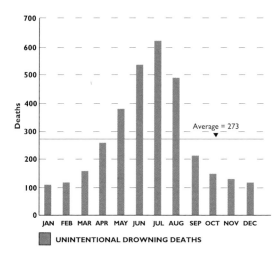

UNINTENTIONAL DROWNING DEATHS

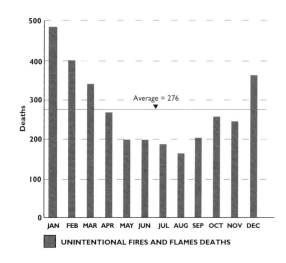

UNINTENTIONAL FIRES AND FLAMES DEATHS

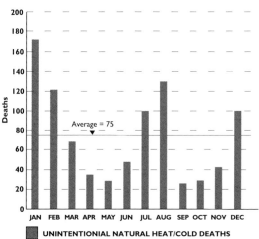

UNINTENTIONIAL NATURAL HEAT/COLD DEATHS

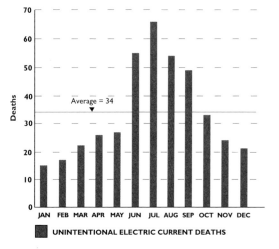

UNINTENTIONAL ELECTRIC CURRENT DEATHS

See page 98 for motor-vehicle deaths by month.

THE NATIONAL HEALTH INTERVIEW SURVEY

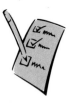

The National Health Interview Survey, conducted by the National Center for Health Statistics, is a continuous, personal-interview sampling of households to obtain information about the health status of household members, including injuries experienced during the 3 months prior to the interview. Responsible family members residing in the household supplied the information found in the survey. Of the nation's 108,209,000 households in 2001, 39,932 households containing 100,760 persons were interviewed. See page 23 for definitions and comparability with other injury figures published in *Injury Facts*®.

NUMBER OF LEADING EXTERNAL CAUSES OF INJURY AND POISONING EPISODES BY SEX AND AGE, UNITED STATES, 2001[a]

Sex and Age	Population (000)	External Cause of Injury and Poisoning (number in thousands)						
		Fall	Struck By or Against Person or Object	Transportation[b]	Overexertion	Cutting-Piercing Instruments	Other Injury Causes[b]	Poisoning[b]
Total[d]	285,094	7,957	3,112	3,459	3,232	1,928	3,989	874
Both sexes								
Under 12 years	48,089	1,542	624	277	79[c]	317	679	318
12–17 years	24,471	700	867	364	324	218	350	66[c]
18–44 years	112,715	2,257	1,100	1,873	1,686	875	1,909	317
45–64 years	64,494	1,785	386	774	937	436	721	82[c]
65–74 years	18,308	710	104[c]	94[c]	111[c]	36[c]	207	36[c]
75 years and over	17,017	964	32[c]	78[c]	95[c]	47[c]	123[c]	55[c]
Male								
Under 12 years	24,611	839	423	95[c]	44[c]	216	382	204
12–17 years	12,552	395	628	193	167[c]	132	225	42[c]
18–44 years	56,807	1,074	736	969	962	585	1,182	72[c]
45–64 years	31,388	755	217	421	436	213	402	20[c]
65 years and over	14,608	504	27[c]	81[c]	101[c]	63[c]	147[c]	12[c]
Female								
Under 12 years	23,478	703	201	182	34[c]	101[c]	297	114[c]
12–17 years	11,918	305	239	171[c]	158	86[c]	125[c]	23[c]
18–44 years	55,908	1,182	363	904	725	290	726	245[c]
45–64 years	33,106	1,029	169	353	501	223	318	62[c]
65 years and over	20,718	1,169	109[c]	91[c]	105[c]	20[c]	183	80[c]

Source: Barnes, P.M., Adams, P.F., & Schiller, J.S. (2003, December). Summary health statistics for the U.S. population: National Health Interview Survey, 2001. Vital and Health Statistics, Series 10 (No. 217). Hyattsville, MD: National Center for Health Statistics.
[a]Latest official figures.
[b]Transportation includes motor vehicle, bicycle, motorcycle, pedestrian, train, boat, or airplane. "Other" includes fire/burn/scald related, animal or insect bites, machinery, and unknown causes. Poisoning does not include food poisoning or allergic reaction.
[c]Figure does not meet standard of reliability or precision.
[d]Numbers and percents may not sum to respective totals due to rounding.

According to the 2001 National Health Interview Survey (NHIS), nearly 11 million men and women suffered injuries that were serious enough to require medical attention. Forty-four percent of all injuries occurred inside or outside the home environment.

Injuries among males accounted for 53% of the total number of medically attended injuries. The most common place of occurrence for injuries among men was in or around the home (37%), followed by sport/recreational settings (16%), the street (15%), and industrial facilities (10%).

Injuries inside the home accounted for the greatest share, 33%, of medically attended injuries among women. More than half of all injuries among women occurred in or around the home. Injuries at sport facilities or other recreational areas made up an additional 15% of the total for women.

The NHIS injury definitions are listed below for comparability with other injury figures published in *Injury Facts*®.

NUMBER AND PERCENT OF INJURY EPISODES BY PLACE OF OCCURRENCE AND SEX, UNITED STATES, 2001[a]

Place of Occurrence of Injury Episode[b]	Both Sexes		Male		Female	
	Number of Episodes (000)	Percent	Number of Episodes (000)	Percent	Number of Episodes (000)	Percent
Total episodes[c]	24,551	100.0%	12,966	100.0%	11,585	100.0%
Home (inside)	6,296	26.0	2,425	18.7	3,871	33.4
Home (outside)	4,457	18.2	2,329	18.0	2,128	18.4
School/child care center/preschool	1,463	6.0	835	6.4	628	5.4
Hospital/residential institution	584	2.4	101[d]	1.0	483	4.2
Street/highway/parking lot	3,767	15.3	1,984	15.3	1,783	15.4
Sport facility/recreation area/lake/river/pool	3,074	12.5	2,091	16.1	982	8.5
Industrial/construction/farm/mine/quarry	1,449	5.9	1,297	10.0	153	1.3
Trade/service area	1,065	4.3	549	4.2	516	4.5
Other public building	487	2.0	203	1.6	283	2.4
Other unspecified	1,761	7.2	1,081	8.3	680	5.9

Source: Barnes, P.M., Adams, P.F., & Schiller, J.S. (2003, December). Summary health statistics for the U.S. population: National Health Interview Survey, 2001. Vital and Health Statistics, Series 10 (No. 217). Hyattsville, MD: National Center for Health Statistics.
[a]Latest official figures.
[b]Place of occurrence of injury and poisoning episodes is based on the question, "Where was [person] when the injury/poisoning happened?" Respondents could indicate up to two places.
[c]Numbers and percents may not sum to respective totals due to rounding.
[d]Figure does not meet standard of reliability or precision.

Injury definitions

National Health Interview Survey definitions. The National Health Interview Survey (NHIS) figures include injuries due to intentional violence as well as unintentional injuries. An injury episode refers to a traumatic event in which the person was injured one or more times from an external cause. Poisoning episodes include ingestion of or contact with harmful substances and also overdoses or wrong use of any drug or medication, but exclude illnesses such as food poisoning or poison ivy. An injury or poisoning is included in the NHIS totals if it is *medically attended*. A *medically attended* injury or poisoning is one for which a physician has been consulted (in person or by telephone) for advice or treatment. Calls to poison control centers are considered contact with a health care professional and are included in this definition of medical attendance.

National Safety Council definition of injury. A disabling injury is defined as one that results in death, some degree of permanent impairment, or renders the injured person unable to effectively perform their regular duties or activities for a full day beyond the day of the injury. This definition applies to all unintentional injuries. All injury totals labeled "disabling injuries" in *Injury Facts*® are based on this definition. Some *rates* in the Work section are based on OSHA definitions of recordable cases (see Glossary).

Numerical differences between NHIS and National Safety Council injury totals are due mainly to the duration of disability. The Council's injury estimating procedure was revised for the 1993 edition of *Accident Facts*®. See the Technical Appendix for more information.

INJURY-RELATED HOSPITAL EMERGENCY DEPARTMENT VISITS, 2002

About 39.2 million visits to hospital emergency departments in 2002 were due to injuries.

About 36% of all hospital emergency department visits in the United States were injury related, according to information from the 2002 National Hospital Ambulatory Medical Care Survey conducted for the National Center for Health Statistics. There were approximately 110.2 million visits made to emergency departments, of which about 39.2 million were injury related. This resulted in an annual rate of about 38.9 emergency department visits per 100 persons, of which about 13.8 visits per 100 persons were injury related.

Males had a higher rate of injury-related visits than females. For males, about 15.4 visits per 100 males were recorded; for females the rate was 12.3 per 100 females. Those aged 15 to 24 had the highest rate of injury-related visits for males, and those aged 75 and over had the highest rate for females.

Falls and motor-vehicle accidents were the leading causes of injury-related emergency department visits,

accounting for about 18% and 12% of the total, respectively. In total, about 7.0 million visits to emergency departments were made in 2002 due to accidental falls, and about 4.6 million were made due to motor-vehicle accidents. The next leading types were struck against or struck accidentally by objects or persons with 4.5 million visits (over 11% of the total), and accidents caused by cutting or piercing instruments, which accounted for about 2.5 million visits (over 6% of the total).

By intentionality of the injury, about 68% of the injury-related emergency department visits were due to unintentional injuries, while about 4% were due to assault, over 1% were due to self-inflicted injuries, and 23% were due to unknown or blank causes. About 8% of the injury-related emergency department visits were work-related, 64% were due to nonwork-related causes, and work-relatedness was unknown or blank for 28% of the injuries.

NUMBER AND PERCENT DISTRIBUTION OF EMERGENCY DEPARTMENT VISITS BY CAUSE OF INJURY, UNITED STATES, 2002

Cause of Injury and E-code[a]	Number of Visits (000)	Percent
All Injury-Related Visits	**39,157**	**100.0%**
Unintentional Injuries, E800–E869, E880–E929	**26,622**	**68.0**
Accidental Falls, E880.0–E886.9, E888	7,034	18.0
Total Motor-Vehicle Accidents, E810–E825	4,645	11.9
Motor-vehicle traffic, E810–E819	*4,216*	*10.8*
Motor-vehicle, nontraffic, E820-E825(.0–.5, .7–.9)	*429*	*1.1*
Striking Against or Struck Accidentally by Objects or Persons, E916–E917	4,513	11.5
Accidents Caused by Cutting or Piercing Instruments, E920	2,518	6.4
Overexertion and Strenuous Movements, E927	1,521	3.9
Accidents Due to Natural and Environmental Factors, E900-E909, E928.0–E928.2	1,505	3.8
Accidental Poisoning by Drugs, Medicinal Substances, Biologicals, Other Solid and Liquid Substances, Gases and Vapors, E850–E869	700	1.8
Accidents Caused by Fire and Flames, Hot Substances or Object, Caustic or Corrosive Material, and Steam, E890–E899, E924	564	1.4
Pedalcycle, Nontraffic and Other, E800–E807(.3), E820–E825(.6), E826.1, E826.9	411	1.0
Machinery, E919	305	0.8

Cause of Injury and E-code[a]	Number of Visits (000)	Percent
Other Transportation, E800–E807(.0–.2, .8–.9), E826(.0, .2–.8), E827–E829, E831, E83–E845	139	0.4
Other Mechanism,[b] E830, E832, E846–E848, E910–E915, E918, E921–E923, E925–E926, E928.8, E929.0–E929.5	1,931	4.9
Mechanism Unspecified, E887, E928.9, E929.8, E929.9	838	2.1
Intentional Injuries, E950–E959, E960–E969, E970–E978,E990–E999	**2,176**	**5.6**
Assault, E960–E969	1,568	4.0
Unarmed Fight or Brawl and Striking by Blunt or Thrown Object, E960.0, E968.2	868	2.2
Assault by Cutting or Piercing Instrument, E966	145	0.4
Assault by Other and Unspecified Mechanism,[c] E960.1, E962–964, E965.5–E965.9, E967–E968.1, E968.3–E969	555	1.4
Self-inflicted Injury, E950–E959	509	1.3
Poisoning by Solid or Liquid Substances, Gases or Vapors, E950–E952	387	1.0
Other and Unspecified Mechanism,[d] E953–E959	122	0.3
Other Causes of Violence, E970–E978, E990–E999	99	0.3
Adverse Effects of Medical Treatment, E870–E879, E930–E949	**1,377**	**3.5**
Other and Unknown[e]	8,982	22.9

Source: McCaig, L.F. & Burt, C.W. (2004). National Hospital Ambulatory Medical Care Survey: 2002 Emergency Department Summary (Advance Data, Number 340, March 18, 2004). Hyattsville, MD: National Center for Health Statistics.
Note: Sum of parts may not add to total due to rounding.
[a] *Based on the International Classification of Diseases, 9th Revision, Clinical Modification (ICD-9-CM).*
[b] *Includes drowning, suffocation, firearm missile, and other mechanism.*
[c] *Includes assault by firearms and explosives, and other mechanism.*
[d] *Includes injury by cutting or piercing instrument, suffocation, and other and unspecified mechanism.*
[e] *Includes all other major E-code categories where the estimate was too low to be reliable and uncodable, illegible, and blank E-codes.*

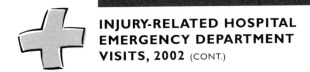

NUMBER AND PERCENT DISTRIBUTION OF INJURY-RELATED EMERGENCY DEPARTMENT VISITS BY CHARACTERISTIC OF THE INJURY AND AGE, UNITED STATES, 2002

Characteristic of the Injury	All Ages		Under 18		18–64 Years		65 Years & Over	
	Number of Visits (000)	Percent	Number of Visits (000)	Percent	Number of Visits (000)	Percent	Number of Visits (000)	Percent
Total	39,157	100.0%	10,285	100.0%	24,378	100.0%	4,495	100.0%
Intentionality								
Self-inflicted	1,059	2.7	123	1.2	926	3.8	(a)	(a)
Assault	1,463	3.7	275	2.7	1,147	4.7	(a)	(a)
Unintentional	30,481	77.8	8,428	81.9	18,195	74.6	3,858	85.8
Unknown or blank	6,154	15.7	1,459	14.2	4,110	16.9	585	13.0
Work-related								
Yes	3,032	7.7	(a)	(a)	2,919	12.0	(a)	(a)
No	25,077	64.0	7,958	77.4	14,035	57.6	3,084	68.6
Unknown or blank	11,048	28.2	2,265	22.0	7,424	30.5	1,360	30.3

See source on page 24.
Note: Sum of parts may not add to total due to rounding.
aEstimate did not meet standard of reliability or precision.

RATE OF INJURY-RELATED VISITS TO EMERGENCY DEPARTMENTS BY PATIENT AGE AND SEX, 2002

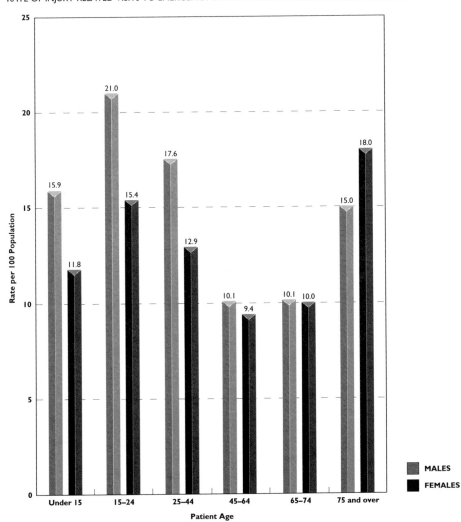

RACE AND HISPANIC ORIGIN

The rank of unintentional-injuries as a cause of death varies with race and Hispanic origin. While ranking fifth overall, following heart disease, cancer, stroke, and chronic lower respiratory diseases, unintentional injuries rank third for Hispanics after heart disease and cancer.

By race, unintentional injuries rank fifth for whites and fourth (after heart disease, cancer, and stroke) for blacks and Asians, Pacific Islanders, American Indians, and Alaskan Natives.

UNINTENTIONAL-INJURY DEATHS RANK, NUMBER, AND RATE BY RACE, HISPANIC ORIGIN, AND SEX, UNITED STATES, 2001

| Race | Total | | | Hispanic Origin | | | | | |
| | | | | Non-Hispanic Origin | | | Hispanic Origin | | |
	Rank	Number	Rate	Rank	Number	Rate	Rank	Number	Rate
All Races	5	101,537	35.6	5	91,522	36.9	3	9,523	25.7
Males	3	66,060	47.2	4	58,528	48.4	3	7,157	37.6
Females	7	35,477	24.4	8	32,994	25.9	5	2,666	14.8
White	5	85,964	36.9	5	76,262	38.4	3	9,325	27.1
Males	3	55,493	48.3	5	48,180	49.6	3	7,024	39.6
Females	7	30,471	25.8	7	28,082	27.7	5	2,301	13.8
Black	4	12,462	33.4	4	12,239	34.3	3	116	7.4
Males	3	8,537	48.1	3	8,381	49.4	3	75	9.8
Females	6	3,925	20.1	6	3,858	20.6	4	41	5.1
Not White or Black[a]	4	3,111	20.4	4	3,021	21.3	3	82	7.5
Males	3	2,030	27.2	4	1,967	28.5	3	58	10.4
Females	4	1,081	13.8	4	1,054	14.5	4	24	4.5

Source: National Center for Health Statistics, Centers for Disease Control and Prevention, and National Safety Council.
Note: Rates are deaths per 100,000 population in each race/sex/Hispanic origin group. Total column includes 492 deaths for which Hispanic origin was not determined.
[a]Includes American Indian, Alaskan Native, Asian, and Pacific Islander.

LEADING UNINTENTIONAL-INJURY CAUSES OF DEATH BY RACE, HISPANIC ORIGIN, AND SEX, UNITED STATES, 2001

| Cause of Death | All Races | | | White | | | Black | | | Not White or Black | | |
	Both	Male	Female	Both	Male	Female	Both	Male	Female	Both	Male	Female
Motor vehicle	43,788	30,064	13,724	36,576	25,084	11,492	5,506	3,900	1,606	1,706	1,080	626
Fall	15,019	8,089	6,930	13,827	7,331	6,496	854	547	307	338	211	127
Poisoning	14,078	9,885	4,193	11,662	8,232	3,430	2,169	1,490	679	247	163	84
Suffocation by inhalation or ingestion	4,185	2,133	2,072	3,550	1,762	1,788	559	308	251	76	43	33
Fires, flames, smoke	3,309	1,998	1,311	2,387	1,436	951	846	511	335	76	51	25
Drowning	3,281	2,560	721	2,515	1,936	579	579	478	101	187	146	41

| Cause of Death | Non-Hispanic | | | Hispanic | | |
	Both	Male	Female	Both	Male	Female
Motor vehicle	38,362	25,962	12,400	5,272	3,987	1,285
Fall	14,204	7,527	6,677	757	525	232
Poisoning	12,631	8,720	3,911	1,324	1,061	263
Suffocation by inhalation or ingestion	4,000	2,003	1,997	168	99	69
Fires, flames, smoke	3,106	1,873	1,233	176	109	67
Drowning	2,832	2,188	644	421	348	73

Source: National Safety Council tabulations of National Center for Health Statistics mortality data.

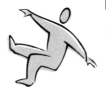
UNINTENTIONAL-INJURY DEATH RATES BY RACE, SEX, AND HISPANIC ORIGIN, UNITED STATES, 2001

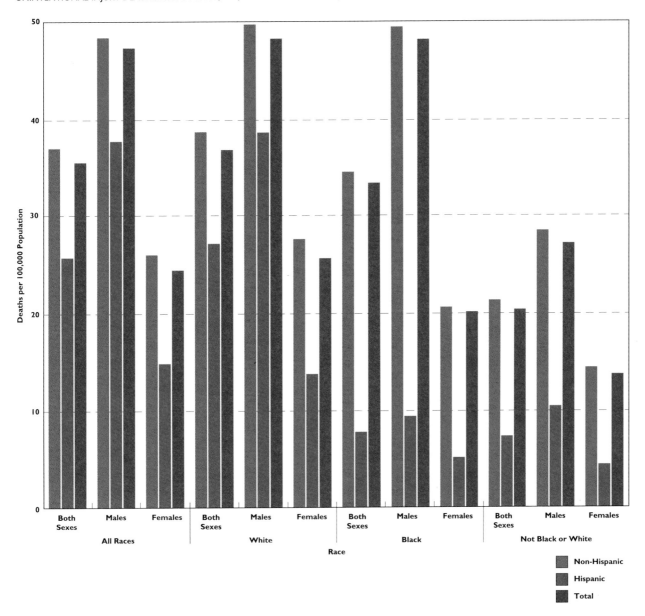

PRINCIPAL CLASSES BY STATE

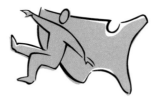

The states listed below participate in the Injury Mortality Tabulations reporting system. Reports from these states are used to make current year estimates. See the Technical Appendix for more information.

The estimated total number of unintentional-injury deaths for 2003 decreased 2% from 2002. The number of unintentional-injury deaths in the Home class was down 6%, while the Work and Public Nonmotor-

Vehicle classes also showed decreases of 5% and 1%, respectively. The Motor-Vehicle class showed an increase of 2%. The population death rate for the Home class decreased 7%, the rate for the Work class decreased 6%, and the rates for the Total and Public Nonmotor-Vehicle classes were each down 3%. The rate for the Motor-Vehicle class increased 1% from 2002 to 2003.

PRINCIPAL CLASSES OF UNINTENTIONAL-INJURY DEATHS BY STATE, 2003

State	Total[a]		Motor-Vehicle[b]		Work[c]		Home		Public Nonmotor-Vehicle	
	Deaths	Rate[d]	Deaths	Rate[d]	Deaths	Rate[d]	Deaths	Rate[d]	Deaths	Rate[d]
Total U.S.	101,500	34.9	44,800	15.4	4,500	1.5	33,100	11.4	21,300	7.3
Colorado	1,796	39.5	687	15.1	67	1.5	546	12.0	535	11.8
Delaware	257	31.4	172	21.0	4	0.5	47	5.7	39	4.8
Florida	6,229	36.6	3,165	18.6	239	1.4	1,419	8.3	1,268	7.5
Idaho	650	47.6	299	21.9	36	2.6	165	12.1	168	12.3
Kansas	1,005	36.9	439	16.1	50	1.8	293	10.8	243	8.9
Kentucky	1,987	48.3	819	19.9	85	2.1	312	7.8	799	19.4
Missouri	2,584	45.3	1,253	22.0	71	1.2	780	13.7	480	8.4
South Dakota	410	53.6	215	28.1	22	2.9	73	9.6	104	13.6
Virginia	2,196	29.7	829	11.2	78	1.1	643	8.7	259	3.5

Source: Provisional reports of vital statistics registrars; deaths are by place of occurrence. U.S. totals are National Safety Council estimates.

[a] The all-class total may not equal the sum of the separate class totals because Motor-Vehicle and other transportation deaths occurring to persons in the course of their employment are included in the Work death totals as well as the Motor-Vehicle and Public Nonmotor-Vehicle totals and also because unclassified deaths are included in the total.

[b] Differences between the figures given above and those on pages 162 and 163 are due in most cases to the inclusion of nontraffic deaths in this table.

[c] Work death totals may be too low where incomplete information on death certificates results in the deaths being included in the Public class. The Work totals may include some cases that are not compensable. For compensable cases only, see page 53.

[d] Deaths per 100,000 population.

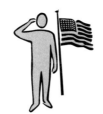

WAR DEATHS

From World War I through the Gulf War, 667,655 military personnel died during the years of major conflicts involving the United States. About 64% of the deaths (426,202) were battle-related. Another 1,132,902 incurred nonfatal wounds.

U.S. MILITARY CASUALTIES IN PRINCIPAL WARS

War	Service Members		Battle Deaths	Other Deaths		Nonfatal Wounds
	World-wide	In Theater		In Theater	Non-Theater	
Total (during war)	**42,348,460**	**—**	**650,954**	**13,853**	**229,661**	**1,431,290**
American Revolution (1775–1783)	217,000	—	4,435	—		6,188
War of 1812 (1812–1815)	286,730	—	2,260	—		4,505
Indian Wars (approx. 1817–1898)	106,000[a]	—	1,000[a]	—		—
Mexican War (1846–1848)	78,718	—	1,733	11,550		4,152
Civil War (1861–1865)						
Union	2,213,363	—	140,414	224,097		281,881
Confederate	1,050,000	—	74,524	59,297[b]		—
Spanish-American War (1898–1902)	306,760	—	385	2,061		1,662
World War I (1917–1918)	4,734,991	—	53,402	63,114		204,002
World War II (1941–1945)	16,112,566	—	291,557	113,842		671,846
Korean War (1950–1953)	5,720,000	—	33,686	2,830	17,730	103,284
Vietnam War (1964–1975)	9,200,000	3,100,000	47,410	10,788	32,000	153,303
Gulf War (1990–1991)	2,322,332	1,136,658	147	235	914	467

Source: U.S. Department of Veterans Affairs from U.S. Department of Defense data.
Note: Dash (—) indicates data not available.
[a]VA estimate.
[b]Does not include 26,000 to 31,000 who died in Union prisons.

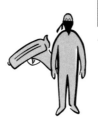

TERRORISM

There were 208 acts of international terrorism in 2003 that killed 625 people and wounded 3,646. None of the attacks occurred in the United States. Thirty-five U.S. citizens, however, died in terrorist attacks in other countries in 2003. Sixty of the acts were classified as "anti-U.S." attacks. One third (20) of the 60 occurred in the Middle East, 17 in Western Europe, and 14 in Latin America.

U.S. CITIZEN CASUALTIES DUE TO INTERNATIONAL TERRORIST ACTS, 1998–2003

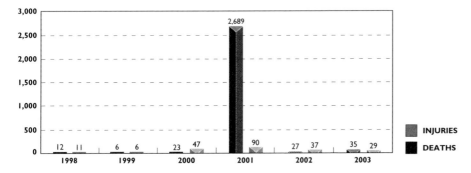

Source: Office of the Coordinator for Counterterrorism. (2004). Patterns of Global Terrorism, 2003 (revised June 22, 2004). Washington: U.S. Department of State.

MAJOR DISASTERS, 2003

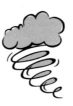

Disasters are front-page news even though the lives lost in the United States are relatively few when compared to the day-to-day life losses from injuries. The National Safety Council tracks major disasters resulting in unintentional-injury deaths. Listed below are the major U.S. disasters taking 25 or more lives during 2003.

Type and Location	No. of Deaths	Date of Disaster
Nightclub fire, Warwick, Rhode Island	100	February 20, 2003
Tornadoes in Kansas, Missouri, Arkansas, and Tennessee	38	May 4, 2003
Hurricane Isabel, North Carolina and Virginia	40	September 18, 2003

Source: National Climatic Data Center and infoplease.com.

LARGEST U.S. DISASTERS, 1984–2003

Year	Date	Type and Location	No. of Deaths
		Air Transportation	
2001	November 12	Crash of scheduled plane near Belle Harbor, N.Y.	265
1996	July 17	Crash of scheduled plane near East Moriches, N.Y.	230
1987	August 16	Crash of scheduled plane in Detroit, Mich.	156
1985	August 2	Crash of scheduled plane in Ft. Worth/Dallas, Texas, Airport	135
1994	September 8	Crash of scheduled plane in Aliquippa, Pa.	132
1989	July 19	Crash of scheduled plane in Sioux City, Iowa	112
1996	May 11	Crash of scheduled plane near Miami, Fla.	110
2000	January 31	Crash of scheduled plane near Point Mugu, Calif.	88
1986	August 31	Two-plane collision over Los Angeles, Calif.	82
1990	January 25	Crash of scheduled plane in Cove Neck, N.Y.	73
1994	October 31	Crash of scheduled plane in Indiana	68
1994	July 2	Crash of scheduled plane in Charlotte, N.C.	37
		Weather	
1995	July 11–27	Heat wave in Chicago, Ill.	465
1993	March 12–15	Severe snowstorm in Eastern States	270
1999	July 22–31	Heat wave in the Midwest	232
1998	May–July	Drought and heat wave in South and Southeast	200[a]
1996	January	Snow storm and floods in Appalachians, Mid-Atlantic, and Northeast	187
1996	Jan.–Feb.	Cold wave in eastern two-thirds of the U.S.	100[a]
1993	June–July	Heat wave in Southeast	100[a]
1998	January 5	Winter storm and flooding in South and East	90[a]
1999	September 14–18	Hurricane Floyd, North Carolina and other states	78
1985	May 31	Storm and tornadoes in Pennsylvania and Ohio	74
1997	March	Tornadoes and flooding in South and Southeast	67
1985	Nov. 4–5	Floods in W.Va., Va., Pa., and East Coast	65
1984	March 28–29	Storm and tornadoes in N.C., S.C., and East Coast	62
2001	August	Heat wave in Midwest	56
1999	May 3	Tornadoes in Oklahoma, Kansas, Texas, and Tennessee	54
2002	July 1–2	Heat wave in the Midwest and East	48
1994	March 27	Tornado in Southeast	47
2000	July 8–20	Heat wave in the Southeast	46
1998	February 22	Tornadoes across central Florida	42
2001	June 8–15	Tropical storm Allison from Gulf Coast to southern New England	41
2003	September 18	Hurricane Isabel in North Carolina and Virginia	40
2003	May 4	Tornadoes in Kansas, Missouri, Arkansas, and Tennessee	38
2002	November 9–11	Tornadoes in Tennessee and Ohio valleys region	36
1996	September 5	Hurricane Fran in North Carolina and Virginia	36
1998	April 8	Tornado in central Alabama	34
2002	December 4–5	Winter storm in South and Southeast states	29
1997	May 27	Tornadoes in Texas	29
1994	July 4–17	Floods in Georgia	28
		Work	
1987	April 24	Collapse of apartment building under construction in Bridgeport, Conn.	28
1984	December 21	Mine fire in Orangeville, Utah	27
1991	September 3	Fire at food processing plant in Hamlet, N.C.	25
		Other Disasters	
2003	February 20	Nightclub fire, Warwick, R.I.	100
1994	January 17	Earthquake in San Andreas Fault, Calif.	61
1989	October 17	Earthquake in San Francisco, Calif., and surrounding area	61
1993	September 22	Bridge collapse under train, Mobile, Ala.	47

Source: National Safety Council, Accident Facts, 1985–1998 editions, and Injury Facts, 1999–2003 editions.
[a]*Final death toll undetermined.*

While you make a 10-minute safety speech, 2 persons will be killed and about 390 will suffer a disabling injury. Costs will amount to $11,560,000. On the average, there are 12 unintentional-injury deaths and about 2,360 disabling injuries every hour during the year.

Deaths and disabling injuries by class occurred in the nation at the following rates in 2003:

DEATHS AND DISABLING INJURIES BY CLASS, 2003

Class	Severity	One Every —	Number per ...			2003 Total
			Hour	Day	Week	
All	**Deaths**	5 minutes	12	278	1,950	101,500
	Injuries	2 seconds	2,360	56,700	398,100	20,700,000
Motor-Vehicle	Deaths	12 minutes	5	123	860	44,800
	Injuries	13 seconds	270	6,600	46,200	2,400,000
Work	Deaths	117 minutes	1	12	90	4,500
	Injuries	9 seconds	390	9,300	65,400	3,400,000
Workers Off-the-Job	Deaths	12 minutes	5	116	810	42,300
	Injuries	5 seconds	740	17,800	125,000	6,500,000
Home	Deaths	16 minutes	4	91	640	33,100
	Injuries	4 seconds	900	21,600	151,900	7,900,000
Public Nonmotor-Vehicle	Deaths	25 minutes	2	58	410	21,300
	Injuries	4 seconds	810	19,500	136,500	7,100,000

Source: National Safety Council estimates.

DEATHS EVERY HOUR . . .

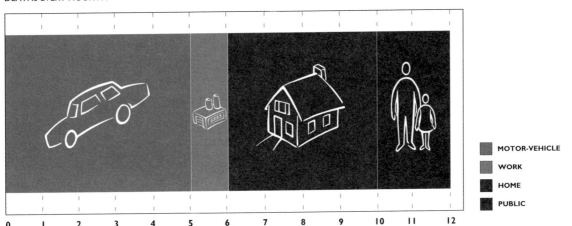

- MOTOR-VEHICLE
- WORK
- HOME
- PUBLIC

AN UNINTENTIONAL-INJURY DEATH EVERY FIVE MINUTES . . .

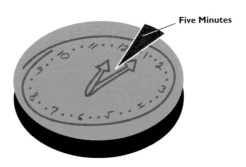

Five Minutes

CHILDREN AND YOUTHS

Unintentional-injury deaths increase seven-fold from age 12 to age 19.

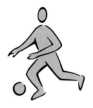

For children and youths aged 1 to 19 years, unintentional injuries are the leading cause of death, accounting for 43% of the 25,947 total deaths of these persons in 2001. Overall, motor-vehicle crashes were the leading cause of unintentional-injury deaths for this age group, followed by drowning, fires and flames, poisonings, mechanical suffocation, falls, and firearms.

While unintentional-injury deaths decrease fairly steadily for those aged 1 to 8, they increase markedly for teenagers—from 242 for those age 10 to 1,795 for those age 19. Injury deaths related to motor-vehicle crashes account for most of this increase.

For infants under 1 year of age, unintentional injuries are the seventh leading cause of death, following congenital anomalies; short gestation and low birth weight; sudden infant death syndrome; maternal complications of pregnancy; complications involving the placenta, cord, and membranes; and respiratory distress (see page 10). Although unintentional injuries only account for about 4% of deaths for those under age 1, the number of unintentional-injury deaths for this age is greater than for any age from 1 to 15.

UNINTENTIONAL-INJURY DEATHS BY EVENT, AGE 0–19, UNITED STATES, 2001

Age	Population (000)	Unintentional-Injury Deaths										
		Total	Rates[a]	Motor-vehicle	Drowning	Poisoning	Fires/Flames	Falls	Firearms	Choking[b]	Mechanical Suffocation	All Other
<1 year	4,027	976	24.2	144	68	15	50	23	0	62	552	62
1–19 years	76,663	11,196	14.6	7,520	1,113	487	553	186	182	126	189	840
1 year	3,865	575	14.9	182	182	11	56	8	1	39	33	63
2 years	3,810	442	11.6	156	140	11	58	6	2	18	10	41
3 years	3,827	361	9.4	139	71	4	56	12	8	7	14	50
4 years	3,819	336	8.8	149	65	5	55	6	4	10	7	35
5 years	3,921	277	7.1	137	42	3	49	9	2	7	7	21
6 years	3,957	264	6.7	150	25	2	41	8	5	5	7	21
7 years	4,026	261	6.5	148	32	5	33	3	3	2	7	28
8 years	4,099	235	5.7	134	37	5	22	3	5	1	2	26
9 years	4,190	246	5.9	149	32	3	19	10	3	1	5	24
10 years	4,260	242	5.7	140	28	5	20	5	2	3	9	30
11 years	4,288	278	6.5	155	47	5	21	5	5	2	12	26
12 years	4,189	269	6.4	160	21	3	25	3	12	5	7	33
13 years	4,091	323	7.9	208	28	11	11	8	13	4	10	30
14 years	4,066	441	10.8	305	41	8	11	12	7	3	13	41
15 years	4,057	606	14.9	420	59	25	11	8	16	3	12	52
16 years	4,049	1,116	27.6	902	55	55	15	7	19	2	6	55
17 years	4,018	1,417	35.3	1,133	64	62	18	19	18	7	9	87
18 years	4,050	1,712	42.3	1,382	72	103	10	22	29	5	12	77
19 years	4,081	1,795	44.0	1,371	72	161	22	32	28	2	7	100
0–4 years	19,348	2,690	13.9	770	526	46	275	55	15	136	616	251
5–9 years	20,193	1,283	6.4	718	168	18	164	33	18	16	28	120
10–14 years	20,894	1,553	7.4	968	165	32	88	33	39	17	51	160
15–19 years	20,255	6,646	32.8	5,208	322	406	76	88	110	19	46	371

Source: National Safety Council tabulations of National Center for Health Statistics mortality data.
Note: Data does not include "age unknown" cases, which totaled 120 in 2001.
[a]Deaths per 100,000 population in each age group.
[b]Suffocation by inhalation or ingestion of food or other object.

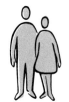

ADULTS

Falls account for more than one-third of unintentional-injury deaths of the elderly.

33

More than 89,000 adults aged 20 and older died as a result of unintentional injuries in 2001, with motor vehicles accounting for over 40% of these deaths. Data for five-year age groups indicate that motor-vehicle crashes are the most common type of unintentional-injury death through age 74. Poisoning is the second most common type for age groups 20 through 59, and falls are the second most common type from age 60 through age 74, at which point it becomes the primary cause of fatal injury for those aged 75 and older. Falls account for more than one third of the unintentional-injury deaths in this age group. Choking is the second

leading cause of unintentional-injury deaths for the most elderly (age 90 and older).

Among adults between ages 20 and 69, younger persons aged 20–24 have the highest unintentional-injury death rate—39.4 deaths per 100,000 population. Injury death rates remain relatively stable for those aged 25–69, averaging about 32.9 deaths per 100,000 population, and then increase with age. The death rate for those aged 100 and older is nearly 17 times higher than the average rate for those aged 25–69. All age groups older than 65 have death rates higher than the all-ages rate of 35.6.

UNINTENTIONAL-INJURY DEATHS BY EVENT, AGES 20 AND OLDER, UNITED STATES, 2001

Age	Population (000)	Unintentional-Injury Deaths											
		Total	Rates[a]	Motor-vehicle	Drowning	Poisoning	Fires/Flames	Falls	Firearms	Choking[b]	Mechanical Suffocation	Natural Heat/Cold	All Other
20–24	19,696	7,765	39.4	5,517	274	956	133	168	96	36	44	14	527
25–29	19,008	5,935	31.2	3,710	212	1,078	114	160	71	23	47	14	506
30–34	20,775	5,904	28.4	3,227	162	1,429	133	180	51	34	52	24	612
35–39	22,300	7,589	34.0	3,545	221	2,307	190	272	70	73	80	47	784
40–44	22,805	8,356	36.6	3,538	241	2,729	251	375	76	103	88	56	899
45–49	20,782	7,469	35.9	3,011	214	2,266	213	520	61	163	73	64	884
50–54	18,415	5,875	31.9	2,553	145	1,281	206	504	42	180	45	88	615
55–59	14,185	4,159	29.3	1,939	109	530	215	463	44	167	30	47	632
60–64	11,111	3,499	31.5	1,526	97	268	163	541	25	163	21	63	603
65–69	9,531	3,506	36.8	1,409	78	161	190	747	19	221	22	56	603
70–74	8,777	4,329	49.3	1,581	81	130	221	1,086	14	318	34	63	801
75–79	7,424	5,972	80.4	1,823	85	153	225	1,873	24	535	32	80	1,142
80–84	5,149	6,716	130.4	1,489	72	126	198	2,567	17	658	23	85	1,481
85–89	2,880	6,266	217.6	868	56	91	159	2,647	6	669	18	72	1,680
90–94	1,192	4,074	341.8	294	15	47	72	1,850	2	430	15	46	1,303
95–99	317	1,519	479.2	59	4	12	18	718	0	181	5	12	510
100 and older	56	312	557.1	2	0	2	2	135	0	43	0	2	126
20 and older	204,403	89,245	43.7	36,091	2,066	13,566	2,703	14,806	618	3,997	629	833	13,936
25 and older	184,707	81,480	44.1	30,574	1,792	12,610	2,570	14,638	522	3,961	585	819	13,409
35 and older	144,924	69,641	48.1	23,637	1,418	10,103	2,323	14,298	400	3,904	486	781	12,291
45 and older	99,819	53,696	53.8	16,554	956	5,067	1,882	13,651	254	3,728	318	678	10,608
55 and older	60,622	40,352	66.6	10,990	597	1,520	1,463	12,627	151	3,385	200	526	8,893
65 and older	35,326	32,694	92.5	7,525	391	722	1,085	11,623	82	3,055	149	416	7,646
75 and older	17,018	24,859	146.1	4,535	232	431	674	9,790	49	2,516	93	297	6,242

Source: National Safety Council tabulations of National Center for Health Statistics mortality data.
Note: Data does not include "age unknown" cases, which totaled 120 in 2001.
[a]Deaths per 100,000 population in each age group.
[b]Suffocation by inhalation or ingestion of food or other object.

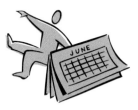

Age-adjusted rates, which eliminate the effect of shifts in the age distribution of the population, have decreased 62% from 1912 to 2003. The adjusted rates, which are shown in the graph on the opposite page, are standardized to the year 2000 standard U.S. population. The break in the lines at 1948 shows the estimated effect of changes in the International Classification of Diseases (ICD). The break in the lines at 1992 resulted from the adoption of the Bureau of Labor Statistics Census of Fatal Occupational Injuries for work-related deaths. Another change in the ICD in 1999 also affects the trends. See the Technical Appendix for comparability.

The table below shows the change in the age distribution of the population since 1910.

The age-adjusted death rate for all unintentional-injuries increased and decreased significantly several times during the period from 1910 to 1940. Since 1940, there have been some setbacks, such as in the early 1960s, but the overall trend has been positive. The age-adjusted death rates for unintentional-injury deaths in the work and home classes have declined fairly steadily since they became available in the late 1920s, although the home class rates have increased since the early 1990s. The rates in the public class declined for three decades, rose in the 1960s and then continued declining. The age-adjusted motor-vehicle death rate rose steadily from 1910 to the late 1930s as the automobile became more widely used. A sharp drop in use occurred during World War II and a sharp rise in rates occurred in the 1960s, with death rates reflecting economic cycles and a long-term downward trend since then.

UNITED STATES POPULATION, SELECTED YEARS

Year	All Ages	0–14	15–24	25–44	45–64	65 & Older
Number (in thousands)						
1910	91,973[a]	29,499	18,121	26,810	13,424	3,950
2000[b]	274,634	58,964	38,077	81,892	60,991	34,710
2003	290,810	60,920	41,191	83,940	68,795	35,964
Percent						
1910	100.0%	32.1%	19.7%	29.2%	14.6%	4.3%
2000[b]	100.0%	21.5%	13.9%	29.8%	22.2%	12.6%
2003	100.0%	20.9%	14.2%	28.9%	23.7%	12.4%

Source: For 1910: U.S. Bureau of the Census. (1960). Historical Statistics of the United States, Colonial Times to 1957. Series A 71–85. Washington, DC: U.S. Government Printing Office. For 2000: Anderson, R.N., & Rosenberg, H.M. (1998). Age standardization of death rates: Implementation of the year 2000 standard. National Vital Statistics Reports, 47(3), 13. For 2003: National Safety Council estimates based on U.S. Census Bureau data.
[a] Includes 169,000 persons with age unknown.
[b] This is the population used for standardization (age-adjustment) and differs slightly from the actual 2000 population which totaled 275,306,000.

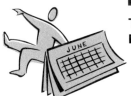

AGE-ADJUSTED DEATH RATES BY CLASS OF INJURY, UNITED STATES, 1910–2003

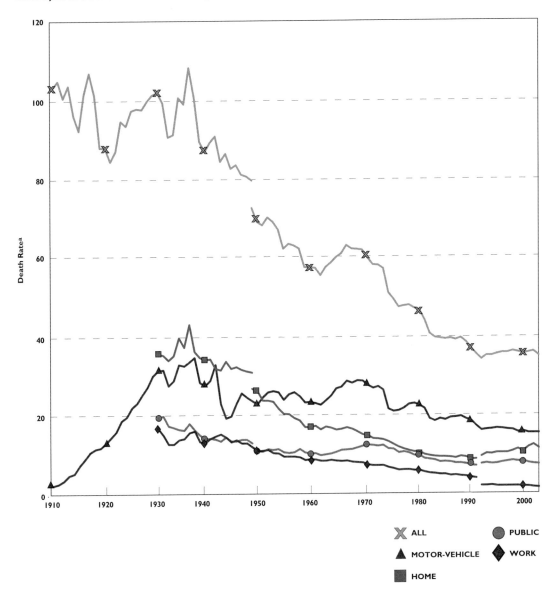

^{a}Deaths per 100,000 population, adjusted to 2000 standard population. The break at 1948 shows the estimated effect of classification changes.
The break at 1992 is due to the adoption of the Bureau of Labor Statistics' Census of Fatal Occupational Injuries for work-related deaths.

PRINCIPAL CLASSES OF UNINTENTIONAL-INJURY DEATHS

100 years of data.

PRINCIPAL CLASSES OF UNINTENTIONAL-INJURY DEATHS, UNITED STATES, 1903–2003

Year	Total[a] Deaths	Rate[b]	Motor-Vehicle Deaths	Rate[b]	Work Deaths	Rate[b]	Home Deaths	Rate[b]	Public Nonmotor-Vehicle Deaths	Rate[b]
1903	70,600	87.2	(c)	—	(c)	—	(c)	—	(c)	—
1904	71,500	86.6	(c)	—	(c)	—	(c)	—	(c)	—
1905	70,900	84.2	(c)	—	(c)	—	(c)	—	(c)	—
1906	80,000	93.2	400	0.5	(c)	—	(c)	—	(c)	—
1907	81,900	93.6	700	0.8	(c)	—	(c)	—	(c)	—
1908	72,300	81.2	800	0.9	(c)	—	(c)	—	(c)	—
1909	72,700	80.1	1,300	1.4	(c)	—	(c)	—	(c)	—
1910	77,900	84.4	1,900	2.0	(c)	—	(c)	—	(c)	—
1911	79,300	84.7	2,300	2.5	(c)	—	(c)	—	(c)	—
1912	78,400	82.5	3,100	3.3	(c)	—	(c)	—	(c)	—
1913	82,500	85.5	4,200	4.4	(c)	—	(c)	—	(c)	—
1914	77,000	78.6	4,700	4.8	(c)	—	(c)	—	(c)	—
1915	76,200	76.7	6,600	6.6	(c)	—	(c)	—	(c)	—
1916	84,800	84.1	8,200	8.1	(c)	—	(c)	—	(c)	—
1917	90,100	88.2	10,200	10.0	(c)	—	(c)	—	(c)	—
1918	85,100	82.1	10,700	10.3	(c)	—	(c)	—	(c)	—
1919	75,500	71.9	11,200	10.7	(c)	—	(c)	—	(c)	—
1920	75,900	71.2	12,500	11.7	(c)	—	(c)	—	(c)	—
1921	74,000	68.4	13,900	12.9	(c)	—	(c)	—	(c)	—
1922	76,300	69.4	15,300	13.9	(c)	—	(c)	—	(c)	—
1923	84,400	75.7	18,400	16.5	(c)	—	(c)	—	(c)	—
1924	85,600	75.6	19,400	17.1	(c)	—	(c)	—	(c)	—
1925	90,000	78.4	21,900	19.1	(c)	—	(c)	—	(c)	—
1926	91,700	78.7	23,400	20.1	(c)	—	(c)	—	(c)	—
1927	92,700	78.4	25,800	21.8	(c)	—	(c)	—	(c)	—
1928	95,000	79.3	28,000	23.4	19,000	15.8	30,000	24.9	21,000	17.4
1929	98,200	80.8	31,200	25.7	20,000	16.4	30,000	24.6	20,000	16.4
1930	99,100	80.5	32,900	26.7	19,000	15.4	30,000	24.4	20,000	16.3
1931	97,300	78.5	33,700	27.2	17,500	14.1	29,000	23.4	20,000	16.1
1932	89,000	71.3	29,500	23.6	15,000	12.0	29,000	23.2	18,000	14.4
1933	90,932	72.4	31,363	25.0	14,500	11.6	29,500	23.6	18,500	14.7
1934	100,977	79.9	36,101	28.6	16,000	12.7	34,000	26.9	18,000	14.2
1935	99,773	78.4	36,369	28.6	16,500	13.0	32,000	25.2	18,000	14.2
1936	110,052	85.9	38,089	29.7	18,500	14.5	37,000	28.9	19,500	15.2
1937	105,205	81.7	39,643	30.8	19,000	14.8	32,000	24.8	18,000	14.0
1938	93,805	72.3	32,582	25.1	16,000	12.3	31,000	23.9	17,000	13.1
1939	92,623	70.8	32,386	24.7	15,500	11.8	31,000	23.7	16,000	12.2
1940	96,885	73.4	34,501	26.1	17,000	12.9	31,500	23.9	16,500	12.5
1941	101,513	76.3	39,969	30.0	18,000	13.5	30,000	22.5	16,500	12.4
1942	95,889	71.6	28,309	21.1	18,000	13.4	30,500	22.8	16,000	12.0
1943	99,038	73.8	23,823	17.8	17,500	13.0	33,500	25.0	17,000	12.7
1944	95,237	71.7	24,282	18.3	16,000	12.0	32,500	24.5	16,000	12.0
1945	95,918	72.4	28,076	21.2	16,500	12.5	33,500	25.3	16,000	12.1
1946	98,033	70.0	33,411	23.9	16,500	11.8	33,000	23.6	17,500	12.5
1947	99,579	69.4	32,697	22.8	17,000	11.9	34,500	24.1	18,000	12.6
1948 (5th Rev.)[d]	98,001	67.1	32,259	22.1	16,000	11.0	35,000	24.0	17,000	11.6
1948 (6th Rev.)[d]	93,000	63.7	32,259	22.1	16,000	11.0	31,000	21.2	16,000	11.0
1949	90,106	60.6	31,701	21.3	15,000	10.1	31,000	20.9	15,000	10.1
1950	91,249	60.3	34,763	23.0	15,500	10.2	29,000	19.2	15,000	9.9
1951	95,871	62.5	36,996	24.1	16,000	10.4	30,000	19.6	16,000	10.4
1952	96,172	61.8	37,794	24.3	15,000	9.6	30,500	19.6	16,000	10.3
1953	95,032	60.1	37,955	24.0	15,000	9.5	29,000	18.3	16,500	10.4
1954	90,032	55.9	35,586	22.1	14,000	8.7	28,000	17.4	15,500	9.6
1955	93,443	56.9	38,426	23.4	14,200	8.6	28,500	17.3	15,500	9.4
1956	94,780	56.6	39,628	23.7	14,300	8.5	28,000	16.7	16,000	9.6
1957	95,307	55.9	38,702	22.7	14,200	8.3	28,000	16.4	17,500	10.3
1958	90,604	52.3	36,981	21.3	13,300	7.7	26,500	15.3	16,500	9.5
1959	92,080	52.2	37,910	21.5	13,800	7.8	27,000	15.3	16,500	9.3
1960	93,806	52.1	38,137	21.2	13,800	7.7	28,000	15.6	17,000	9.4
1961	92,249	50.4	38,091	20.8	13,500	7.4	27,000	14.8	16,500	9.0
1962	97,139	52.3	40,804	22.0	13,700	7.4	28,500	15.3	17,000	9.2
1963	100,669	53.4	43,564	23.1	14,200	7.5	28,500	15.1	17,500	9.3
1964	105,000	54.9	47,700	25.0	14,200	7.4	28,000	14.6	18,500	9.7
1965	108,004	55.8	49,163	25.4	14,100	7.3	28,500	14.7	19,500	10.1
1966	113,563	58.1	53,041	27.1	14,500	7.4	29,500	15.1	20,000	10.2
1967	113,169	57.3	52,924	26.8	14,200	7.2	29,000	14.7	20,500	10.4
1968	114,864	57.6	54,862	27.5	14,300	7.2	28,000	14.0	21,500	10.8
1969	116,385	57.8	55,791	27.7	14,300	7.1	27,500	13.7	22,500	11.2
1970	114,638	56.2	54,633	26.8	13,800	6.8	27,000	13.2	23,500	11.5
1971	113,439	54.8	54,381	26.3	13,700	6.6	26,500	12.8	23,500	11.4
1972	115,448	55.2	56,278	26.9	14,000	6.7	26,500	12.7	23,500	11.2
1973	115,821	54.8	55,511	26.3	14,300	6.8	26,500	12.5	24,500	11.6

See source and footnotes on page 37.

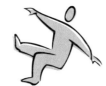
PRINCIPAL CLASSES OF UNINTENTIONAL-INJURY DEATHS, UNITED STATES, 1903–2003, Cont.

Year	Total[a] Deaths	Total[a] Rate[b]	Motor-Vehicle Deaths	Motor-Vehicle Rate[b]	Work Deaths	Work Rate[b]	Home Deaths	Home Rate[b]	Public Nonmotor-Vehicle Deaths	Public Nonmotor-Vehicle Rate[b]
1974	104,622	49.0	46,402	21.8	13,500	6.3	26,000	12.2	23,000	10.8
1975	103,030	47.8	45,853	21.3	13,000	6.0	25,000	11.6	23,000	10.6
1976	100,761	46.3	47,038	21.6	12,500	5.7	24,000	11.0	21,500	10.0
1977	103,202	47.0	49,510	22.5	12,900	5.9	23,200	10.6	22,200	10.1
1978	105,561	47.5	52,411	23.6	13,100	5.9	22,800	10.3	22,000	9.9
1979	105,312	46.9	53,524	23.8	13,000	5.8	22,500	10.0	21,000	9.4
1980	105,718	46.5	53,172	23.4	13,200	5.8	22,800	10.0	21,300	9.4
1981	100,704	43.9	51,385	22.4	12,500	5.4	21,700	9.5	19,800	8.6
1982	94,082	40.6	45,779	19.8	11,900	5.1	21,200	9.2	19,500	8.4
1983	92,488	39.6	44,452	19.0	11,700	5.0	21,200	9.1	19,400	8.3
1984	92,911	39.4	46,263	19.6	11,500	4.9	21,200	9.0	18,300	7.8
1985	93,457	39.3	45,901	19.3	11,500	4.8	21,600	9.1	18,800	7.9
1986	95,277	39.7	47,865	19.9	11,100	4.6	21,700	9.0	18,700	7.8
1987	95,020	39.2	48,290	19.9	11,300	4.7	21,400	8.8	18,400	7.6
1988	97,100	39.7	49,078	20.1	11,000	4.5	22,700	9.3	18,400	7.5
1989	95,028	38.5	47,575	19.3	10,900	4.4	22,500	9.1	18,200	7.4
1990	91,983	36.9	46,814	18.8	10,100	4.0	21,500	8.6	17,400	7.0
1991	89,347	35.4	43,536	17.3	9,800	3.9	22,100	8.8	17,600	7.0
1992	86,777	34.0	40,982	16.1	4,968[e]	1.9[e]	24,000[e]	9.4[e]	19,000[e]	7.4[e]
1993	90,523	35.1	41,893	16.3	5,035	2.0	26,100	10.1	19,700	7.6
1994	91,437	35.1	42,524	16.3	5,338	2.1	26,300	10.1	19,600	7.5
1995	93,320	35.5	43,363	16.5	5,018	1.9	27,200	10.3	20,100	7.6
1996	94,948	35.8	43,649	16.5	5,058	1.9	27,500	10.4	21,000	7.9
1997	95,644	35.7	43,458	16.2	5,162	1.9	27,700	10.3	21,700	8.1
1998	97,835	36.2	43,501	16.1	5,120	1.9	29,000	10.7	22,600	8.4
1999[f]	97,860	35.9	42,401	15.5	5,185	1.9	30,500	11.2	22,200	8.1
2000	97,900	35.6	43,354	15.7	5,022	1.8	29,200	10.6	22,700	8.2
2001[g]	101,537	35.6	43,788	15.4	5,042	1.8	33,200	11.6	21,800	7.6
2002[g]	103,500	35.9	44,100	15.3	4,716	1.6	35,300	12.3	21,600	7.5
2003[h]	101,500	34.9	44,800	15.4	4,500	1.5	33,100	11.4	21,300	7.3
Changes										
1993 to 2003	+12%	−1%	+7%	−6%	−11%	−25%	+27%	+13%	+8%	−4%
2002 to 2003	−2%	−3%	+2%	+1%	−5%	−6%	−6%	−7%	−1%	−3%

Source: Total and motor-vehicle deaths, 1903–1932 based on National Center for Health Statistics death registration states; 1933–1948 (5th Rev.), 1949–1963, 1965–2001 are NCHS totals for the U.S. Work deaths for 1992–2002 are from the Bureau of Labor Statistics, Census of Fatal Occupational Injuries. All other figures are National Safety Council estimates.
[a] Duplications between Motor-Vehicle, Work, and Home are eliminated in the Total column.
[b] Rates are deaths per 100,000 population.
[c] Data insufficient to estimate yearly totals.
[d] In 1948 a revision was made in the International Classification of Diseases. The first figures for 1948 are comparable with those for earlier years, the second with those for later years.
[e] Adoption of the Census of Fatal Occupational Injuries figure for the Work class necessitated adjustments to the Home and Public classes. See the Technical Appendix for details.
[f] In 1999 a revision was made in the International Classification of Diseases. See the Technical Appendix for comparability with earlier years.
[g] Revised.
[h] Preliminary.

UNINTENTIONAL-INJURY DEATHS BY AGE

100 years of data.

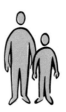

UNINTENTIONAL-INJURY DEATHS BY AGE, UNITED STATES, 1903–2003

Year	All Ages	Under 5 Years	5–14 Years	15–24 Years	25–44 Years	45–64 Years	65–74 Years	75 Years & Over[a]
1903	70,600	9,400	8,200	10,300	20,100	12,600	10,000	
1904	71,500	9,700	9,000	10,500	19,900	12,500	9,900	
1905	70,900	9,800	8,400	10,600	19,600	12,600	9,900	
1906	80,000	10,000	8,400	13,000	24,000	13,600	11,000	
1907	81,900	10,500	8,300	13,400	24,900	14,700	10,100	
1908	72,300	10,100	7,600	11,300	20,500	13,100	9,700	
1909	72,700	9,900	7,400	10,700	21,000	13,300	10,400	
1910	77,900	9,900	7,400	11,900	23,600	14,100	11,000	
1911	79,300	11,000	7,500	11,400	22,400	15,100	11,900	
1912	78,400	10,600	7,900	11,500	22,200	14,700	11,500	
1913	82,500	9,800	7,400	12,200	24,500	16,500	12,100	
1914	77,000	10,600	7,900	11,000	21,400	14,300	11,800	
1915	76,200	10,300	8,200	10,800	20,500	14,300	12,100	
1916	84,800	11,600	9,100	7,700	24,900	17,800	13,700	
1917	90,100	11,600	9,700	11,700	24,400	18,500	14,200	
1918	85,100	10,600	10,100	10,600	21,900	17,700	14,200	
1919	75,500	10,100	10,000	10,200	18,600	13,800	12,800	
1920	75,900	10,200	9,900	10,400	18,100	13,900	13,400	
1921	74,000	9,600	9,500	9,800	18,000	13,900	13,200	
1922	76,300	9,700	9,500	10,000	18,700	14,500	13,900	
1923	84,400	9,900	9,800	11,000	21,500	16,900	15,300	
1924	85,600	10,200	9,900	11,900	20,900	16,800	15,900	
1925	90,000	9,700	10,000	12,400	22,200	18,700	17,000	
1926	91,700	9,500	9,900	12,600	22,700	19,200	17,800	
1927	92,700	9,200	9,900	12,900	22,900	19,700	18,100	
1928	95,000	8,900	9,800	13,100	23,300	20,600	19,300	
1929	98,200	8,600	9,800	14,000	24,300	21,500	20,000	
1930	99,100	8,200	9,100	14,000	24,300	22,200	21,300	
1931	97,300	7,800	8,700	13,500	23,100	22,500	21,700	
1932	89,000	7,100	8,100	12,000	20,500	20,100	21,200	
1933	90,932	6,948	8,195	12,225	21,005	20,819	21,740	
1934	100,977	7,034	8,272	13,274	23,288	24,197	24,912	
1935	99,773	6,971	7,808	13,168	23,411	23,457	24,958	
1936	110,052	7,471	7,866	13,701	24,990	26,535	29,489	
1937	105,205	6,969	7,704	14,302	23,955	24,743	27,532	
1938	93,805	6,646	6,593	12,129	20,464	21,689	26,284	
1939	92,628	6,668	6,378	12,066	20,164	20,842	26,505	
1940	96,885	6,851	6,466	12,763	21,166	21,840	27,799	
1941	101,513	7,052	6,702	14,346	22,983	22,509	27,921	
1942	95,889	7,220	6,340	13,732	21,141	20,764	26,692	
1943	99,038	8,039	6,636	15,278	20,212	20,109	28,764	
1944	95,237	7,912	6,704	14,750	19,115	19,097	27,659	
1945	95,918	7,741	6,836	12,446	19,393	20,097	29,405	
1946	98,033	7,949	6,545	13,366	20,705	20,249	29,219	
1947	99,579	8,219	6,069	13,166	21,155	20,513	30,457	
1948 (5th Rev.)[b]	98,001	8,387	5,859	12,595	20,274	19,809	31,077	
1948 (6th Rev.)[b]	93,000	8,350	5,850	12,600	20,300	19,300	9,800	16,800
1949	90,106	8,469	5,539	11,522	19,432	18,302	9,924	16,918
1950	91,249	8,389	5,519	12,119	20,663	18,665	9,750	16,144
1951	95,871	8,769	5,892	12,366	22,363	19,610	10,218	16,653
1952	96,172	8,871	5,980	12,787	21,950	19,892	10,026	16,667
1953	95,032	8,678	6,136	12,837	21,422	19,479	9,927	16,553
1954	90,032	8,380	5,939	11,801	20,023	18,299	9,652	15,938
1955	93,443	8,099	6,099	12,742	29,911	19,199	9,929	16,464
1956	94,780	8,173	6,319	13,545	20,986	19,207	10,160	16,393
1957	95,307	8,423	6,454	12,973	20,949	19,495	10,076	16,937
1958	90,604	8,789	6,514	12,744	19,658	18,095	9,431	15,373
1959	92,080	8,748	6,511	13,269	19,666	18,937	9,475	15,474
1960	93,806	8,950	6,836	13,457	19,600	19,385	9,689	15,829
1961	92,249	8,622	6,717	13,431	19,273	19,134	9,452	15,620
1962	97,139	8,705	6,751	14,557	19,955	20,335	10,149	16,687
1963	100,669	8,688	6,962	15,889	20,529	21,262	10,194	17,145
1964	100,500	8,670	7,400	17,420	22,080	22,100	10,400	16,930
1965	108,004	8,586	7,391	18,688	22,228	22,900	10,430	17,781
1966	113,563	8,507	7,958	21,030	23,134	24,022	10,706	18,206
1967	113,169	7,825	7,874	21,645	23,255	23,826	10,645	18,099
1968	114,864	7,263	8,369	23,012	23,684	23,896	10,961	17,679
1969	116,385	6,973	8,186	24,668	24,410	24,192	10,643	17,313
1970	114,638	6,594	8,203	24,336	23,979	24,164	10,644	16,718
1971	113,439	6,496	8,143	24,733	23,535	23,240	10,494	16,798
1972	115,448	6,142	8,242	25,762	23,852	23,658	10,446	17,346
1973	115,821	6,037	8,102	26,550	24,750	23,059	10,243	17,080

See source and footnotes on page 39.

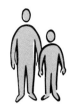

UNINTENTIONAL-INJURY DEATHS BY AGE, UNITED STATES, 1903–2003, Cont.

Year	All Ages	Under 5 Years	5–14 Years	15–24 Years	25–44 Years	45–64 Years	65–74 Years	75 Years & Over[a]
1974	104,622	5,335	7,037	24,200	22,547	20,334	9,323	15,846
1975	103,030	4,948	6,818	24,121	22,877	19,643	9,220	15,403
1976	100,761	4,692	6,308	24,316	22,399	19,000	8,823	15,223
1977	103,202	4,470	6,305	25,619	23,460	19,167	9,006	15,175
1978	105,561	4,766	6,118	26,622	25,024	18,774	9,072	15,185
1979	105,312	4,429	5,689	26,574	26,097	18,346	9,013	15,164
1980	105,718	4,479	5,224	26,206	26,722	18,140	8,997	15,950
1981	100,704	4,130	4,866	23,582	26,928	17,339	8,639	15,220
1982	94,082	4,108	4,504	21,306	25,135	15,907	8,224	14,898
1983	92,488	3,999	4,321	19,756	24,996	15,444	8,336	15,636
1984	92,911	3,652	4,198	19,801	25,498	15,273	8,424	16,065
1985	93,457	3,746	4,252	19,161	25,940	15,251	8,583	16,524
1986	95,277	3,843	4,226	19,975	27,201	14,733	8,499	16,800
1987	95,020	3,871	4,198	18,695	27,484	14,807	8,686	17,279
1988	97,100	3,794	4,215	18,507	28,279	15,177	8,971	18,157
1989	95,028	3,770	4,090	16,738	28,429	15,046	8,812	18,143
1990	91,983	3,496	3,650	16,241	27,663	14,607	8,405	17,921
1991	89,347	3,626	3,660	15,278	26,526	13,693	8,137	18,427
1992	86,777	3,286	3,388	13,662	25,808	13,882	8,165	18,586
1993	90,523	3,488	3,466	13,966	27,277	14,434	8,125	19,767
1994	91,437	3,406	3,508	13,898	27,012	15,200	8,279	20,134
1995	93,320	3,067	3,544	13,842	27,660	16,004	8,400	20,803
1996	94,948	2,951	3,433	13,809	27,092	16,717	8,780	22,166
1997	94,644	2,770	3,371	13,367	27,129	17,521	8,578	22,908
1998	97,835	2,689	3,254	13,349	27,172	18,286	8,892	24,193
1999[c]	97,860	2,743	3,091	13,656	27,121	18,924	8,208	24,117
2000	97,900	2,707	2,979	14,113	27,182	19,783	7,698	23,438
2001[d]	101,537	2,690	2,836	14,411	27,784	21,002	7,835	24,979
2002[d]	103,500	2,500	2,700	14,900	28,700	22,400	8,000	24,300
2003[e]	101,500	2,500	2,600	14,100	26,000	22,000	8,400	25,900
Changes								
1993 to 2003	+12%	−28%	−25%	+1%	−5%	+52%	+3%	+31%
2002 to 2003	−2%	0%	−4%	−5%	−9%	−2%	+5%	+7%

Source: 1903 to 1932 based on National Center for Health Statistics data for registration states; 1933–1948 (5th Rev.), 1949–1963, 1965–2001 are NCHS totals. All other figures are National Safety Council estimates. See Technical Appendix for comparability.
[a] *Includes age unknown. In 2001, these deaths numbered 120.*
[b] *In 1948, a revision was made in the International Classification of Diseases. The first figures for 1948 are comparable with those for earlier years, the second with those for later years.*
[c] *In 1999, a revision was made in the International Classification of Diseases. See the Technical Appendix for comparability with earlier years.*
[d] *Revised.*
[e] *Preliminary.*

UNINTENTIONAL-INJURY DEATH RATES BY AGE

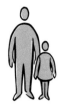

100 years of data.

UNINTENTIONAL-INJURY DEATH RATES[a] BY AGE, UNITED STATES, 1903–2003

Year	Standardized Rate[b]	All Ages	Under 5 Years	5–14 Years	15–24 Years	25–44 Years	45–64 Years	65–74 Years	75 Years & Over[c]
1903	99.4	87.2	98.7	46.8	65.0	87.4	111.7	299.8	
1904	103.4	86.6	99.1	50.9	64.9	84.6	108.1	290.0	
1905	98.4	84.2	98.6	47.0	64.1	81.4	106.2	282.5	
1906	114.2	93.2	99.1	46.5	77.1	97.3	111.7	306.0	
1907	112.4	93.6	102.7	45.5	78.0	98.8	117.8	274.2	
1908	99.7	81.2	97.5	41.2	64.4	79.5	102.2	256.7	
1909	97.4	80.1	94.2	39.6	59.9	79.6	101.0	268.2	
1910	103.0	84.4	92.8	39.1	65.3	87.3	104.0	276.0	
1911	104.7	84.7	101.9	39.3	62.1	81.4	108.7	292.1	
1912	100.4	82.5	97.1	40.5	62.3	79.2	103.2	275.8	
1913	103.5	85.5	88.4	37.4	65.2	85.6	112.5	281.7	
1914	95.9	78.6	94.3	38.9	58.5	73.2	94.6	268.1	
1915	92.1	76.7	90.8	39.7	57.3	69.0	92.1	268.8	
1916	101.4	84.1	101.4	43.3	40.8	82.5	112.1	297.6	
1917	106.7	88.2	108.4	45.3	62.1	79.8	113.8	301.2	
1918	101.2	82.1	91.0	46.5	58.7	72.2	106.3	294.2	
1919	87.7	71.9	87.2	45.9	55.3	60.1	81.8	262.0	
1920	87.8	71.2	87.4	44.9	55.5	56.9	85.6	289.5	
1921	84.3	68.4	80.8	42.4	51.4	55.5	79.4	259.8	
1922	86.9	69.4	80.6	41.5	51.4	57.1	81.4	265.1	
1923	94.5	75.7	82.0	42.4	55.6	64.5	92.6	282.8	
1924	93.3	75.6	82.9	42.4	58.6	61.7	90.2	283.5	
1925	97.2	78.4	78.6	42.3	59.7	64.7	97.8	293.9	
1926	97.7	78.7	77.9	41.4	59.9	65.4	98.2	298.7	
1927	97.5	78.4	75.9	41.0	60.2	65.2	98.0	295.4	
1928	99.6	79.3	74.4	40.4	59.9	65.6	99.9	306.2	
1929	101.2	80.8	73.3	40.0	63.1	67.7	102.1	308.9	
1930	101.8	80.5	71.8	36.9	62.3	67.0	102.9	317.9	
1931	99.2	78.5	69.9	35.2	59.7	63.0	102.1	313.3	
1932	90.5	71.3	65.1	32.8	52.7	55.6	89.3	296.9	
1933	91.1	72.4	65.5	33.4	53.6	56.3	90.8	295.3	
1934	100.5	79.9	68.1	33.9	57.8	61.8	103.3	328.5	
1935	97.9	78.4	68.5	32.2	56.9	61.6	98.0	319.8	
1936	108.1	85.9	74.4	32.9	58.8	65.3	108.6	367.4	
1937	100.7	81.7	69.6	32.7	60.9	62.1	99.3	333.4	
1938	89.4	72.3	65.3	28.5	51.3	52.5	85.4	308.9	
1939	86.7	70.8	62.9	28.2	50.7	51.2	81.0	300.0	
1940	89.1	73.4	64.8	28.8	53.5	53.2	83.4	305.7	
1941	90.7	76.3	65.0	29.7	60.9	57.2	84.8	297.4	
1942	84.3	71.6	63.9	27.9	59.8	52.4	77.1	275.5	
1943	86.3	73.8	66.9	29.0	69.7	50.3	73.6	287.8	
1944	82.5	71.7	63.2	29.1	72.9	48.9	68.9	268.6	
1945	83.4	72.4	59.8	29.5	64.5	50.5	71.6	277.6	
1946	81.0	70.0	60.2	28.1	61.7	48.8	70.9	267.9	
1947	80.5	69.4	57.4	25.8	59.6	49.0	70.6	270.7	
1948 (5th Rev.)[d]	79.5	67.1	56.3	24.6	56.8	46.2	66.8	267.4	
1948 (6th Rev.)[d]	72.5	63.7	56.0	24.5	56.8	46.2	65.1	122.4	464.3
1949	69.0	60.6	54.4	23.0	52.2	43.5	60.6	120.4	450.7
1950	68.1	60.3	51.4	22.6	55.0	45.6	60.5	115.8	414.7
1951	70.1	62.5	50.8	23.6	57.7	49.0	62.7	117.1	413.6
1952	69.0	61.8	51.5	22.5	60.9	47.7	62.7	111.1	399.8
1953	67.0	60.1	49.5	22.1	61.4	46.4	60.5	106.7	383.6
1954	62.2	55.9	46.7	20.5	56.4	43.0	55.9	100.7	354.4
1955	63.4	56.9	43.9	20.7	60.1	44.7	57.7	100.8	350.2
1956	63.0	56.6	43.3	20.2	63.3	44.7	56.7	100.6	335.6
1957	62.2	55.9	43.5	19.9	59.5	44.6	56.6	97.5	333.3
1958	57.5	52.3	44.5	19.6	56.2	42.0	51.7	89.3	292.6
1959	57.4	52.2	43.6	18.9	56.5	42.1	53.2	87.7	284.7
1960	57.3	52.1	44.0	19.1	55.6	42.0	53.6	87.6	281.4
1961	55.4	50.4	42.0	18.1	54.0	41.2	52.1	83.8	267.9
1962	57.5	52.3	42.6	18.0	55.0	42.7	54.6	88.5	277.7
1963	58.6	53.4	42.8	18.2	57.2	44.0	56.3	87.9	277.0
1964	60.0	54.9	43.1	19.1	59.9	47.3	57.6	88.9	263.9
1965	61.9	55.8	43.4	18.7	61.6	47.7	58.8	88.5	268.7
1966	63.0	58.1	44.4	19.9	66.9	49.6	60.7	89.8	267.4
1967	62.1	57.3	42.2	19.4	66.9	49.7	59.2	88.5	257.4
1968	62.0	57.6	40.6	20.5	69.2	50.1	58.5	90.2	244.0
1969	61.8	57.8	40.2	20.0	71.8	51.2	58.4	86.6	232.0
1970	59.8	56.2	38.4	20.1	68.0	49.8	57.6	85.2	219.6
1971	58.1	54.8	37.7	20.1	66.1	48.4	54.7	82.7	213.2
1972	58.0	55.2	35.9	20.6	67.6	47.5	55.2	80.8	214.2
1973	57.1	54.8	35.8	20.6	68.2	48.0	53.3	77.3	206.3

See source and footnotes on page 41.

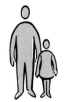

UNINTENTIONAL-INJURY DEATH RATES[a] BY AGE, UNITED STATES, 1903–2003, Cont.

Year	Standardized Rate[b]	All Ages	Under 5 Years	5–14 Years	15–24 Years	25–44 Years	45–64 Years	65–74 Years	75 Years & Over[c]
1974	50.9	49.0	32.4	18.2	60.9	42.7	46.7	68.7	186.7
1975	49.3	47.8	30.7	17.8	59.5	42.3	44.9	66.2	175.5
1976	47.3	46.3	30.0	16.7	58.9	40.3	43.2	62.0	168.4
1977	47.6	47.0	28.7	17.0	61.3	40.9	43.4	61.5	164.0
1978	47.8	47.5	30.3	16.9	63.1	42.3	42.4	60.5	159.7
1979	47.0	46.9	27.6	16.1	62.6	42.7	41.3	58.8	154.8
1980	46.5	46.5	27.2	15.0	61.7	42.3	40.8	57.5	158.6
1981	44.0	43.9	24.4	14.2	55.9	41.2	39.0	54.4	147.4
1982	40.6	40.6	23.8	13.2	51.2	37.3	35.8	50.9	140.0
1983	39.6	39.6	22.8	12.7	48.2	36.0	34.7	50.8	142.8
1984	39.4	39.4	20.6	12.4	48.9	35.7	34.3	50.7	142.8
1985	39.2	39.3	21.0	12.6	47.9	35.3	34.2	50.9	143.0
1986	39.4	39.7	21.4	12.6	50.5	36.1	33.0	49.6	141.5
1987	39.0	39.2	21.4	12.4	48.1	35.7	33.0	49.8	141.6
1988	39.5	39.7	20.9	12.3	48.5	36.1	33.4	50.9	145.3
1989	38.4	38.5	20.4	11.8	44.8	35.7	32.8	49.3	141.5
1990	36.7	36.9	18.5	10.4	44.0	34.2	31.6	46.4	136.5
1991	35.3	35.4	18.9	10.2	42.0	32.3	29.3	44.5	136.7
1992	34.0	34.0	16.8	9.3	37.8	31.3	28.7	44.2	134.5
1993	35.0	35.1	17.7	9.4	38.8	33.0	29.1	43.6	139.9
1994	35.0	35.1	17.3	9.4	38.4	32.5	29.9	44.3	139.2
1995	35.4	35.5	15.7	9.3	38.2	33.2	30.6	44.8	140.6
1996	35.7	35.8	15.3	8.9	38.1	32.3	31.1	47.0	145.9
1997	35.7	35.7	14.5	8.7	36.5	32.5	31.6	46.3	146.2
1998	36.1	36.2	14.2	8.3	35.9	32.6	31.9	48.3	151.1
1999[e]	35.8	35.9	14.5	7.8	36.1	32.7	32.0	45.0	147.7
2000	35.5	35.6	14.3	7.5	36.7	33.0	32.3	42.3	140.8
2001[f]	35.7	35.6	13.9	6.9	36.1	32.7	32.6	42.8	146.8
2002[f]	36.0	35.9	12.7	6.6	36.7	34.0	33.6	43.7	140.4
2003[g]	34.9	34.9	12.5	6.4	34.2	31.0	32.0	45.7	147.2

Changes									
1993 to 2003		−1%	−29%	−32%	−12%	−6%	+10%	+5%	+5%
2002 to 2003		−3%	−2%	−3%	−7%	−9%	−5%	+5%	+5%

2003 Population (Millions)									
Total		290.810[h]	19.976	40.944	41.191	83.940	68.794	18.371	17.593
Male		142.760	10.210	20.963	21.102	42.073	33.488	8.364	6.559
Female		148.049	9.766	19.981	20.089	41.867	35.306	10.007	11.034

Source: All figures are National Safety Council estimates. See Technical Appendix for comparability.
[a] Rates are deaths per 100,000 resident population in each age group.
[b] Adjusted to the year 2000 standard population to remove the influence of changes in age distribution between 1903 and 2001.
[c] Includes age unknown.
[d] In 1948, a revision was made in the International Classification of Diseases. The first figures for 1948 are comparable with those for earlier years, the second with those for later years.
[e] In 1999, a revision was made in the International Classification of Diseases. See the Technical Appendix for comparability.
[f] Revised.
[g] Preliminary.
[h] Sum of parts may not equal total due to rounding.

PRINCIPAL TYPES OF UNINTENTIONAL-INJURY DEATHS

100 years of data.

PRINCIPAL TYPES OF UNINTENTIONAL-INJURY DEATHS, UNITED STATES, 1903–1998

Year	Total	Motor-Vehicle	Falls	Drowning[a]	Fires/Burns[b]	Ingest. of Food/Object	Firearms	Poison (Solid, Liquid)	Poison (Gas, Vapor)	All Other
1903	70,600	[c]	[c]	9,200	[c]	[c]	2,500	[c]	[c]	58,900
1904	71,500	[c]	[c]	9,300	[c]	[c]	2,800	[c]	[c]	59,400
1905	70,900	[c]	[c]	9,300	[c]	[c]	2,000	[c]	[c]	59,600
1906	80,000	400	[c]	9,400	[c]	[c]	2,100	[c]	[c]	68,100
1907	81,900	700	[c]	9,000	[c]	[c]	1,700	[c]	[c]	70,500
1908	72,300	800	[c]	9,300	[c]	[c]	1,900	[c]	[c]	60,300
1909	72,700	1,300	[c]	8,500	[c]	[c]	1,600	[c]	[c]	61,300
1910	77,900	1,900	[c]	8,700	[c]	[c]	1,900	[c]	[c]	65,400
1911	79,300	2,300	[c]	9,000	[c]	[c]	2,100	[c]	[c]	65,900
1912	78,400	3,100	[c]	8,600	[c]	[c]	2,100	[c]	[c]	64,600
1913	82,500	4,200	15,100	10,300	8,900	[c]	2,400	3,200	[c]	38,400
1914	77,000	4,700	15,000	8,700	9,100	[c]	2,300	3,300	[c]	33,900
1915	76,200	6,600	15,000	8,600	8,400	[c]	2,100	2,800	[c]	32,700
1916	84,800	8,200	15,200	8,900	9,500	[c]	2,200	2,900	[c]	37,900
1917	90,100	10,200	15,200	7,600	10,800	[c]	2,300	2,800	[c]	41,200
1918	85,100	10,700	13,200	7,000	10,200	[c]	2,500	2,700	[c]	38,800
1919	75,500	11,200	11,900	9,100	9,100	[c]	2,800	3,100	[c]	28,300
1920	75,900	12,500	12,600	6,100	9,300	[c]	2,700	3,300	[c]	29,400
1921	74,000	13,900	12,300	7,800	7,500	[c]	2,800	2,900	[c]	26,800
1922	76,300	15,300	13,200	7,000	8,300	[c]	2,900	2,800	[c]	26,800
1923	84,400	18,400	14,100	6,800	9,100	[c]	2,900	2,800	2,700	27,600
1924	85,600	19,400	14,700	7,400	7,400	[c]	2,900	2,700	2,900	28,200
1925	90,000	21,900	15,500	7,300	8,600	[c]	2,800	2,700	2,800	28,400
1926	91,700	23,400	16,300	7,500	8,800	[c]	2,800	2,600	3,200	27,100
1927	92,700	25,800	16,500	8,100	8,200	[c]	3,000	2,600	2,700	25,800
1928	95,000	28,000	17,000	8,600	8,400	[c]	2,900	2,800	2,800	24,500
1929	98,200	31,200	17,700	7,600	8,200	[c]	3,200	2,600	2,800	24,900
1930	99,100	32,900	18,100	7,500	8,100	[c]	3,200	2,600	2,500	24,200
1931	97,300	33,700	18,100	7,600	7,100	[c]	3,100	2,600	2,100	23,000
1932	89,000	29,500	18,600	7,500	7,100	[c]	3,000	2,200	2,100	19,000
1933	90,932	31,363	18,962	7,158	6,781	[c]	3,014	2,135	1,633	19,886
1934	100,977	36,101	20,725	7,077	7,456	[c]	3,033	2,148	1,643	22,794
1935	99,773	36,369	21,378	6,744	7,253	[c]	2,799	2,163	1,654	21,413
1936	110,052	38,089	23,562	6,659	7,939	[c]	2,817	2,177	1,665	27,144
1937	105,205	39,643	22,544	7,085	7,214	[c]	2,576	2,190	1,675	22,278
1938	93,805	32,582	23,239	6,881	6,491	[c]	2,726	2,077	1,428	18,381
1939	92,623	32,386	23,427	6,413	6,675	[c]	2,618	1,963	1,440	17,701
1940	96,885	34,501	23,356	6,202	7,521	[c]	2,375	1,847	1,583	19,500
1941	101,513	39,969	22,764	6,389	6,922	[c]	2,396	1,731	1,464	19,878
1942	95,889	28,309	22,632	6,696	7,901	[c]	2,678	1,607	1,741	24,325
1943	99,038	23,823	24,701	7,115	8,726	921	2,282	1,745	2,014	27,711
1944	95,237	24,282	22,989	6,511	8,372	896	2,392	1,993	1,860	25,942
1945	95,918	28,076	23,847	6,624	7,949	897	2,385	1,987	2,120	22,033
1946	98,033	33,411	23,109	6,442	7,843	1,076	2,801	1,961	1,821	19,569
1947	99,579	32,697	24,529	6,885	8,033	1,206	2,439	1,865	1,865	14,060
1948 (5th Rev.)[d]	98,001	32,259	24,836	6,428	7,743	1,315	2,191	1,753	2,045	19,611
1948 (6th Rev.)[d]	93,000	32,259	22,000	6,500	6,800	1,299	2,330	1,600	2,020	17,192
1949	90,106	31,701	22,308	6,684	5,982	1,341	2,326	1,634	1,617	16,513
1950	91,249	34,763	20,783	6,131	6,405	1,350	2,174	1,584	1,769	16,290
1951	95,871	36,996	21,376	6,489	6,788	1,456	2,247	1,497	1,627	17,395
1952	96,172	37,794	20,945	6,601	6,922	1,434	2,210	1,440	1,397	17,429
1953	95,032	37,955	20,631	6,770	6,579	1,603	2,277	1,391	1,223	16,603
1954	90,032	35,586	19,771	6,334	6,083	1,627	2,271	1,339	1,223	15,798
1955	93,443	38,426	20,192	6,344	6,352	1,608	2,120	1,431	1,163	15,807
1956	94,780	39,628	20,282	6,263	6,405	1,760	2,202	1,422	1,213	15,605
1957	95,307	38,702	20,545	6,613	6,269	2,043	2,369	1,390	1,143	16,233
1958	90,604	36,981	18,248	6,582[e]	7,291[e]	2,191[e]	2,172	1,429	1,187	14,523
1959	92,080	37,910	18,774	6,434	6,898	2,189	2,258	1,661	1,141	14,815
1960	93,806	38,137	19,023	6,529	7,645	2,397	2,334	1,679	1,253	14,809
1961	92,249	38,091	18,691	6,525	7,102	2,499	2,204	1,804	1,192	14,141
1962	97,139	40,804	19,589	6,439	7,534	1,813	2,092	1,833	1,376	15,659
1963	100,669	43,564	19,335	6,347	8,172	1,949	2,263	2,061	1,489	15,489
1964	105,000	47,700	18,941	6,709	7,379	1,865	2,275	2,100	1,360	16,571
1965	108,004	49,163	19,984	6,799	7,347	1,836	2,344	2,110	1,526	16,895
1966	113,563	53,041	20,066	7,084	8,084	1,831	2,558	2,283	1,648	16,968
1967	113,169	52,924	20,120	7,076	7,423	1,980	2,896	2,506	1,574	16,670
1968	114,864	54,862	18,651	7,372[e]	7,335	3,100[e]	2,394[e]	2,583	1,526	17,041
1969	116,385	55,791	17,827	7,699	7,163	3,712	2,309	2,967	1,549	16,368
1970	114,638	54,633	16,926	7,860	6,718	2,753	2,406	3,679	1,620	18,043
1971	113,439	54,381	16,755	7,396	6,776	2,877	2,360	3,710	1,646	17,538
1972	115,448	56,278	16,744	7,586	6,714	2,830	2,442	3,728	1,690	17,436
1973	115,821	55,511	16,506	8,725	6,503	3,013	2,618	3,683	1,652	17,610

See source and footnotes on page 43.

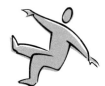

PRINCIPAL TYPES OF UNINTENTIONAL-INJURY DEATHS, UNITED STATES, 1903–1998, Cont.

Year	Total	Motor-Vehicle	Falls	Drowning[a]	Fires/Burns[b]	Ingest. of Food/Object	Firearms	Poison (Solid, Liquid)	Poison (Gas, Vapor)	All Other
1974	104,622	46,402	16,339	7,876	6,236	2,991	2,513	4,016	1,518	16,731
1975	103,030	45,853	14,896	8,000	6,071	3,106	2,380	4,694	1,577	16,453
1976	100,761	47,038	14,136	6,827	6,338	3,033	2,059	4,161	1,569	15,600
1977	103,202	49,510	13,773	7,126	6,357	3,037	1,982	3,374	1,596	16,447
1978	105,561	52,411	13,690	7,026	6,163	3,063	1,806	3,035	1,737	16,630
1979	105,312	53,524	13,216	6,872	5,991	3,243	2,004	3,165	1,472	15,825
1980	105,718	53,172	13,294	7,257	5,822	3,249	1,955	3,089	1,242	16,638
1981	100,704	51,385	12,628	6,277	5,697	3,331	1,871	3,243	1,280	14,992
1982	94,082	45,779	12,077	6,351	5,210	3,254	1,756	3,474	1,259	14,922
1983	92,488	44,452	12,024	6,353	5,028	3,387	1,695	3,382	1,251	14,916
1984	92,911	46,263	11,937	5,388	5,010	3,541	1,668	3,808	1,103	14,193
1985	93,457	45,901	12,001	5,316	4,938	3,551	1,649	4,091	1,079	14,931
1986	95,277	47,865	11,444	5,700	4,835	3,692	1,452	4,731	1,009	14,549
1987	95,020	48,290	11,733	5,100	4,710	3,688	1,440	4,415	900	14,744
1988	97,100	49,078	12,096	4,966	4,965	3,805	1,501	5,353	873	14,463
1989	95,028	47,575	12,151	4,015	4,716	3,578	1,489	5,603	921	14,980
1990	91,983	46,814	12,313	4,685	4,175	3,303	1,416	5,055	748	13,474
1991	89,347	43,536	12,662	4,818	4,120	3,240	1,441	5,698	736	13,096
1992	86,777	40,982	12,646	3,542	3,958	3,182	1,409	6,449	633	13,976
1993	90,523	41,893	13,141	3,807	3,900	3,160	1,521	7,877	660	14,564
1994	91,437	42,524	13,450	3,942	3,986	3,065	1,356	8,309	685	14,120
1995	93,320	43,363	13,986	4,350	3,761	3,185	1,225	8,461	611	14,378
1996	94,948	43,649	14,986	3,959	3,741	3,206	1,134	8,872	638	14,763
1997	95,644	43,458	15,447	4,051	3,490	3,275	981	9,587	576	14,779
1998	97,835	43,501	16,274	4,406	3,255	3,515	866	10,255	546	15,217

PRINCIPAL TYPES OF UNINTENTIONAL-INJURY DEATHS, UNITED STATES, 1999–2003

Year	Total	Motor-Vehicle	Falls	Poisoning	Ingest. of Food/Object	Drowning[f]	Fires, Flames, Smoke[b]	Mechanical Suffocation	Firearms	All Other
1999[g]	97,860	42,401	13,162	12,186	3,885	3,529	3,348	1,618	824	16,907
2000	97,900	43,354	13,322	12,757	4,313	3,482	3,377	1,335	776	15,184
2001[h]	101,537	43,788	15,019	14,078	4,185	3,281	3,309	1,370	802	15,705
2002[h]	103,500	44,100	15,300	16,100	4,400	3,000	2,800	1,500	800	15,500
2003[i]	101,500	44,800	16,200	13,900	4,300	2,900	2,600	1,200	700	14,900

Changes										
1992 to 2003	+12%	+7%	(j)	(j)	+36%	(j)	−33%	(j)	−54%	(j)
2001 to 2003	−2%	+2%	+6%	−14%	−2%	−3%	−7%	−20%	−13%	−4%

Source: National Center for Health Statistics and National Safety Council. See Technical Appendix for comparability.
[a] Includes drowning in water transport accidents.
[b] Includes burns by fire, and deaths resulting from conflagration regardless of nature of injury.
[c] Comparable data not available.
[d] In 1948, a revision was made in the International Classification of Diseases. The first figures for 1948 are comparable with those for earlier years, the second with those for later years.
[e] Data are not comparable to previous years shown due to classification changes in 1958 and 1968.
[f] Excludes water transport drownings.
[g] In 1999, a revision was made in the International Classification of Diseases. See the Technical Appendix for comparability.
[h] Revised.
[i] Preliminary.
[j] Comparison not valid because of change in classifications (see footnote "g").

UNINTENTIONAL-INJURY DEATH RATES FOR PRINCIPAL TYPES

100 years of data.

UNINTENTIONAL-INJURY DEATH RATES[a] FOR PRINCIPAL TYPES, UNITED STATES, 1903–1998

Year	Total	Motor-Vehicle	Falls	Drowning[b]	Fires/Burns[c]	Ingest. of Food/Object	Firearms	Poison (Solid, Liquid)	Poison (Gas, Vapor)	All Other
1903	87.2	(d)	(d)	11.4	(d)	(d)	3.1	(d)	(d)	72.7
1904	86.6	(d)	(d)	11.3	(d)	(d)	3.4	(d)	(d)	71.9
1905	84.2	(d)	(d)	11.1	(d)	(d)	2.4	(d)	(d)	70.7
1906	93.2	0.5	(d)	11.0	(d)	(d)	2.4	(d)	(d)	79.3
1907	93.6	0.8	(d)	10.4	(d)	(d)	2.0	(d)	(d)	80.4
1908	81.2	0.9	(d)	10.5	(d)	(d)	2.1	(d)	(d)	67.7
1909	80.1	1.4	(d)	9.4	(d)	(d)	1.8	(d)	(d)	67.5
1910	84.4	2.0	(d)	9.4	(d)	(d)	2.1	(d)	(d)	70.9
1911	84.7	2.5	(d)	9.6	(d)	(d)	2.2	(d)	(d)	70.4
1912	82.5	3.3	(d)	9.0	(d)	(d)	2.2	(d)	(d)	68.0
1913	85.5	4.4	15.5	10.6	9.1	(d)	2.5	3.3	(d)	40.1
1914	78.6	4.8	15.1	8.8	9.1	(d)	2.3	3.3	(d)	35.2
1915	76.7	6.6	14.9	8.6	8.4	(d)	2.1	2.8	(d)	33.3
1916	84.1	8.1	14.9	8.7	9.3	(d)	2.2	2.8	(d)	38.1
1917	88.2	10.0	14.7	7.4	10.5	(d)	2.2	2.7	(d)	40.7
1918	82.1	10.3	12.8	6.8	9.9	(d)	2.4	2.6	(d)	37.3
1919	71.9	10.7	11.4	6.9	8.7	(d)	2.7	3.0	(d)	28.5
1920	71.2	11.7	11.8	5.7	8.7	(d)	2.5	3.1	(d)	27.7
1921	68.4	12.9	11.3	7.2	6.9	(d)	2.6	2.7	(d)	24.8
1922	69.4	13.9	12.0	6.4	7.5	(d)	2.6	2.5	(d)	24.5
1923	75.7	16.5	12.6	6.1	8.1	(d)	2.6	2.5	2.4	24.9
1924	75.6	17.1	12.9	6.5	8.4	(d)	2.5	2.4	2.5	23.3
1925	78.4	19.1	13.4	6.3	7.4	(d)	2.4	2.3	2.4	25.1
1926	78.7	20.1	13.9	6.4	7.5	(d)	2.4	2.2	2.7	23.5
1927	78.4	21.8	13.9	6.8	6.9	(d)	2.5	2.2	2.3	22.0
1928	79.3	23.4	14.1	7.1	7.0	(d)	2.4	2.3	2.3	20.7
1929	80.8	25.7	14.5	6.2	6.7	(d)	2.6	2.1	2.3	20.7
1930	80.5	26.7	14.7	6.1	6.6	(d)	2.6	2.1	2.0	19.7
1931	78.5	27.2	14.6	6.1	5.7	(d)	2.5	2.1	1.7	18.6
1932	71.3	23.6	14.9	6.0	5.7	(d)	2.4	1.8	1.7	15.2
1933	72.4	25.0	15.1	5.7	5.4	(d)	2.4	1.7	1.3	15.8
1934	79.9	28.6	16.4	5.6	5.9	(d)	2.4	1.7	1.3	18.0
1935	78.4	28.6	16.8	5.3	5.7	(d)	2.2	1.7	1.3	16.8
1936	85.9	29.7	18.4	5.2	6.2	(d)	2.2	1.7	1.3	21.2
1937	81.7	30.8	17.5	5.5	5.6	(d)	2.0	1.7	1.3	17.3
1938	72.3	25.1	17.9	5.3	5.0	(d)	2.1	1.6	1.1	14.2
1939	70.8	24.7	17.9	4.9	5.1	(d)	2.0	1.5	1.1	13.6
1940	73.4	26.1	17.7	4.7	5.7	(d)	1.8	1.4	1.2	14.8
1941	76.3	30.0	17.1	4.8	5.2	(d)	1.8	1.3	1.1	15.0
1942	71.6	21.1	16.9	5.0	5.9	(d)	2.0	1.2	1.3	18.2
1943	73.8	17.8	18.4	5.3	6.5	0.7	1.7	1.3	1.5	20.6
1944	71.7	18.3	17.3	4.9	6.3	0.7	1.8	1.5	1.4	19.5
1945	72.4	21.2	18.0	5.0	6.0	0.7	1.8	1.5	1.6	16.6
1946	70.0	23.9	16.5	4.6	5.6	0.8	2.0	1.4	1.3	13.9
1947	69.4	22.8	17.1	4.8	5.6	0.8	1.7	1.3	1.3	14.0
1948 (5th Rev.)[e]	67.1	22.1	17.0	4.4	5.3	0.9	1.5	1.2	1.4	13.3
1948 (6th Rev.)[e]	63.7	22.1	15.1	4.5	4.7	0.9	1.6	1.1	1.4	12.3
1949	60.6	21.3	15.0	4.5	4.0	0.9	1.6	1.1	1.1	11.1
1950	60.3	23.0	13.7	4.1	4.2	0.9	1.4	1.1	1.2	10.7
1951	62.5	24.1	13.9	4.2	4.4	1.0	1.5	1.0	1.1	11.3
1952	61.8	24.3	13.5	4.2	4.5	0.9	1.4	0.9	0.9	11.2
1953	60.1	24.0	13.0	4.3	4.2	1.0	1.4	0.9	0.8	10.2
1954	55.9	22.1	12.3	3.9	3.8	1.0	1.4	0.8	0.8	9.8
1955	56.9	23.4	12.3	3.9	3.9	1.0	1.3	0.9	0.7	9.5
1956	56.6	23.7	12.1	3.7	3.8	1.1	1.3	0.8	0.7	9.4
1957	55.9	22.7	12.1	3.9	3.7	1.2	1.4	0.8	0.7	9.4
1958	52.3	21.3	10.5	3.8[f]	4.2[f]	1.3[f]	1.3	0.8	0.7	8.4
1959	52.2	21.5	10.6	3.7	3.9	1.2	1.3	0.9	0.7	8.4
1960	52.1	21.2	10.6	3.6	4.3	1.3	1.3	0.9	0.7	8.2
1961	50.4	20.8	10.2	3.6	3.9	1.4	1.2	1.0	0.7	7.6
1962	52.3	22.0	10.5	3.5	4.1	1.0	1.1	1.0	0.7	8.4
1963	53.4	23.1	10.3	3.4	4.3	1.0	1.2	1.1	0.8	8.2
1964	54.9	25.0	9.9	3.5	3.9	1.0	1.2	1.1	0.7	8.4
1965	55.8	25.4	10.3	3.5	3.8	1.0	1.2	1.1	0.8	8.7
1966	58.1	27.1	10.3	3.6	4.8	0.9	1.3	1.2	0.8	8.1
1967	57.3	26.8	10.2	3.6	3.8	1.0	1.5	1.3	0.8	8.3
1968	57.6	27.5	9.4	3.7[f]	3.7[f]	1.6[f]	1.2[f]	1.3	0.8	8.4
1969	57.8	27.7	8.9	3.8	3.6	1.8	1.2	1.5	0.8	8.5
1970	56.2	26.8	8.3	3.9	3.3	1.4	1.2	1.8	0.8	8.7
1971	54.8	26.3	8.1	3.6	3.3	1.4	1.1	1.8	0.8	8.4
1972	55.2	26.9	8.0	3.6	3.2	1.4	1.2	1.8	0.8	8.3
1973	54.8	26.3	7.8	4.1	3.1	1.4	1.2	1.7	0.8	8.4

See source and footnotes on page 45.

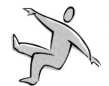

UNINTENTIONAL-INJURY DEATH RATES[a] FOR PRINCIPAL TYPES, UNITED STATES, 1903–1998, Cont.

Year	Total	Motor-Vehicle	Falls	Drowning[b]	Fires/Burns[c]	Ingest. of Food/Object	Firearms	Poison (Solid, Liquid)	Poison (Gas, Vapor)	All Other
1974	49.0	21.8	7.7	3.7	2.9	1.4	1.2	1.8	0.7	7.8
1975	47.8	21.3	6.9	3.7	2.8	1.4	1.1	2.2	0.7	7.7
1976	46.3	21.6	6.5	3.1	2.9	1.4	0.9	1.9	0.7	7.3
1977	47.0	22.5	6.3	3.2	2.9	1.4	0.9	1.5	0.7	7.6
1978	47.5	23.6	6.2	3.2	2.8	1.4	0.8	1.4	0.8	7.3
1979	46.9	23.8	5.9	3.1	2.7	1.4	0.9	1.4	0.7	7.0
1980	46.5	23.4	5.9	3.2	2.6	1.4	0.9	1.4	0.5	7.2
1981	43.9	22.4	5.5	2.7	2.5	1.5	0.8	1.4	0.6	6.5
1982	40.6	19.8	5.2	2.7	2.2	1.4	0.8	1.5	0.5	6.5
1983	39.6	19.0	5.1	2.7	2.2	1.4	0.7	1.4	0.5	6.6
1984	39.4	19.6	5.1	2.3	2.1	1.5	0.7	1.6	0.5	6.0
1985	39.3	19.3	5.0	2.2	2.1	1.5	0.7	1.7	0.5	6.3
1986	39.7	19.9	4.8	2.4	2.0	1.5	0.6	2.0	0.4	6.1
1987	39.2	19.9	4.8	2.1	1.9	1.5	0.6	1.8	0.4	6.2
1988	39.7	20.1	4.9	2.0	2.0	1.6	0.6	2.2	0.4	5.9
1989	38.5	19.3	4.9	1.9	1.9	1.4	0.6	2.3	0.4	5.8
1990	36.9	18.8	4.9	1.9	1.7	1.3	0.6	2.0	0.3	5.4
1991	35.4	17.3	5.0	1.8	1.6	1.3	0.6	2.3	0.3	5.2
1992	34.0	16.1	5.0	1.4	1.6	1.2	0.6	2.5	0.2	5.4
1993	35.1	16.3	5.1	1.5	1.5	1.2	0.6	3.1	0.3	5.5
1994	35.1	16.3	5.2	1.5	1.5	1.2	0.5	3.2	0.3	5.4
1995	35.5	16.5	5.3	1.7	1.4	1.2	0.5	3.2	0.2	5.5
1996	35.8	16.5	5.6	1.5	1.4	1.2	0.4	3.3	0.2	5.7
1997	35.7	16.2	5.8	1.5	1.3	1.2	0.4	3.6	0.2	5.5
1998	36.2	16.1	6.0	1.6	1.2	1.3	0.3	3.8	0.2	5.7

UNINTENTIONAL-INJURY DEATH RATES[a] FOR PRINCIPAL TYPES, UNITED STATES, 1999–2003

Year	Total	Motor-Vehicle	Falls	Poisoning	Ingest. of Food/Object	Drowning[g]	Fires, Flames, Smoke[c]	Mechanical Suffocation	Firearms	All Other
1999[h]	35.9	15.5	4.8	4.5	1.4	1.3	1.2	0.6	0.3	6.3
2000	35.6	15.7	4.8	4.6	1.6	1.3	1.2	0.5	0.3	5.5
2001[i]	35.6	15.4	5.3	4.9	1.5	1.2	1.2	0.5	0.3	5.5
2002[i]	35.9	15.3	5.3	5.6	1.5	1.0	1.0	0.5	0.3	5.4
2003[j]	34.9	15.4	5.6	4.8	1.5	1.0	0.9	0.4	0.2	5.1

Changes										
1993 to 2003	–1%	–6%	(k)	(k)	+25%	(k)	–40%	(k)	–67%	(k)
2002 to 2003	–3%	+1%	+6%	–14%	0%	0%	–10%	–20%	–33%	–6%

Source: National Safety Council estimates. See Technical Appendix for comparability.
[a] *Deaths per 100,000 population.*
[b] *Includes drowning in water transport accidents.*
[c] *Includes burns by fire, and deaths resulting from conflagration regardless of nature of injury.*
[d] *Comparable data not available.*
[e] *In 1948, a revision was made in the International Classification of Diseases. The first figures for 1948 are comparable with those for earlier years, the second with those for later years.*
[f] *Data are not comparable to previous years shown due to classification changes in 1958 and 1968.*
[g] *Excludes water transport drownings.*
[h] *In 1999, a revision was made in the International Classification of Diseases. See the Technical Appendix for comparability.*
[i] *Revised.*
[j] *Preliminary.*
[k] *Comparison not valid because of change in classifications (see footnote "h").*

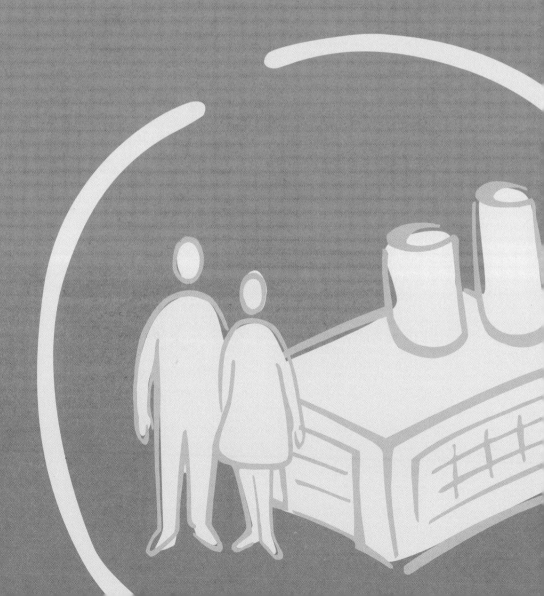

OCCUPATIONAL

INJURY FACTS®

NATIONAL SAFETY COUNCIL

WORK, 2003

Between 1912 and 2003, unintentional work deaths per 100,000 population were reduced 93%, from 21 to 1.5. In 1912, an estimated 18,000 to 21,000 workers' lives were lost. In 2003, in a work force nearly quadrupled in size and producing nine times the goods and services, there were only an estimated 4,500 work deaths.

In addition to unintentional (accidental) fatal work injuries, about 800 homicides and suicides occurred in the workplace in 2002. These intentional injuries are not included in the unintentional-injury estimates.

The State Data section, which begins on page 150, shows fatal occupational injuries and nonfatal injury and illness incidence rates by state.

Unintentional-Injury Deaths **4,500**
Unintentional-Injury Deaths per 100,000 Workers **3.2**
Disabling Injuries **3,400,000**
Workers **138,988,000**
Costs . . . . **$156.2 billion**

UNINTENTIONAL INJURIES AT WORK BY INDUSTRY, UNITED STATES, 2003

| Industry Division | Workers[a] (000) | Deaths[a] | | Deaths per 100,000 Workers[a] | | Disabling Injuries |
		2003	Change from 2002	2003	Change from 2002	
All Industries	**138,988**	**4,500**	**–5%**	**3.2**	**–5%**	**3,400,000**
Agriculture[b]	3,340	710	–6%	20.9	–4%	110,000
Mining, quarrying[b]	539	120	+1%	22.3	–4%	20,000
Construction	9,268	1,060	–3%	11.4	–4%	390,000
Manufacturing	17,708	490	–6%	2.8	–4%	460,000
Transportation and public utilities	7,721	770	–9%	10.0	–5%	320,000
Trade[b]	29,240	380	0%	1.3	–4%	710,000
Services[b]	50,310	550	–3%	1.1	–4%	890,000
Government	20,862	420	–3%	2.0	–3%	500,000

Source: National Safety Council estimates based on data from the Bureau of Labor Statistics, National Center for Health Statistics, state vital statistics departments, and state industrial commissions.
Note: The National Safety Council adopted the Bureau of Labor Statistics' Census of Fatal Occupational Injuries (CFOI), beginning with the 1992 data year, as the authoritative count of work-related deaths. See the Technical Appendix for additional information.
[a] Deaths include persons of all ages. Workers and death rates include persons 16 years and older.
[b] Agriculture includes forestry, fishing, and agricultural services. Mining includes oil and gas extraction. Trade includes wholesale and retail trade. Services includes finance, insurance, and real estate.

OCCUPATIONAL UNINTENTIONAL-INJURY DEATHS AND DEATH RATES BY INDUSTRY, UNITED STATES, 2003

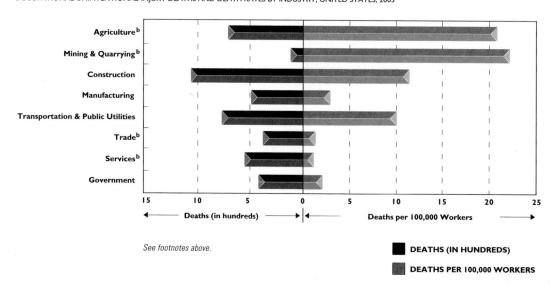

See footnotes above.

■ DEATHS (IN HUNDREDS)
■ DEATHS PER 100,000 WORKERS

UNINTENTIONAL WORK-INJURY DEATHS AND DEATH RATES, UNITED STATES, 1992–2003

Year	Deaths[a]	Workers[b]	Death Rate[c]
1992	4,965	119,168,000	4.2
1993	5,034	120,778,000	4.2
1994	5,338	124,470,000	4.3
1995	5,015	126,248,000	4.0
1996	5,069	127,997,000	4.0
1997	5,160	130,810,000	3.9
1998	5,117	132,772,000	3.9
1999	5,184	134,688,000	3.8
2000	5,022	136,402,000	3.7
2001[d]	5,042	136,246,000	3.7
2002[d]	4,716	137,731,000	3.4
2003[e]	4,500	138,988,000	3.2

Source: Deaths through 2002 are from the Bureau of Labor Statistics, Census of Fatal Occupational Injuries. Employment is from the Bureau of Labor Statistics and is based on the Current Population Survey. All other data are National Safety Council estimates.
[a] *Deaths include persons of all ages. Workers and death rates include persons 16 years and older. Because of adoption of the Census of Fatal Occupational Injuries, deaths and rates from 1992 to the present are not comparable to prior years. See Technical Appendix for change in estimating procedure.*
[b] *Workers are persons ages 16 and older gainfully employed, including owners, managers, other paid employees, the self-employed, unpaid family workers, and active duty resident military personnel. Due to changes in procedures, estimates of workers from 1992 to the present are not comparable to prior years.*
[c] *Deaths per 100,000 workers.*
[d] *Revised.*
[e] *Preliminary.*

WORKERS, UNINTENTIONAL-INJURY DEATHS, AND DEATH RATES, UNITED STATES, 1992–2003

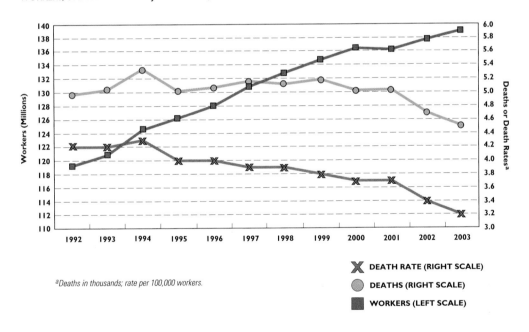

[a] *Deaths in thousands; rate per 100,000 workers.*

✕ DEATH RATE (RIGHT SCALE)
⬤ DEATHS (RIGHT SCALE)
■ WORKERS (LEFT SCALE)

WORK, 2003 (CONT.)

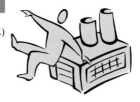

OCCUPATIONAL-INJURY DEATHS AND DEATH RATES, UNITED STATES, 1992–2003

Year	Total	Homicide & Suicide	Unintentional								
			All Industries[a]	Agri-culture[b]	Mining, Quarrying[c]	Construc-tion	Manufac-turing	Transpor-tation & Public Utilities	Trade[d]	Services[e]	Govern-ment
Deaths											
1992	6,217	1,252	4,965	779	175	889	707	767	415	601	586
1993	6,331	1,297	5,034	842	169	895	698	753	450	631	527
1994	6,632	1,294	5,338	814	177	1,000	734	819	492	676	534
1995	6,275	1,260	5,015	769	155	1,021	640	784	461	608	528
1996	6,202	1,133	5,069	762	151	1,025	660	883	451	615	321
1997	6,238	1,078	5,160	799	156	1,075	678	882	451	593	504
1998	6,055	938	5,117	808	143	1,136	631	830	443	634	465
1999	6,054	870	5,184	776	122	1,168	671	918	425	623	451
2000	5,920	898	5,022	693	153	1,114	624	872	447	643	460
2001[f]	5,915	873[h]	5,042	714	169	1,183	546	844	431	636	507
2002[f]	5,524	808	4,716	757	119	1,088	522	843	380	566	435
2003[g]	—	—	4,500	710	120	1,060	490	770	380	550	420
Deaths per 100,000 Workers											
1992	5.2	1.0	4.2	23.1	26.4	13.7	3.6	11.5	1.7	1.6	3.0
1993	5.2	1.0	4.2	26.0	25.3	13.3	3.6	11.0	1.8	1.6	2.6
1994	5.3	1.0	4.3	22.8	26.5	14.4	3.7	11.6	1.9	1.7	2.7
1995	4.9	1.0	4.0	21.4	24.8	14.3	3.1	11.0	1.8	1.5	2.7
1996	4.8	0.9	4.0	21.2	26.6	13.7	3.2	12.2	1.7	1.4	1.6
1997	4.8	0.8	3.9	22.5	24.7	13.7	3.3	11.6	1.7	1.3	2.6
1998	4.5	0.7	3.9	22.7	23.1	14.1	3.1	10.8	1.6	1.4	2.4
1999	4.5	0.6	3.8	22.6	21.7	13.8	3.4	11.5	1.5	1.3	2.2
2000	4.3	0.7	3.7	20.1	29.4	12.4	3.1	10.8	1.6	1.4	2.3
2001[f]	4.3	0.6[h]	3.7	22.0	29.9	13.0	2.9	10.4	1.6	1.3	2.5
2002[f]	4.0	0.6	3.4	21.8	23.1	11.9	2.9	10.5	1.4	1.1	2.1
2003[g]	—	—	3.2	20.9	22.3	11.4	2.8	10.0	1.3	1.1	2.0

Source: Deaths are from Bureau of Labor Statistics, Census of Fatal Occupational Injuries, except 2003 which are National Safety Council estimates. Rates are National Safety Council estimates based on Bureau of Labor Statistics employment data. Deaths include persons of all ages. Death rates include persons 16 years and older. Dashes (—) indicate data not available.
[a] *Includes deaths with industry unknown.*
[b] *Agriculture includes forestry, fishing, and agricultural services.*
[c] *Mining includes oil and gas extraction.*
[d] *Trade includes wholesale and retail trade.*
[e] *Services includes finance, insurance, and real estate.*
[f] *Revised.*
[g] *Preliminary.*
[h] *Excludes 2,886 homicides of workers on September 11, 2001.*

WORK INJURY COSTS

The true cost to the nation, to employers, and to individuals of work-related deaths and injuries is much greater than the cost of workers' compensation insurance alone. The figures presented below show the National Safety Council's estimates of the total economic costs of occupational deaths and injuries. Cost-estimating procedures were revised for the 1993 edition of *Accident Facts*®. In general, cost estimates are not comparable from year to year. As additional or more precise data become available, they are used from that year forward. Previously estimated figures are not revised.

TOTAL COST IN 2003 . . . . **$156.2 billion**
Includes wage and productivity losses of $78.3 billion, medical costs of $30.9 billion, and administrative expenses of $28.7 billion. Includes uninsured employer costs of $13.7 billion such as the money value of time lost by workers other than those with disabling injuries,

who are directly or indirectly involved in injuries, and the cost of time required to investigate injuries, write up injury reports, etc. Also includes damage to motor vehicles in work injuries of $2.0 billion and fire losses of $2.6 billion.

Cost per Worker **$1,120**
This figure indicates the value of goods or services each worker must produce to offset the cost of work injuries. It is *not* the average cost of a work injury.

Cost per Death **$1,110,000**
Cost per Disabling Injury **$38,000**

These figures include estimates of wage losses, medical expenses, administrative expenses, and employer costs, and exclude property damage costs except to motor-vehicles.

TIME LOST BECAUSE OF WORK INJURIES

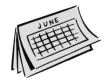

DAYS LOST
TOTAL TIME LOST IN 2003 . . . . **115,000,000**
Due to Injuries in 2003 . . . . **70,000,000**
Includes primarily the actual time lost during the year from disabling injuries, except that it does not include time lost on the day of the injury or time required for further medical treatment or checkup following the injured person's return to work.

Fatalities are included at an average loss of 150 days per case, and permanent impairments are included at actual days lost plus an allowance for lost efficiency resulting from the impairment.

Not included is time lost by persons with nondisabling injuries or other persons directly or indirectly involved in the incidents.

DAYS LOST
Due to Injuries in Prior Years **45,000,000**
This is an indicator of the productive time lost in 2003 due to permanently disabling injuries that occurred in prior years.

DAYS LOST
TIME LOSS IN FUTURE YEARS
FROM 2003 INJURIES **55,000,000**
Includes time lost in future years due to on-the-job deaths and permanently disabling injuries that occurred in 2003.

WORKER DEATHS AND INJURIES
ON AND OFF THE JOB

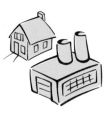

Nine out of 10 deaths and about two thirds of the disabling injuries suffered by workers in 2003 occurred off the job. The ratios of off-the-job deaths and injuries to on-the-job were 9.4 to 1 and 1.9 to 1, respectively. Production time lost due to off-the-job injuries totaled about 160,000,000 days in 2003, compared with 70,000,000 days lost by workers injured on the job. Production time lost in future years due to off-the-job injuries in 2003 will total an estimated 405,000,000 days, more than seven times the 55,000,000 days lost in

future years from 2003's on-the-job injuries. Off-the-job injuries to workers cost the nation at least $205.3 billion in 2003.

The basis of the rates shown in the table below was changed from 1,000,000 hours to 200,000 hours beginning with the 1998 edition. This change was made so that the rates would be on the same basis as the occupational injury and illness incidence rates shown elsewhere in *Injury Facts®*.

ON- AND OFF-THE-JOB INJURIES, UNITED STATES, 2003

Place	Deaths		Disabling Injuries	
	Number	Rate[a]	Number	Rate[a]
On- and off-the-job	**46,800**	**0.011**	**9,900,000**	**2.4**
On-the-job	4,500	0.003	3,400,000	2.3
Off-the-job	42,300	0.016	6,500,000	2.4
Motor-vehicle	*23,100*	*0.083*	*1,200,000*	*4.3*
Public nonmotor-vehicle	*7,200*	*0.017*	*2,400,000*	*5.6*
Home	*12,000*	*0.006*	*2,900,000*	*1.5*

Source: National Safety Council estimates. Procedures for allocating time spent on and off the job were revised for the 1990 edition. Rate basis changed to 200,000 hours for the 1998 edition. Death and injury rates are not comparable to rate estimates prior to the 1998 edition.
[a] Per 200,000 hours exposure by place.

WORKERS' ON- AND OFF-THE-JOB INJURIES, 2003

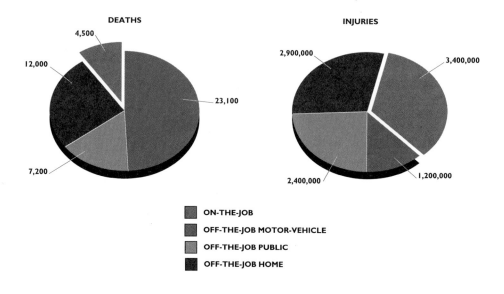

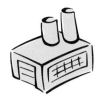

According to the National Academy of Social Insurance, an estimated $49.4 billion, including benefits under deductible provisions, was paid out under workers' compensation in 2001 (the latest year for which data were available), an increase of about 3.5% from 2000. Of this total, $27.4 billion was for income benefits, and $22.0 billion was for medical and hospitalization costs. Private carriers paid about $27.1 billion of the total workers' compensation benefits in 2001. In 2001,

approximately 127.0 million workers were covered by workers' compensation — a decrease of 0.1% over the 127.1 million in 2000.

The table below shows the trend in the number of compensated or reported cases in each reporting state. Due to the differences in population, industries, and coverage of compensation laws, comparison among states should not be made.

WORKERS' COMPENSATION CASES, UNITED STATES, 2001–2003

State	Deaths[a]			Cases[a]			2001 Compensation Paid ($000)
	2003	2002	2001	2003	2002	2001	
Alabama[b]	83	99	107	19,739	21,972	22,994	562,773
Alaska	17	24	39	24,742	26,365	28,621	171,248
Arkansas[b]	—	72	73	—	12,377	12,940	201,136
Colorado[c]	—	—	111	—	—	31,896	581,266
Connecticut	59	99	61	56,524	72,982	68,149	661,471
Delaware	6	11	10	20,981	22,685	21,505	144,588
Hawaii[b]	—	31	34	—	29,757	30,179	252,041
Iowa	55	40	69	22,060	23,587	28,957	395,981
Kentucky	52	—	—	35,016	—	—	524,566
Louisiana[d]	54	53	70	10,419	13,161	15,824	501,662
Maine	—	30	23	16,362	16,891	18,158	263,852
Massachusetts	60	46	62	36,641	36,122	41,195	763,795
Minnesota[d]	34	53	60	—	141,000	154,000	908,100
Mississippi	—	96	105	—	13,682	14,790	271,163
Missouri	95	142	147	143,245	156,079	166,567	1,108,464
Montana[d]	6	13	18	8,682	9,494	11,114	172,725
Nevada[d]	—	40	49	—	83,999	85,303	380,756
New Mexico[d]	21	29	28	19,440	20,534	22,852	162,022
North Carolina	186	183	163	60,050	62,656	63,318	867,965
North Dakota	15	14	13	18,753	19,950	20,320	79,633
Ohio	167	147	155	230,186	236,344	263,911	2,249,200
Oregon[d,e]	41	52	34	21,829[f]	23,482	24,645	455,625
Pennsylvania[b]	140	146	134	99,161	95,206	90,405	2,440,407
South Dakota[d,g]	20	15	13	24,254	26,498	29,204	74,950
Washington	64	91	92	200,688	217,125	232,708	1,637,714
Wisconsin[b]	49	51	66	48,336	51,843	56,063	921,857

Source: Deaths and Cases — State workers' compensation authorities for calendar or fiscal year. States not listed did not respond to the survey. Compensation Paid — Thompson-Williams, C., Reno, V. P., & Burton, J. F., Jr., (July, 2003). Workers' compensation: benefits, coverage, and costs, 2001. Washington DC: National Academy of Social Insurance.
Note: Dash (—) indicates data not available.

Definitions:
 Reported case — a reported case may or may not be work-related and may not receive compensation.
 Compensated case — a case determined to be work-related and for which compensation was paid.

[a]Reported cases involving medical and indemnity benefits, unless otherwise noted.
[b]Reported cases involving indemnity benefits only.
[c]Reported and closed or compensated cases.
[d]Closed or compensated cases.
[e]Accepted disabling claims, including lost-time claims in which the worker misses 3 or more days of work, has a validated hospital admittance, or a fatal injury.
[f]Preliminary.
[g]Cases first closed in the calendar year involving indemnity benefits only.

WORKERS' COMPENSATION CLAIMS COSTS, 2001–2002

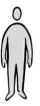

Motor-vehicle crashes are the most costly workers' compensation claims.

The data in the graphs on this and the next page are from the National Council on Compensation Insurance's (NCCI) Detailed Claim Information (DCI) file, a stratified random sample of lost-time claims in 41 states. Total incurred costs consist of medical and indemnity payments plus case reserves on open claims, and are calculated as of the second report (18 months after the initial report of injury). Injuries that result in medical payments only, without lost time, are not included. For open claims, costs include all payments as of the second report plus case reserves for future payments. Because the estimates are based on a sample, they can be volatile from year to year due to the influence of a small but variable number of large claims.

The average cost for all claims combined in 2001–2002 was $15,865, up 16% from the 2000–2001 average of $13,719.

Cause of Injury. The most costly lost-time workers' compensation claims by cause of injury, according to the NCCI data, are for those resulting from motor-vehicle crashes. These injuries averaged more than

$27,500 per workers' compensation claim filed in 2001 and 2002. The other causes with above average costs were those involving a fall or slip ($18,838) and miscellaneous causes ($16,243).

Nature of Injury. The most costly lost-time workers' compensation claims by the nature of the injury are for those resulting from amputation. These injuries averaged $31,546 per workers' compensation claim filed in 2001 and 2002. The next highest costs were for injuries resulting in fracture ($21,476), other trauma ($18,524), and carpal tunnel syndrome ($17,202).

Part of Body. The most costly lost-time workers' compensation claims are for those involving the head or central nervous system. These injuries averaged $40,392 per workers' compensation claim filed in 2001 and 2002. The next highest costs were for injuries involving multiple body parts ($23,903) and the neck ($23,862). Injuries to the arm/shoulder; hip, thigh, and pelvis; knee; leg; and lower back also had above-average costs.

AVERAGE TOTAL INCURRED COSTS PER CLAIM BY CAUSE OF INJURY, 2001–2002

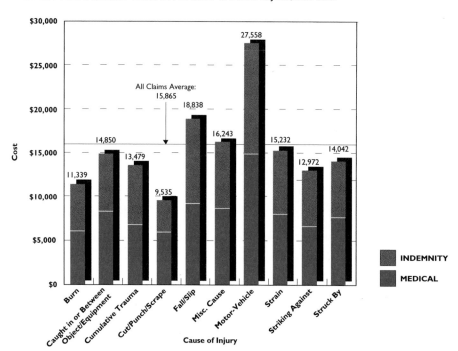

AVERAGE TOTAL INCURRED COSTS PER CLAIM BY NATURE OF INJURY, 2001–2002

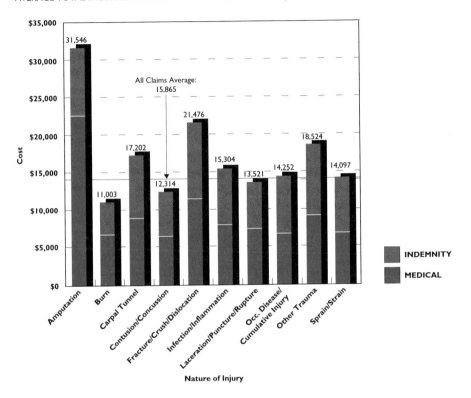

AVERAGE TOTAL INCURRED COSTS PER CLAIM BY PART OF BODY, 2001–2002

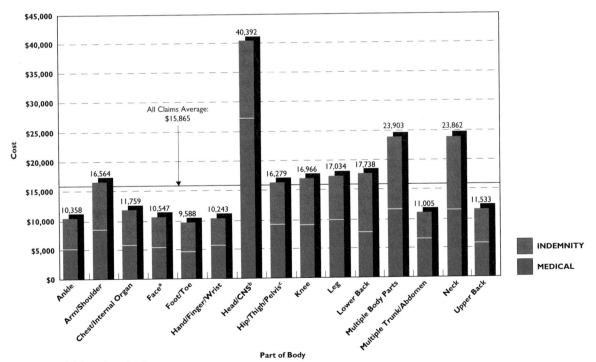

^aIncludes teeth, mouth, and eyes.
^bCentral nervous system.
^cIncludes sacrum and coccyx.
 Please note that these are estimates based on a sample of claims reported to NCCI and can be volatile from year to year due to the influence
 of a small but variable number of large claims.

RELATIVE RISK BY AGE AND SEX

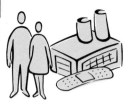

The risk of fatal and nonfatal injury and illness varies greatly by age and sex of the worker. Relative risk was calculated by dividing the fatal or nonfatal injury rate for each sex/age combination by the corresponding both sexes/all ages rate. Ratios greater than 1.00 indicate persons in that sex/age group are at greater risk of injury/illness than the average for all ages and both sexes. The table below shows that male workers ages 65 and older are at greatest risk of fatal injury on the job — 4.64 times more likely than workers of all ages and both sexes. Males ages 25–34 are at greatest risk of nonfatal injury with days away from work.

Severity of work injuries, as measured by median days away from work, increases steadily with age. The median time away from work to recuperate was 12 days for workers 55 and older compared to 7 days for all workers and only 4 days for teenage workers.

SEVERITY AND RELATIVE RISK OF OCCUPATIONAL INJURY AND ILLNESS BY AGE AND SEX, UNITED STATES, 2002

Age and Sex	Severity (Median Days away from Work)			Nonfatal Case with Days away from Work, Private Industry			Fatal Injuries, All Industries		
	Both Sexes	Males	Females	Both Sexes	Males	Females	Both Sexes	Males	Females
Total, 16 and older	7	8	6	1.00	1.18	0.78	1.00	1.73	0.17
16–19	4	4	4	0.50	0.64	0.36	0.44	0.76	0.13
20–24	5	5	4	1.05	1.37	0.70	0.80	1.43	0.12
25–34	6	6	5	1.13	1.40	0.80	0.86	1.45	0.17
35–44	8	9	7	1.07	1.25	0.83	0.97	1.67	0.15
45–54	10	11	8	0.99	1.11	0.84	0.99	1.72	0.19
55–64	12	14	8	0.92	0.98	0.85	1.25	2.19	0.18
65 and older	12	13	11	0.55	0.54	0.55	2.86	4.64	0.45

Source: National Safety Council estimates based on Bureau of Labor Statistics data.

ESTIMATES OF NONFATAL OCCUPATIONAL INJURIES

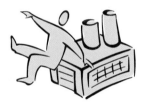

The national estimates of occupational injuries produced by the Survey of Occupational Injuries and Illnesses (SOII), conducted annually by the Bureau of Labor Statistics, cover only private sector employees. In 1999, the survey of approximately 174,000 establishments resulted in an estimate of 5.3 million OSHA-recordable nonfatal injuries to private sector employees.

A recent study examined the issue of cases not included in the SOII estimate due to coverage and underreporting. By law or regulation, the SOII does not cover farms with fewer than 11 employees; the self-employed; federal, state, and local government workers; private household workers; and workers regulated by other federal safety and health laws. These categories of workers accounted for at least 22% of the workforce. There is also reliable evidence of underreporting, both intentional and unintentional.

The study estimated that complete coverage of the workforce (disregarding underreporting) would have resulted in an estimate of 7.1 million injuries in 1999, or about 34% more than the SOII estimate. Various credible studies indicate that underreporting accounted for 0% to 59% of injuries, which resulted in estimates (including complete coverage) of 7.1 million to 23.7 million injuries in 1999.

Source: Leigh, J.P., Marcin, J.P., & Miller, T.R. (2004). An estimate of the U.S. Government's undercount of nonfatal occupational injuries. Journal of Occupational and Environmental Medicine, 46(1), 10–18.

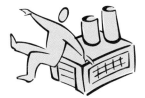

PART OF BODY

According to the Bureau of Labor Statistics, the back was the body part most frequently affected in injuries involving days away from work in 2002, accounting for 24% of the total 1,436,194 injuries in private industry. Multiple-part injuries were the second most common, followed by finger, knee, and head injuries. Overall, the services and manufacturing industries had the highest number of injuries, combining to make up over 45% of the total.

NUMBER OF NONFATAL OCCUPATIONAL INJURIES INVOLVING DAYS AWAY FROM WORK[a] BY PART OF BODY AFFECTED AND INDUSTRY DIVISION, PRIVATE INDUSTRY, UNITED STATES, 2002

| Part of Body Affected | Private Industry[b] | Goods Producing | | | | Service Producing | | | | |
		Agriculture[b,c]	Mining[c]	Construction	Manufacturing	Trans. & Public Utilities[d]	Wholesale Trade	Retail Trade	Finance, Insurance, & Real Estate	Services
Total[e]	1,436,194	31,520	11,355	163,641	280,005	168,632	108,791	263,401	36,689	372,159
Head	90,228	2,779	676	11,322	20,347	9,204	6,044	16,285	1,601	21,970
Eye	42,286	1,556	274	6,281	12,420	3,536	2,554	6,799	465	8,401
Neck	22,885	500	236	2,198	3,689	3,288	2,438	3,680	433	6,423
Trunk	522,055	10,035	4,062	54,277	94,694	67,100	42,211	93,833	11,119	144,724
Shoulder	83,924	1,725	574	7,872	18,598	12,416	6,443	13,307	1,517	21,474
Back	345,294	6,235	2,475	34,663	55,695	42,612	28,302	64,056	7,672	103,584
Upper extremities	328,274	7,182	2,496	40,007	88,454	27,340	21,143	65,987	8,642	67,023
Wrist	69,187	1,064	468	5,813	19,043	6,418	3,989	12,003	3,279	17,112
Hand, except finger	55,894	1,547	327	7,682	14,576	4,827	3,600	11,352	1,114	10,869
Finger	121,562	2,638	1,264	16,715	36,542	7,890	8,296	26,908	2,146	19,162
Lower extremities	304,453	7,005	2,770	39,459	49,353	39,826	25,174	55,649	8,063	77,155
Knee	113,035	2,193	1,025	14,930	18,721	14,682	8,308	18,775	2,957	31,445
Foot, except toe	46,180	1,086	402	6,186	8,194	6,071	4,302	9,577	1,146	9,216
Toe	14,548	297	42	2,195	2,748	1,276	1,166	3,934	344	2,546
Body systems	19,933	695	89	1,340	3,220	2,082	727	2,823	1,680	7,279
Multiple parts	139,445	2,777	1,007	13,802	18,547	18,967	10,300	23,458	5,026	45,561

Source: Bureau of Labor Statistics. (2004). Occupational Injuries and Illnesses in the United States—Profiles Data 1992–2002, CD-ROM Disk 2 (National and Atlanta, Dallas, and San Francisco Regions), Version 10.3.
[a]Days-away-from-work cases include those that result in days away from work with or without restricted work activity.
[b]Excludes farms with less than 11 employees.
[c]Agriculture includes forestry and fishing; mining includes quarrying and oil and gas extraction.
[d]Data for transportation and public utilities do not reflect the changes OSHA made to its recordkeeping requirements effective January 1, 2002; therefore, estimates for these industries are not comparable with estimates for other industries.
[e]Data may not sum to column totals because of rounding and exclusion of nonclassifiable responses.

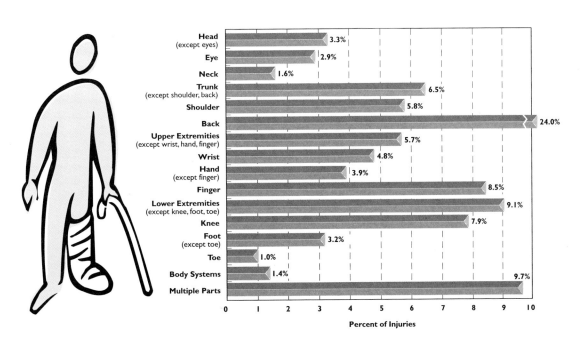

Safety professionals in business and industry often want to compare, or benchmark, the occupational injury and illness incidence rates of their establishments with the national average rates compiled by the U.S. Bureau of Labor Statistics (BLS) through its annual Survey of Occupational Injuries and Illnesses.[a] The incidence rates published on the following pages are for 2002 and were compiled under the revised OSHA record-keeping requirements that became effective that year.

Step 1.

The first step in benchmarking is to calculate the incidence rates for the establishment. The basic formula for computing incidence rates is $(N \times 200,000)/EH$, or, the number of cases (N) multiplied by $200,000$ then divided by the number of hours worked (EH) by all employees during the time period, where $200,000$ is the base for 100 full-time workers (working 40 hours per week, 50 weeks per year). Because the BLS rates are based on reports from entire establishments, both the OSHA 300 Log and the number of hours worked should cover the whole establishment being benchmarked. The hours worked and the log also should cover the same time period, (e.g., a month, quarter, or full year). The following rates may be calculated.

Total Cases — the incidence rate of total OSHA-recordable cases per 200,000 hours worked. For this rate, N is the total number of cases on the OSHA 300 Log.

Cases with Days Away from Work or Job Transfer or Restriction — the incidence rate of cases with days away from work, or job transfer, or restriction. N is the count of cases with a check in column H or column I of the OSHA 300 Log.

Cases with Days Away from Work — the incidence rate of cases with days away from work. N is the count of cases with a check in column H of the OSHA 300 Log.

Cases with Job Transfer or Restriction — the incidence rate of cases with job transfer or restriction, but no days away from work. N is the count of cases with a check in column I of the OSHA 300 Log.

Other Recordable Cases — the incidence rate of recordable cases without days away from work or job transfer or restriction. N is the count of cases with a check in column J of the OSHA 300 Log.

Step 2.

After computing one or more of the rates, the next step is to determine the Standard Industrial Classification (SIC) code for the establishment.[b] This code is used to find the appropriate BLS rate for comparison. A convenient way to find an SIC code is to use the search feature on the OSHA Internet site (www.osha.gov/oshstats/sicser.html). Otherwise, call a regional BLS office for assistance.

Step 3.

Once the SIC code is known, the national average incidence rates may be found by (a) consulting the table of rates on pages 62–64, (b) visiting the BLS Internet site (www.bls.gov/iif), or (c) calling a regional BLS office. Note that some tables on the Internet site provide incidence rates by size of establishment and rate quartiles within each SIC code. These rates may be useful for a more precise comparison. Note that the incidence rates for 2001 and earlier years were compiled under the old OSHA record-keeping requirements in effect at that time. Caution must be used in comparing rates computed for 2002 with rates published for 2001 — keeping in mind the differences in record-keeping requirements.

An alternative way of benchmarking is to compare the current incidence rates for an establishment to its own prior historical rates to determine if the rates are improving and if progress is satisfactory (using criteria set by the organization).

[a]*Bureau of Labor Statistics. (1997). BLS Handbook of Methods. Washington, DC: U.S. Government Printing Office.* (Or on the Internet at http://www.bls.gov/opub/hom/home.htm)
[b]*Executive Office of the President, Office of Management and Budget. (1987). Standard Industrial Classification Manual. Springfield, VA: National Technical Information Service.*

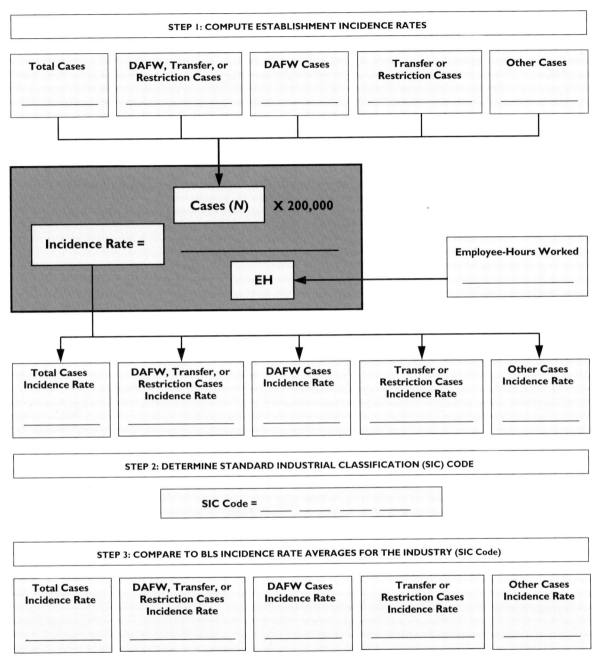

STEP 1: COMPUTE ESTABLISHMENT INCIDENCE RATES

Total Cases	DAFW, Transfer, or Restriction Cases	DAFW Cases	Transfer or Restriction Cases	Other Cases
_____	_____	_____	_____	_____

Incidence Rate =

$$\text{Cases } (N) \text{ X 200,000}$$

Employee-Hours Worked _____

EH

Total Cases Incidence Rate	DAFW, Transfer, or Restriction Cases Incidence Rate	DAFW Cases Incidence Rate	Transfer or Restriction Cases Incidence Rate	Other Cases Incidence Rate
_____	_____	_____	_____	_____

STEP 2: DETERMINE STANDARD INDUSTRIAL CLASSIFICATION (SIC) CODE

SIC Code = _____ _____ _____ _____

STEP 3: COMPARE TO BLS INCIDENCE RATE AVERAGES FOR THE INDUSTRY (SIC Code)

Total Cases Incidence Rate	DAFW, Transfer, or Restriction Cases Incidence Rate	DAFW Cases Incidence Rate	Transfer or Restriction Cases Incidence Rate	Other Cases Incidence Rate
_____	_____	_____	_____	_____

See page 58 for detailed instructions.
DAFW = Days Away From Work

TRENDS IN OCCUPATIONAL INCIDENCE RATES

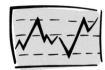

Revisions to the Occupational Safety and Health Administration's (OSHA) recordkeeping requirements for recording occupational injuries and illnesses became effective January 1, 2002, and are, therefore, reflected in the 2002 survey. Due to the revised requirements, the estimates from the 2002 survey are not comparable with those from prior years. The incidence rate for total recordable cases was 5.3 per 100 full-time workers in 2002, while the rate for total cases with days away from

work, job transfer, or restriction was 2.8. The incidence rate for cases with days away from work was 1.6 in 2002 and the rate for cases with job transfer or restriction was 1.2. The incidence rate in 2002 for other recordable cases was 2.5.

Beginning with 1992 data, the Bureau of Labor Statistics revised its annual survey to include only nonfatal cases and stopped publishing the incidence rate of lost workdays.

OCCUPATIONAL INJURY AND ILLNESS INCIDENCE RATES, BUREAU OF LABOR STATISTICS, UNITED STATES, 1982–2002

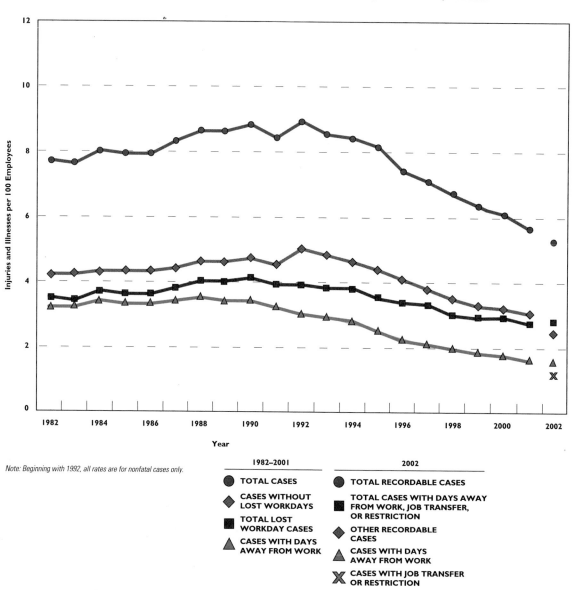

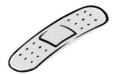

OCCUPATIONAL INJURIES AND ILLNESSES

The tables below and on pages 62-64 present the results of the 2002 Survey of Occupational Injuries and Illnesses conducted by the Bureau of Labor Statistics (BLS), U.S. Department of Labor. The survey collects data on injuries and illnesses (from the OSHA 300 Log) and employee-hours worked from a nationwide sample of about 182,800 establishments representing the private sector of the economy. The survey excludes public employees, private households, the self-

employed, and farms with fewer than 11 employees. The incidence rates give the number of cases per 100 full-time workers per year using 200,000 employee-hours as the equivalent. Definitions of the terms are given in the Glossary on page 183.

Beginning with 1992 data, the BLS revised its annual survey to include only nonfatal cases and stopped publishing incidence rates of lost workdays.

BLS ESTIMATES OF NONFATAL OCCUPATIONAL INJURY AND ILLNESS INCIDENCE RATES AND NUMBER OF INJURIES AND ILLNESSES BY INDUSTRY DIVISION, 2002

Industry Division	Total Recordable Cases	Cases With Days Away from Work, Job Transfer, or Restriction			Other Recordable Cases
		Total	Cases With Days Away from Work	Cases With Job Transfer or Restriction	
Incidence Rate per 100 Full-Time Workers[c]					
Private Sector[d]	**5.3**	**2.8**	**1.6**	**1.2**	**2.5**
Agriculture, Forestry, and Fishing[d]	6.4	3.3	2.1	1.2	3.1
Mining	4.0	2.6	2.0	0.7	1.4
Construction	7.1	3.8	2.8	1.1	3.2
Manufacturing	7.2	4.1	1.7	2.3	3.1
Transportation and Public Utilities	6.1	4.0	2.7	1.3	2.1
Wholesale and Retail Trade	5.3	2.7	1.6	1.1	2.6
Finance, Insurance, and Real Estate	1.7	0.8	0.5	0.2	0.9
Services	4.6	2.2	1.3	0.9	2.4
Number of Injuries and Illnesses (in thousands)					
Private Sector[d]	**4,700.6**	**2,494.3**	**1,436.2**	**1,058.2**	**2,206.3**
Agriculture, Forestry, and Fishing[d]	96.3	49.3	31.5	17.7	47.0
Mining	23.0	15.1	11.4	3.7	7.9
Construction	417.7	226.8	163.7	63.1	190.9
Manufacturing	1,159.5	656.4	280.0	376.4	503.1
Transportation and Public Utilities	382.7	251.8	168.6	83.2	130.9
Wholesale and Retail Trade	1,227.7	625.6	372.2	253.4	602.1
Finance, Insurance, and Real Estate	115.4	52.3	36.7	15.6	63.1
Services	1,278.4	617.1	372.2	244.9	661.3

Source: Bureau of Labor Statistics.
[a] Industry Division and 2- and 3-digit SIC code totals on pages 62–64 include data for industries not shown separately.
[b] Standard Industrial Classification Manual, 1987 Edition, for industries shown on pages 62–64.
[c] Incidence Rate = $\dfrac{\text{Number of injuries \& illnesses} \times 200,000}{\text{Total hours worked by all employees during period covered}}$

where 200,000 is the base for 100 full-time workers (working 40 hours per week, 50 weeks per year). The "Total Recordable Cases" rate is based on the number of cases with check marks in columns (G), (H), (I), and (J) of the OSHA 300 Log. The "Cases With Days Away From Work, Job Transfer, or Restriction—Total" rate is based on columns (H) and (I). The "Cases With Days Away From Work" rate is based on column (H). The "Cases With Job Transfer or Restriction" rate is based on column (I). The "Other Recordable Cases" rate is based on column (J).
[d] Excludes farms with less than 11 employees.
[e] Standard error of estimate exceeded publication guidelines.

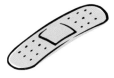

62

BLS ESTIMATES OF NONFATAL OCCUPATIONAL INJURY AND ILLNESS INCIDENCE RATES FOR SELECTED INDUSTRIES, 2002

Industry[a]	SIC Code[b]	Total Recordable Cases	Cases With Days Away from Work, Job Transfer, or Restriction			Other Recordable Cases
			Total	Cases With Days Away from Work	Cases With Job Transfer or Restriction	
PRIVATE SECTOR[d]	—	5.3	2.8	1.6	1.2	2.5
Agriculture, Forestry, and Fishing[d]	—	6.4	3.3	2.1	1.2	3.1
Agricultural production	01–02	7.0	3.8	2.2	1.6	3.2
Agricultural services	07	6.1	3.0	2.1	0.9	3.1
Forestry	08	5.2	2.4	1.4	0.9	2.8
Fishing, hunting, and trapping	09	4.5	1.2	1.1	0.1	3.4
Mining	—	4.0	2.6	2.0	0.7	1.4
Metal mining	10	4.1	2.3	1.6	0.7	1.7
Coal mining	12	6.8	4.9	4.6	0.3	1.9
Oil and gas extraction	13	3.4	2.2	1.5	0.7	1.3
Crude petroleum and natural gas	131	1.6	0.6	0.4	0.2	1.0
Oil and gas field services	138	4.5	3.0	2.1	0.9	1.5
Nonmetallic minerals, except fuels	14	3.8	2.6	1.7	0.9	1.2
Construction	—	7.1	3.8	2.8	1.1	3.2
General building contractors	15	6.2	3.2	2.3	0.9	2.9
Residential building construction	152	5.7	3.2	2.5	0.6	2.5
Nonresidential building construction	154	6.9	3.4	2.2	1.2	3.5
Heavy construction, except building	16	6.4	3.4	2.4	1.3	2.7
Highway and street construction	161	6.8	4.0	2.3	1.7	2.8
Heavy construction, except highway	162	6.2	3.5	2.4	1.1	2.6
Special trade contractors	17	7.5	4.1	3.0	1.1	3.5
Plumbing, heating, air-conditioning	171	8.9	4.3	3.1	1.2	4.5
Electrical work	173	6.4	3.1	2.4	0.7	3.3
Masonry, stonework and plastering	174	8.1	4.9	3.7	1.3	3.2
Carpentry and floor work	175	7.9	4.8	3.7	1.1	3.0
Roofing, siding, and sheet metal work	176	9.5	5.4	4.0	1.4	4.0
Concrete work	177	7.2	4.3	3.0	1.2	2.9
Miscellaneous special trade contractors	179	6.9	3.8	2.7	1.1	3.1
Manufacturing	—	7.2	4.1	1.7	2.3	3.1
Durable goods	—	7.9	4.3	1.9	2.4	3.6
Lumber and wood products	24	10.1	5.7	2.9	2.8	4.4
Logging	241	6.8	4.1	3.5	0.5	2.7
Sawmills and planing mills	242	10.4	5.8	3.1	2.6	4.6
Millwork, plywood and structural members	243	10.0	5.9	2.7	3.2	4.1
Wood containers	244	9.5	5.7	3.7	2.0	3.8
Wood buildings and mobile homes	245	15.8	7.8	3.5	4.3	8.0
Furniture and fixtures	25	9.9	6.0	2.2	3.8	3.9
Household furniture	251	9.7	6.1	2.1	4.0	3.6
Office furniture	252	8.8	5.1	1.9	3.2	3.7
Public building and related furniture	253	13.5	8.5	2.6	5.8	5.0
Stone, clay, and glass products	32	9.4	5.4	2.6	2.8	4.0
Flat glass	321	9.4	4.4	1.7	2.6	5.0
Glass and glassware, pressed or blown	322	9.0	4.9	2.2	2.8	4.0
Products of purchased glass	323	9.4	4.6	1.6	3.1	4.7
Structural clay products	325	10.9	6.0	2.6	3.4	4.8
Pottery and related products	326	11.1	6.9	2.2	4.6	4.3
Concrete, gypsum, and plaster products	327	10.0	6.0	3.4	2.6	4.0
Miscellaneous nonmetallic mineral products	329	7.1	4.5	1.9	2.6	2.7
Primary metal industries	33	10.3	5.5	2.5	3.0	4.8
Blast furnace and basic steel products	331	8.6	4.4	2.3	2.1	4.1
Iron and steel foundries	332	15.8	7.2	3.0	4.1	8.6
Primary nonferrous metals	333	7.6	4.5	1.6	2.8	3.1
Nonferrous rolling and drawing	335	7.5	4.4	2.1	2.3	3.1
Nonferrous foundries (castings)	336	13.5	8.5	3.7	4.8	5.0
Fabricated metal products	34	9.8	5.1	2.4	2.7	4.7
Metal cans and shipping containers	341	7.1	3.3	1.2	2.1	3.8
Cutlery, hand tools, and hardware	342	8.5	4.6	2.0	2.7	3.8
Plumbing and heating, except electric	343	10.3	5.3	1.7	3.6	4.9
Fabricated structural metal products	344	10.9	5.6	3.1	2.6	5.3
Screw machine products, bolts, etc.	345	7.7	3.7	1.7	2.1	4.0
Metal forgings and stampings	346	11.2	6.0	2.4	3.6	5.2
Metal services, n.e.c.	347	9.2	4.8	2.4	2.4	4.4
Ordnance and accessories, n.e.c.	348	4.5	2.5	0.9	1.6	2.0
Miscellaneous fabricated metal products	349	8.9	4.8	2.1	2.7	4.2
Industrial machinery and equipment	35	6.7	3.3	1.6	1.7	3.4
Farm and garden machinery	352	10.1	5.1	3.0	2.1	5.0
Construction and related machinery	353	7.8	3.7	2.1	1.7	4.1
Metalworking machinery	354	7.5	3.4	1.7	1.8	4.0
Special industry machinery	355	5.7	2.5	1.4	1.1	3.2
General industrial machinery	356	7.4	3.8	1.9	1.9	3.6
Computer and office equipment	357	1.9	1.1	0.5	0.6	0.8
Refrigeration and service machinery	358	8.2	4.6	1.8	2.8	3.7

See source and footnotes on page 61.
n.e.c. = not elsewhere classified.
Dash indicates data not available.

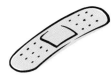

BLS ESTIMATES OF NONFATAL OCCUPATIONAL INJURY AND ILLNESS INCIDENCE RATES FOR SELECTED INDUSTRIES, 2002, Cont.

Industry[a]	SIC Code[b]	Total Recordable Cases	Cases With Days Away from Work, Job Transfer, or Restriction			Other Recordable Cases
			Total	Cases With Days Away from Work	Cases With Job Transfer or Restriction	
Industrial machinery, n.e.c.	359	7.4	3.3	1.9	1.4	4.1
Electronic and other electric equipment	36	4.5	2.4	1.0	1.3	2.1
Electric distribution equipment	361	6.9	3.8	1.7	2.1	3.1
Electrical industrial apparatus	362	5.9	2.9	1.3	1.6	3.1
Household appliances	363	9.3	4.6	1.8	2.8	4.7
Electric lighting and wiring equipment	364	6.1	3.4	1.4	2.0	2.7
Household audio and video equipment	365	5.3	3.1	1.7	1.4	2.2
Electronic components and accessories	367	3.1	1.6	0.7	0.8	1.5
Misc. electrical equipment and supplies	369	5.7	3.2	1.1	2.1	2.5
Transportation equipment	37	10.1	5.8	1.9	3.9	4.3
Motor vehicles and equipment	371	12.1	7.1	2.0	5.1	5.0
Aircraft and parts	372	5.7	3.1	1.4	1.7	2.6
Ship and boat building and repairing	373	14.6	8.1	3.4	4.7	6.5
Railroad equipment	374	6.9	4.0	2.3	1.6	3.0
Motorcycles, bicycles, and parts	375	11.6	6.1	2.7	3.4	5.6
Guided missiles, space vehicles, parts	376	1.6	0.9	0.4	0.6	0.7
Miscellaneous transportation equipment	379	11.3	6.3	2.7	3.6	5.1
Instruments and related products	38	3.3	1.9	0.8	1.1	1.5
Search and navigation equipment	381	1.5	0.8	0.3	0.5	0.7
Measuring and controlling devices	382	3.2	1.6	0.8	0.9	1.5
Medical instruments and supplies	384	4.2	2.4	0.9	1.5	1.7
Photographic equipment and supplies	386	4.1	2.6	0.8	1.8	1.5
Miscellaneous manufacturing industries	39	6.2	3.4	1.7	1.7	2.8
Musical instruments	393	7.7	3.6	1.9	1.7	4.1
Toys and sporting goods	394	7.3	3.7	1.7	2.0	3.6
Pens, pencils, office, and art supplies	395	5.0	2.4	1.3	1.2	2.6
Costume jewelry and notions	396	3.6	2.3	1.2	1.1	1.3
Nondurable goods	—	6.2	3.8	1.6	2.2	2.5
Food and kindred products	20	9.3	6.1	2.2	3.9	3.2
Meat products	201	11.5	7.9	1.8	6.1	3.6
Dairy products	202	9.4	6.0	2.9	3.1	3.4
Preserved fruits and vegetables	203	7.6	4.7	1.8	2.9	2.9
Grain mill products	204	7.0	4.1	1.8	2.3	2.8
Bakery products	205	8.2	5.6	2.4	3.2	2.6
Sugar and confectionery products	206	8.6	5.7	2.5	3.2	3.0
Fats and oils	207	9.1	5.5	3.0	2.5	3.5
Beverages	208	9.5	6.1	3.0	3.1	3.4
Miscellaneous foods and kindred products	209	7.9	4.7	2.3	2.4	3.2
Tobacco products	21	4.0	2.1	1.3	0.7	1.9
Textile mill products	22	5.2	3.0	0.9	2.1	2.2
Broadwoven fabric mills, cotton	221	4.0	2.5	0.5	2.0	1.6
Broadwoven fabric mills, manmade	222	3.1	2.0	0.5	1.5	1.1
Narrow fabric mills	224	4.2	2.6	1.4	1.1	1.6
Knitting mills	225	4.1	2.1	0.8	1.3	1.9
Textile finishing, except wool	226	5.5	3.2	1.4	1.8	2.4
Carpets and rugs	227	7.3	4.8	0.7	4.0	2.5
Yarn and thread mills	228	5.2	2.7	0.7	2.0	2.4
Miscellaneous textile goods	229	7.3	4.1	1.6	2.5	3.2
Apparel and other textile products	23	4.6	2.7	1.2	1.6	1.8
Men's and boys' furnishings	232	6.4	3.7	1.8	1.9	2.6
Women's and misses' outerware	233	1.5	0.9	0.5	0.4	0.6
Hats, caps, and millinery	235	3.7	1.6	0.7	0.9	2.1
Miscellaneous apparel and accessories	238	3.6	2.2	0.8	1.4	1.4
Miscellaneous fabricated textile products	239	6.1	3.8	1.4	2.4	2.3
Paper and allied products	26	5.6	3.1	1.7	1.5	2.4
Pulp mills	261	2.7	1.4	0.6	0.7	1.3
Paper mills	262	4.3	2.4	1.6	0.8	2.0
Paperboard mills	263	3.9	2.1	1.4	0.7	1.8
Paperboard containers and boxes	265	6.1	3.3	1.6	1.7	2.7
Printing and publishing	27	4.0	2.2	1.2	1.1	1.8
Newspapers	271	4.2	2.3	1.5	0.8	1.9
Periodicals	272	1.4	0.8	0.3	0.4	0.6
Books	273	3.2	1.9	0.8	1.1	1.3
Commercial printing	275	4.9	2.7	1.3	1.4	2.2
Blankbooks and bookbinding	278	5.5	3.4	1.4	1.9	2.1
Printing trade services	279	2.4	1.5	0.6	0.9	0.9
Chemicals and allied products	28	3.3	1.9	0.8	1.1	1.4
Industrial inorganic chemicals	281	2.8	1.8	0.6	1.2	1.0
Plastics materials and synthetics	282	3.1	1.8	0.8	1.0	1.3
Drugs	283	3.0	1.7	0.7	1.0	1.4
Soap, cleaners, and toilet goods	284	4.0	2.1	0.9	1.2	1.9
Paints and allied products	285	5.4	3.6	1.4	2.2	1.8
Industrial organic chemicals	286	2.2	1.2	0.6	0.6	1.1
Agricultural chemicals	287	4.1	2.4	1.2	1.1	1.7

See source and footnotes on page 61.
n.e.c. = not elsewhere classified.
Dash indicates data not available.

OCCUPATIONAL INJURIES AND ILLNESSES (CONT.)

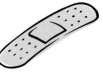

BLS ESTIMATES OF NONFATAL OCCUPATIONAL INJURY AND ILLNESS INCIDENCE RATES FOR SELECTED INDUSTRIES, 2002, Cont.

Industry Division[a]	SIC Code[b]	Total Recordable Cases	Incidence Rates[c] Cases With Days Away from Work, Job Transfer, or Restriction — Total	Cases With Days Away from Work	Cases With Job Transfer or Restriction	Other Recordable Cases
Miscellaneous chemical products	289	4.0	2.2	0.7	1.5	1.8
Petroleum and coal products	29	3.6	2.2	1.3	0.8	1.4
Petroleum refining	291	1.8	1.1	0.6	0.5	0.7
Asphalt paving and roofing materials	295	7.6	4.7	3.2	1.5	2.9
Rubber and miscellaneous plastics products	30	8.8	5.1	2.2	2.9	3.6
Tires and inner tubes	301	9.4	6.1	2.4	3.8	3.3
Hose and belting and gaskets and packing	305	6.6	4.2	1.8	2.4	2.4
Fabricated rubber products, n.e.c.	306	8.4	4.8	2.1	2.7	3.6
Miscellaneous plastic products, n.e.c.	308	9.0	5.2	2.2	2.9	3.8
Leather and leather products	31	7.3	4.3	1.7	2.7	3.0
Footwear, except rubber	314	8.3	4.3	1.7	2.6	4.1
Transportation and Public Utilities	—	**6.1**	**4.0**	**2.7**	**1.3**	**2.1**
Railroad transportation	40	3.0	2.3	2.1	0.2	0.7
Local and interurban passenger transit	41	7.9	4.3	3.3	1.3	3.4
Local and suburban transportation	411	9.9	5.8	3.9	1.9	4.1
School buses	415	5.8	2.9	2.3	0.6	2.9
Trucking and warehousing	42	7.0	4.6	3.3	1.3	2.4
Trucking & courier services, except air	421	6.8	4.5	3.3	1.2	2.3
Public warehousing and storage	422	7.9	5.3	2.7	2.5	2.6
Water transportation	44	6.8	4.4	3.2	(e)	(e)
Transportation by air	45	11.8	8.4	5.2	3.2	3.4
Air transportation, scheduled	451	12.3	8.8	5.8	3.1	3.5
Transportation services	47	2.9	1.7	1.0	0.7	1.2
Communications	48	3.0	2.0	1.4	0.5	1.0
Telephone communications	481	2.8	2.0	1.6	0.4	0.9
Cable and other pay television services	484	4.8	3.3	1.7	1.6	1.5
Electric, gas, and sanitary services	49	5.0	2.8	1.5	1.3	2.2
Electric services	491	3.7	2.0	1.1	0.9	1.7
Gas production and distribution	492	5.0	3.0	1.4	1.6	2.0
Combination utility services	493	4.7	2.3	1.3	1.0	2.4
Water supply	494	8.2	4.4	3.0	1.4	3.8
Sanitary services	495	7.3	4.5	2.5	2.0	2.8
Wholesale and Retail Trade	—	**5.3**	**2.7**	**1.6**	**1.1**	**2.6**
Wholeale trade	—	*5.2*	*3.1*	*1.7*	*1.3*	*2.1*
Wholesale trade-durable goods	50	4.5	2.5	1.5	1.0	2.0
Lumber and construction materials	503	6.7	4.0	2.3	1.8	2.7
Electrical goods	506	2.9	1.4	1.0	0.4	1.5
Machinery, equipment, and supplies	508	4.6	2.3	1.5	0.8	2.3
Wholesale trade-nondurable goods	51	6.1	3.9	2.2	1.7	2.2
Groceries and related products	514	8.6	5.9	3.1	2.8	2.7
Petroleum and petroleum products	517	4.4	2.3	1.7	0.6	2.0
Retail trade	—	*5.3*	*2.5*	*1.5*	*1.0*	*2.7*
Building materials and garden supplies	52	7.2	4.3	2.5	1.8	2.9
General merchandise stores	53	7.7	4.7	2.2	2.5	2.9
Food stores	54	6.8	3.4	2.1	1.2	3.4
Automotive dealers and service stations	55	5.1	2.2	1.6	0.6	2.8
Apparel and accessory stores	56	3.0	1.3	0.8	0.5	1.6
Home furniture, furnishings, and equipment	57	4.2	2.3	1.4	0.9	1.9
Eating and drinking places	58	4.6	1.6	1.1	0.5	3.0
Miscellaneous retail	59	3.6	1.9	1.1	0.8	1.7
Finance, Insurance, and Real Estate	—	**1.7**	**0.8**	**0.5**	**0.2**	**0.9**
Depository institutions	60	1.5	0.6	0.4	0.1	0.9
Insurance agents, brokers, and service	64	0.9	0.3	0.2	0.1	0.6
Real estate	65	3.5	1.9	1.3	0.7	1.6
Services	—	**4.6**	**2.2**	**1.3**	**0.9**	**2.4**
Hotels and other lodging places	70	6.6	3.4	1.8	1.5	3.2
Personal services	72	3.0	1.8	1.1	0.7	1.2
Business services	73	2.7	1.3	0.9	0.4	1.4
Services to buildings	734	5.1	2.5	2.0	0.6	2.6
Auto repair, services, and parking	75	4.5	2.2	1.6	0.6	2.3
Miscellaneous repair services	76	4.9	2.7	2.0	0.8	2.2
Amusement and recreation services	79	6.3	3.2	1.7	1.5	3.1
Health services	80	7.4	3.4	2.0	1.5	4.0
Nursing and personal care facilities	805	12.6	7.6	4.1	3.5	5.0
Hospitals	806	9.7	4.1	2.3	1.7	5.6
Legal services	81	0.8	0.3	0.2	0.1	0.4
Educational services	82	2.8	1.3	0.8	0.5	1.5
Social services	83	5.5	2.9	1.8	1.1	2.6
Child day care services	835	2.9	1.6	1.1	0.5	1.3
Engineering and management services	87	1.5	0.7	0.5	0.2	0.8

See source and footnotes on page 61.
n.e.c. = not elsewhere classified.
Dash indicates data not available.

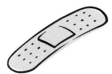

BLS ESTIMATES OF NONFATAL OCCUPATIONAL INJURY AND ILLNESS INCIDENCE RATES FOR SELECTED INDUSTRIES, 2002

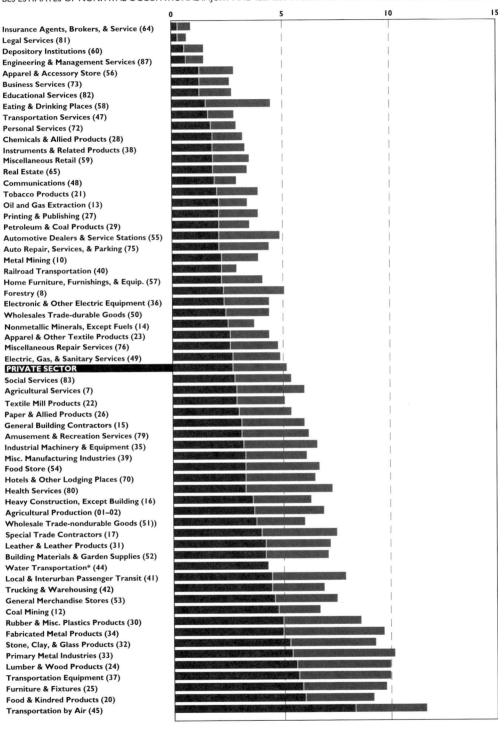

Insurance Agents, Brokers, & Service (64)
Legal Services (81)
Depository Institutions (60)
Engineering & Management Services (87)
Apparel & Accessory Store (56)
Business Services (73)
Educational Services (82)
Eating & Drinking Places (58)
Transportation Services (47)
Personal Services (72)
Chemicals & Allied Products (28)
Instruments & Related Products (38)
Miscellaneous Retail (59)
Real Estate (65)
Communications (48)
Tobacco Products (21)
Oil and Gas Extraction (13)
Printing & Publishing (27)
Petroleum & Coal Products (29)
Automotive Dealers & Service Stations (55)
Auto Repair, Services, & Parking (75)
Metal Mining (10)
Railroad Transportation (40)
Home Furniture, Furnishings, & Equip. (57)
Forestry (8)
Electronic & Other Electric Equipment (36)
Wholesales Trade-durable Goods (50)
Nonmetallic Minerals, Except Fuels (14)
Apparel & Other Textile Products (23)
Miscellaneous Repair Services (76)
Electric, Gas, & Sanitary Services (49)
PRIVATE SECTOR
Social Services (83)
Agricultural Services (7)
Textile Mill Products (22)
Paper & Allied Products (26)
General Building Contractors (15)
Amusement & Recreation Services (79)
Industrial Machinery & Equipment (35)
Misc. Manufacturing Industries (39)
Food Store (54)
Hotels & Other Lodging Places (70)
Health Services (80)
Heavy Construction, Except Building (16)
Agricultural Production (01–02)
Wholesale Trade-nondurable Goods (51))
Special Trade Contractors (17)
Leather & Leather Products (31)
Building Materials & Garden Supplies (52)
Water Transportation* (44)
Local & Interurban Passenger Transit (41)
Trucking & Warehousing (42)
General Merchandise Stores (53)
Coal Mining (12)
Rubber & Misc. Plastics Products (30)
Fabricated Metal Products (34)
Stone, Clay, & Glass Products (32)
Primary Metal Industries (33)
Lumber & Wood Products (24)
Transportation Equipment (37)
Furniture & Fixtures (25)
Food & Kindred Products (20)
Transportation by Air (45)

Total cases with days away from work, job transfer, or restriction plus other recordable cases equals total cases.
Standard error of the estimate for other recordable cases exceeded publication guidelines; total cases rate was 6.8
Note: Industries are shown at the 2-digit SIC level.

■ **TOTAL CASES WITH DAYS AWAY FROM WORK, JOB TRANSFER, OR RESTRICTION**

▮ **OTHER RECORDABLE CASES**

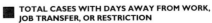

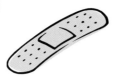
The tables on pages 67 through 77 present data on the characteristics of injured and ill workers and the injuries and illnesses that affected them. These data indicate how many workers are killed by on-the-job injuries and how many are affected by nonfatal injuries and illnesses. The data may be used to help set priorities for safety and health programs and for benchmarking.

The fatality information covers only deaths due to injuries and comes from the Bureau of Labor Statistics (BLS) Census of Fatal Occupational Injuries. The data are **10-year totals** for the calendar years 1993–2002. The 10 years were combined because counts for many of the items would be too small to publish if data for a single year were used.

The data on nonfatal cases cover both injuries and illnesses and come from the BLS Survey of Occupational Injuries and Illnesses for the 2002 reference year. The Survey also is used to produce the incidence rates shown on the preceding pages. The estimates on the following pages are the number of cases involving days away from work (with or without days of restricted work activity).

Data are presented for the sex, age, occupation, and race or ethnic origin of the worker and for the nature of injury/illness, the part of body affected, the source of injury/illness, and the event or exposure that produced the injury/illness.

The text at the top of each page describes the kind of establishments that are included in the industry division, the number of workers in the industry division for 2002, and the annual average number of workers for the 1993–2002 period.

How to Benchmark
Incidence rates, percent distributions, or ranks may be used for benchmarking purposes. The results of the calculations described here may be compared to similar rates, percent distributions, and rankings based on data for a company.

For nonfatal cases incidence rates, multiply the number of cases by 1,000 and then divide by the 2002 employment given in the text at the top of the page. This will give the number of cases with days away from work per 1,000 employees per year. For fatality rates, multiply the 10-year total fatalities by 100 then divide by the 1993–2002 average annual employment given at the top of the page. This will give the number of deaths per 1,000 employees per year.

To compute percent distributions, divide the number of cases for each characteristic by the total number of cases found on the first line of the table. Multiply the quotient by 100 and round to one decimal place. Percent distributions may not add to 100% because of unclassifiable cases not shown.

Ranks are determined by arranging the characteristics from largest to smallest within each group and then numbering consecutively starting with 1 for the largest.

Major Industry Divisions
Page 67 shows nonfatal injury/illness data for the private sector of the economy (excluding government entities) and fatal injury data for all industries (including government). Pages 68 through 76 present the data for private sector industry divisions. Page 77 presents the fatal injury data for the Government industry division (the BLS Survey does not cover government entities nationwide, so no nonfatal case data are available).

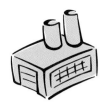

The nonfatal occupational injury and illness data cover only the private sector of the economy and exclude employees in federal, state, and local government entities. The fatal injury data cover employees in both the private sector and government.

There were 137,731,000 people employed in 2002, of which 116,861,000 worked in the private sector and 20,870,000 in government. Over the 10 years from 1993 through 2002, total employment averaged 130,814,000 per year with 110,205,000 in the private sector.

NUMBER OF NONFATAL OCCUPATIONAL INJURIES AND ILLNESSES INVOLVING DAYS AWAY FROM WORK[a] AND FATAL OCCUPATIONAL INJURIES BY SELECTED WORKER AND CASE CHARACTERISTICS, UNITED STATES

Characteristic	Private Industry[b,c] Nonfatal Cases, 2002	All Industries Fatalities, 1993–2002
Total	**1,436,194**	**61,146**
Sex		
Men	930,925	56,308
Women	500,592	4,838
Age		
Under 16	198	252
16 to 19	38,387	1,571
20 to 24	159,229	4,680
25 to 34	358,377	12,922
35 to 44	400,871	15,272
45 to 54	304,970	12,857
55 to 64	143,523	8,275
65 and over	25,103	5,204
Occupation		
Managerial and professional	92,967	6,609
Technical, sales, and administrative support	239,364	7,367
Service	270,251	5,023
Farming, forestry, and fishing	35,629	8,884
Precision production, craft, and repair	242,787	11,009
Operators, fabricators, and laborers	552,886	20,743
Military occupations	N/A	961
Race or ethnic origin[d]		
White, non-Hispanic	688,009	41,138
Black, non-Hispanic	114,453	5,542
Hispanic	180,419	7,160
Asian or Pacific Islander	22,099	1,741
American Indian or Alaskan Native	8,225	355
Not reported	422,989	5,206
Nature of injury, illness		
Sprains, strains	617,186	92
Fractures	99,171	343
Cuts, lacerations, punctures	128,061	9,008
Bruises, contusions	126,986	30
Heat burns	21,468	1,478
Chemical burns	8,257	61
Amputations	8,793	210
Carpal tunnel syndrome	22,651	—
Tendonitis	9,275	—
Multiple injuries	52,496	18,016
Soreness, pain	116,956	10
Back pain	46,504	8
All other	224,896	31,898

Characteristic	Private Industry[b,c] Nonfatal Cases, 2002	All Industries Fatalities, 1993–2002
Part of body affected		
Head	90,228	14,934
Eye	42,286	7
Neck	22,885	1,214
Trunk	522,055	12,003
Back	345,294	767
Shoulder	83,924	27
Upper extremities	328,274	143
Finger	121,562	16
Hand, except finger	55,894	13
Wrist	69,187	9
Lower extremities	304,453	554
Knee	113,035	77
Foot, toe	60,729	30
Body systems	19,933	9,869
Multiple	139,445	22,073
All other	8,921	356
Source of injury, illness		
Chemicals, chemical products	20,652	1,449
Containers	193,146	834
Furniture, fixtures	52,393	175
Machinery	92,560	4,857
Parts and materials	147,553	4,161
Worker motion or position	220,794	28
Floor, ground surfaces	255,548	6,733
Handtools	66,588	1,053
Vehicles	118,569	26,350
Health care patient	69,994	21
All other	198,395	15,485
Event or exposure		
Contact with object, equipment	380,517	9,838
Struck by object	191,607	5,598
Struck against object	99,916	147
Caught in object, equipment, material	63,057	4,058
Fall to lower level	86,946	6,207
Fall on same level	176,019	585
Slips, trips	48,140	15
Overexertion	381,048	63
Overexertion in lifting	208,260	39
Repetitive motion	58,576	—
Exposed to harmful substance	60,044	5,556
Transportation accidents	62,956	25,795
Fires, explosions	2,695	1,946
Assault, violent act	23,903	10,755
by person	18,104	8,271
by other	5,799	2,484
All other	155,349	386

Source: National Safety Council tabulations of Bureau of Labor Statistics data.
Note: Because of rounding and data exclusion of nonclassifiable responses, data may not sum to the totals. Dashes (—) indicate data that do not meet publication guidelines. "N/A" means not applicable.
[a] *Days away from work include those that result in days away from work with or without restricted work activity.*
[b] *Excludes farms with fewer than 11 employees.*

[c] *Data conforming to OSHA definitions for mining operators in coal, metal, and nonmetal mining and for employees in railroad transportation are provided to BLS by the Mine Safety and Health Administration, U.S. Department of Labor; and the Federal Railroad Administration, U.S. Department of Transportation. Independent mining contractors are excluded from the coal, metal, and nonmetal mining industries.*
[d] *In the fatalities column, non-Hispanic categories include cases with Hispanic origin not reported.*

AGRICULTURE, FORESTRY, AND FISHING

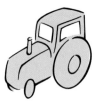

The Agriculture, Forestry, and Fishing industry division includes production of crops and livestock, animal specialties, agricultural services, forestry (but excluding logging, which is in the Manufacturing industry division), and commercial fishing, hunting, and trapping.

Employment in Agriculture, Forestry, and Fishing totaled 3,417,000 in 2002 and averaged 3,397,000 per year from 1993 through 2002. It is the second smallest industry division after Mining.

NUMBER OF NONFATAL OCCUPATIONAL INJURIES AND ILLNESS INVOLVING DAYS AWAY FROM WORK[a] AND FATAL OCCUPATIONAL INJURIES BY SELECTED WORKER AND CASE CHARACTERISTICS, UNITED STATES, AGRICULTURE, FORESTRY, AND FISHING

Characteristic	Nonfatal Cases,[b] 2002	Fatalities, 1993–2002
Total	**31,520**	**8,059**
Sex		
Men	25,116	7,793
Women	6,403	266
Age		
Under 16	—	166
16 to 19	982	224
20 to 24	5,450	490
25 to 34	9,806	1,142
35 to 44	8,307	1,430
45 to 54	4,691	1,273
55 to 64	1,734	1,298
65 and over	453	2,021
Occupation		
Managerial and professional	491	99
Technical, sales, and administrative support	1,413	169
Service	511	32
Farming, forestry, and fishing	22,909	7,361
Precision production, craft, and repair	1,117	53
Operators, fabricators, and laborers	5,078	323
Race or ethnic origin[c]		
White, non-Hispanic	12,697	5,845
Black, non-Hispanic	1,075	296
Hispanic	13,836	1,117
Asian or Pacific Islander	439	102
American Indian or Alaskan Native	93	58
Not reported	3,380	640
Nature of injury, illness		
Sprains, strains	10,524	—
Fractures	2,881	25
Cuts, lacerations, punctures	3,261	341
Bruises, contusions	2,388	—
Heat burns	124	99
Chemical burns	307	—
Amputations	369	44
Carpal tunnel syndrome	216	—
Tendonitis	341	—
Multiple injuries	1,490	1,991
Soreness, pain	2,457	—
Back pain	1,348	—
All other	7,163	5,551

Characteristic	Nonfatal Cases,[b] 2002	Fatalities, 1993–2002
Part of body affected		
Head	2,779	1,573
Eye	1,556	—
Neck	500	176
Trunk	10,035	2,043
Back	6,235	76
Shoulder	1,725	—
Upper extremities	7,182	24
Finger	2,638	—
Hand, except finger	1,547	—
Wrist	1,064	—
Lower extremities	7,005	76
Knee	2,193	—
Foot, toe	1,383	—
Body systems	695	1,937
Multiple	2,777	2,200
All other	548	30
Source of injury, illness		
Chemicals, chemical products	774	117
Containers	2,754	109
Furniture, fixtures	271	—
Machinery	1,920	1,097
Parts and materials	2,160	318
Worker motion or position	4,393	—
Floor, ground surfaces	5,367	556
Handtools	2,186	83
Vehicles	3,145	4,189
Health care patient	—	—
All other	8,534	1,588
Event or exposure		
Contact with object, equipment	9,531	1,869
Struck by object	5,185	1,011
Struck against object	1,968	18
Caught in object, equipment, material	1,754	836
Fall to lower level	2,433	555
Fall on same level	2,866	33
Slips, trips	750	—
Overexertion	5,023	—
Overexertion in lifting	2,745	—
Repetitive motion	689	—
Exposed to harmful substance	1,908	787
Transportation accidents	1,805	4,104
Fires, explosions	56	112
Assault, violent act	1,944	563
by person	57	151
by other	1,887	412
All other	4,515	35

Source: National Safety Council tabulations of Bureau of Labor Statistics data.
Note: Because of rounding and data exclusion of nonclassifiable responses, data may not sum to the totals. Dashes (—) indicate data that do not meet publication guidelines.
[a]Days away from work include those that result in days away from work with or without restricted work activity.

[b]Excludes farms with fewer than 11 employees.
[c]In the fatalities column, non-Hispanic categories include cases with Hispanic origin not reported.

MINING, QUARRYING, AND OIL AND GAS EXTRACTION

The Mining industry division includes metal mining, coal mining, oil and gas extraction, and mining and quarrying of nonmetallic minerals such as stone, sand, and gravel.

Mining is the smallest industry division. Mining employment in 2002 amounted to 515,000 workers. Over the 10 years from 1993 through 2002, employment in Mining averaged 594,000 per year.

NUMBER OF NONFATAL OCCUPATIONAL INJURIES AND ILLNESS INVOLVING DAYS AWAY FROM WORK[a] AND FATAL OCCUPATIONAL INJURIES BY SELECTED WORKER AND CASE CHARACTERISTICS, UNITED STATES, MINING, QUARRYING, AND OIL AND GAS EXTRACTION

Characteristic	Nonfatal Cases,[b] 2002	Fatalities, 1993–2002
Total	11,355	1,537
Sex		
Men	11,115	1,519
Women	241	18
Age		
Under 16	—	—
16 to 19	155	31
20 to 24	1,434	141
25 to 34	2,938	363
35 to 44	2,967	449
45 to 54	2,744	364
55 to 64	914	135
65 and over	59	54
Occupation		
Managerial and professional	199	73
Technical, sales, and administrative support	71	31
Service	22	12
Farming, forestry, and fishing	—	—
Precision production, craft, and repair	5,754	856
Operators, fabricators, and laborers	5,256	559
Race or ethnic origin[c]		
White, non-Hispanic	2,429	1,154
Black, non-Hispanic	207	52
Hispanic	1,284	199
Asian or Pacific Islander	25	6
American Indian or Alaskan Native	10	17
Not reported	7,402	108
Nature of injury, illness		
Sprains, strains	4,540	—
Fractures	1,824	—
Cuts, lacerations, punctures	805	27
Bruises, contusions	1,216	—
Heat burns	137	62
Chemical burns	146	5
Amputations	191	10
Carpal tunnel syndrome	18	—
Tendonitis	—	—
Multiple injuries	494	512
Soreness, pain	409	—
Back pain	109	—
All other	1,573	917

Characteristic	Nonfatal Cases,[b] 2002	Fatalities, 1993–2002
Part of body affected		
Head	676	330
Eye	274	—
Neck	236	29
Trunk	4,062	300
Back	2,475	10
Shoulder	574	—
Upper extremities	2,496	6
Finger	1,264	—
Hand, except finger	327	—
Wrist	468	—
Lower extremities	2,770	10
Knee	1,025	—
Foot, toe	445	—
Body systems	89	274
Multiple	1,007	585
All other	19	
Source of injury, illness		
Chemicals, chemical products	834	81
Containers	586	35
Furniture, fixtures	35	6
Machinery	1,422	295
Parts and materials	2,318	190
Worker motion or position	577	—
Floor, ground surfaces	1,916	101
Handtools	758	8
Vehicles	597	444
Health care patient	—	—
All other	2,314	376
Event or exposure		
Contact with object, equipment	4,795	583
Struck by object	2,794	274
Struck against object	831	8
Caught in object, equipment, material	1,074	300
Fall to lower level	883	112
Fall on same level	1,004	5
Slips, trips	179	—
Overexertion	3,061	—
Overexertion in lifting	1,130	—
Repetitive motion	43	—
Exposed to harmful substance	446	162
Transportation accidents	251	467
Fires, explosions	55	169
Assault, violent act	21	25
by person	—	9
by other	21	16
All other	617	11

Source: National Safety Council tabulations of Bureau of Labor Statistics data.
Note: Because of rounding and data exclusion of nonclassifiable responses, data may not sum to the totals. Dashes (—) indicate data that do not meet publication guidelines.
[a]Days away from work include those that result in days away from work with or without restricted work activity.
[b]Data conforming to OSHA definitions for mining operators in coal, metal, and nonmetal mining are provided to BLS by the Mine Safety and Health Administration, U.S. Department of Labor. Independent mining contractors are excluded from the coal, metal, and nonmetal mining industries.
[c]In the fatalities column, non-Hispanic categories include cases with Hispanic origin not reported.

CONSTRUCTION

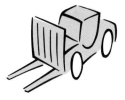

The Construction industry division includes establishments engaged in construction of buildings, heavy construction other than buildings, and special trade contractors such as plumbing, electrical, carpentry, etc.

In 2002, employment in the Construction industry division totaled 9,162,000 workers. Employment over the 1993–2002 period averaged 7,989,000 workers per year.

NUMBER OF NONFATAL OCCUPATIONAL INJURIES AND ILLNESS INVOLVING DAYS AWAY FROM WORK[a] AND FATAL OCCUPATIONAL INJURIES BY SELECTED WORKER AND CASE CHARACTERISTICS, UNITED STATES, CONSTRUCTION

Characteristic	Nonfatal Cases, 2002	Fatalities, 1993–2002
Total	163,641	11,036
Sex		
Men	159,621	10,880
Women	4,020	156
Age		
Under 16	—	16
16 to 19	3,081	357
20 to 24	21,711	1,069
25 to 34	49,727	2,744
35 to 44	49,387	3,092
45 to 54	26,615	2,118
55 to 64	10,448	1,179
65 and over	1,402	445
Occupation		
Managerial and professional	2,661	695
Technical, sales, and administrative support	4,525	110
Service	507	23
Farming, forestry, and fishing	389	30
Precision production, craft, and repair	94,947	5,641
Operators, fabricators, and laborers	60,399	4,510
Race or ethnic origin[b]		
White, non-Hispanic	98,674	7,331
Black, non-Hispanic	7,070	746
Hispanic	26,133	1,890
Asian or Pacific Islander	1,244	109
American Indian or Alaskan Native	988	70
Not reported	29,532	889
Nature of injury, illness		
Sprains, strains	60,259	7
Fractures	17,356	45
Cuts, lacerations, punctures	23,460	287
Bruises, contusions	11,304	7
Heat burns	1,678	199
Chemical burns	643	5
Amputations	931	24
Carpal tunnel syndrome	948	—
Tendonitis	760	—
Multiple injuries	6,490	3,373
Soreness, pain	11,964	—
Back pain	*5,485*	—
All other	27,851	7,088

Characteristic	Nonfatal Cases, 2002	Fatalities, 1993–2002
Part of body affected		
Head	11,322	3,036
Eye	*6,281*	—
Neck	2,198	158
Trunk	54,277	1,669
Back	*34,663*	*91*
Shoulder	*7,872*	—
Upper extremities	40,007	18
Finger	*16,715*	—
Hand, except finger	*7,682*	—
Wrist	*5,813*	—
Lower extremities	39,459	64
Knee	*14,930*	*7*
Foot, toe	*8,381*	*5*
Body systems	1,340	2,385
Multiple	13,802	3,671
All other	1,236	35
Source of injury, illness		
Chemicals, chemical products	1,240	194
Containers	8,643	128
Furniture, fixtures	2,704	47
Machinery	10,158	1,262
Parts and materials	37,541	1,520
Worker motion or position	20,686	—
Floor, ground surfaces	33,558	3,495
Handtools	14,439	138
Vehicles	9,761	2,583
Health care patient	—	—
All other	24,875	1,667
Event or exposure		
Contact with object, equipment	57,368	2,102
Struck by object	*32,281*	*1,046*
Struck against object	*12,336*	*22*
Caught in object, equipment, material	*7,222*	*1,026*
Fall to lower level	22,421	3,494
Fall on same level	12,308	51
Slips, trips	4,736	—
Overexertion	33,799	—
Overexertion in lifting	*17,903*	—
Repetitive motion	2,866	—
Exposed to harmful substance	4,306	1,860
Transportation accidents	6,681	2,844
Fires, explosions	429	292
Assault, violent act	595	332
by person	*206*	*168*
by other	*388*	*164*
All other	18,134	53

Source: National Safety Council tabulations of Bureau of Labor Statistics data.
Note: Because of rounding and data exclusion of nonclassifiable responses, data may not sum to the totals. Dashes (—) indicate data that do not meet publication guidelines.

[a] Days away from work include those that result in days away from work with or without restricted work activity.
[b] In the fatalities column, non-Hispanic categories include cases with Hispanic origin not reported.

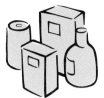

MANUFACTURING

The Manufacturing industry division includes establishments engaged in the mechanical or chemical transformation of materials or substances into new products. It includes durable and nondurable goods such as food, textiles, apparel, lumber, wood products, paper and paper products, printing, chemicals and pharmaceuticals, petroleum and coal products, rubber and plastics products, metals and metal products, machinery, electrical equipment, and transportation equipment.

Manufacturing employment in 2002 was 18,073,000 workers. Average annual employment from 1993 through 2002 was 19,858,000 workers.

NUMBER OF NONFATAL OCCUPATIONAL INJURIES AND ILLNESS INVOLVING DAYS AWAY FROM WORK[a] AND FATAL OCCUPATIONAL INJURIES BY SELECTED WORKER AND CASE CHARACTERISTICS, UNITED STATES, MANUFACTURING

Characteristic	Nonfatal Cases, 2002	Fatalities, 1993–2002
Total	**280,005**	**6,983**
Sex		
Men	214,713	6,580
Women	65,275	403
Age		
Under 16	—	14
16 to 19	4,256	150
20 to 24	24,140	501
25 to 34	65,886	1,416
35 to 44	80,719	1,890
45 to 54	67,920	1,594
55 to 64	32,671	1,058
65 and over	3,304	349
Occupation		
Managerial and professional	4,615	676
Technical, sales, and administrative support	16,662	502
Service	6,046	106
Farming, forestry, and fishing	1,972	1,041
Precision production, craft, and repair	49,405	1,336
Operators, fabricators, and laborers	200,741	3,284
Race or ethnic origin[b]		
White, non-Hispanic	150,204	4,777
Black, non-Hispanic	22,520	756
Hispanic	39,478	687
Asian or Pacific Islander	5,155	114
American Indian or Alaskan Native	1,191	34
Not reported	61,458	615
Nature of injury, illness		
Sprains, strains	105,530	17
Fractures	19,567	40
Cuts, lacerations, punctures	29,748	517
Bruises, contusions	23,543	5
Heat burns	4,823	301
Chemical burns	2,564	29
Amputations	4,227	41
Carpal tunnel syndrome	8,962	—
Tendonitis	3,032	—
Multiple injuries	10,246	1,893
Soreness, pain	17,441	—
Back pain	*6,147*	—
All other	50,322	4,138

Characteristic	Nonfatal Cases, 2002	Fatalities, 1993–2002
Part of body affected		
Head	20,347	1,794
Eye	*12,420*	—
Neck	3,689	120
Trunk	94,694	1,518
Back	*55,695*	*94*
Shoulder	*18,598*	—
Upper extremities	88,454	28
Finger	*36,542*	*5*
Hand, except finger	*14,576*	—
Wrist	*19,043*	—
Lower extremities	49,353	86
Knee	*18,721*	*17*
Foot, toe	*10,942*	*7*
Body systems	3,220	1,009
Multiple	18,547	2,396
All other	1,702	32
Source of injury, illness		
Chemicals, chemical products	5,608	264
Containers	35,029	214
Furniture, fixtures	7,695	27
Machinery	34,297	1,142
Parts and materials	49,060	705
Worker motion or position	54,045	6
Floor, ground surfaces	32,040	536
Handtools	16,072	80
Vehicles	13,639	2,134
Health care patient	—	—
All other	32,516	1,875
Event or exposure		
Contact with object, equipment	95,463	2,585
Struck by object	*41,129*	*1,596*
Struck against object	*20,838*	*28*
Caught in object, equipment, material	*26,202*	*956*
Fall to lower level	9,950	478
Fall on same level	23,922	87
Slips, trips	7,732	6
Overexertion	68,789	18
Overexertion in lifting	*35,562*	*11*
Repetitive motion	23,593	—
Exposed to harmful substance	14,032	639
Transportation accidents	5,816	2,076
Fires, explosions	598	461
Assault, violent act	741	581
by person	*410*	*351*
by other	*331*	*230*
All other	29,369	52

Source: National Safety Council tabulations of Bureau of Labor Statistics data.
Note: Because of rounding and data exclusion of nonclassifiable responses, data may not sum to the totals. Dashes (—) indicate data that do not meet publication guidelines.

[a]*Days away from work include those that result in days away from work with or without restricted work activity.*
[b]*In the fatalities column, non-Hispanic categories include cases with Hispanic origin not reported.*

TRANSPORTATION AND PUBLIC UTILITIES

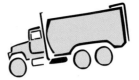

This industry division includes transportation by rail, highway, air, water, or pipeline and associated transportation services; communications by telephone, radio, television, cable, or satellite; and electric, gas, and sanitary services.

Employment in the Transportation and Public Utilities industry division totaled 8,060,000 in 2002 and averaged 7,585,000 workers per year from 1993 through 2002.

NUMBER OF NONFATAL OCCUPATIONAL INJURIES AND ILLNESS INVOLVING DAYS AWAY FROM WORK[a] AND FATAL OCCUPATIONAL INJURIES BY SELECTED WORKER AND CASE CHARACTERISTICS, UNITED STATES, TRANSPORTATION AND PUBLIC UTILITIES[b]

Characteristic	Nonfatal Cases, 2002	Fatalities, 1993–2002
Total	**168,632**	**9,423**
Sex		
Men	129,985	8,980
Women	34,025	443
Age		
Under 16	—	—
16 to 19	1,636	89
20 to 24	11,882	449
25 to 34	41,148	1,950
35 to 44	53,002	2,610
45 to 54	41,054	2,462
55 to 64	17,603	1,392
65 and over	1,694	453
Occupation		
Managerial and professional	3,635	340
Technical, sales, and administrative support	27,744	869
Service	9,891	129
Farming, forestry, and fishing	704	26
Precision production, craft, and repair	27,312	787
Operators, fabricators, and laborers	99,106	7,257
Race or ethnic origin[c]		
White, non-Hispanic	53,420	6,309
Black, non-Hispanic	9,232	1,209
Hispanic	10,803	848
Asian or Pacific Islander	1,268	244
American Indian or Alaskan Native	591	37
Not reported	93,317	776
Nature of injury, illness		
Sprains, strains	81,884	11
Fractures	10,456	24
Cuts, lacerations, punctures	7,377	887
Bruises, contusions	15,749	—
Heat burns	714	340
Chemical burns	614	6
Amputations	849	44
Carpal tunnel syndrome	1,847	—
Tendonitis	807	—
Multiple injuries	7,161	3,732
Soreness, pain	16,144	—
Back pain	6,436	—
All other	25,029	4,376

Characteristic	Nonfatal Cases, 2002	Fatalities, 1993–2002
Part of body affected		
Head	9,204	1,905
Eye	3,536	—
Neck	3,288	171
Trunk	67,100	1,624
Back	42,612	103
Shoulder	12,416	—
Upper extremities	27,340	11
Finger	7,890	—
Hand, except finger	4,827	—
Wrist	6,418	—
Lower extremities	39,826	56
Knee	14,682	9
Foot, toe	7,347	—
Body systems	2,082	1,243
Multiple	18,967	4,348
All other	825	65
Source of injury, illness		
Chemicals, chemical products	1,447	158
Containers	30,443	111
Furniture, fixtures	3,388	9
Machinery	3,876	233
Parts and materials	14,624	424
Worker motion or position	26,898	—
Floor, ground surfaces	29,973	331
Handtools	3,115	73
Vehicles	31,273	6,861
Health care patient	1,387	—
All other	22,207	1,219
Event or exposure		
Contact with object, equipment	35,694	779
Struck by object	17,132	504
Struck against object	11,280	11
Caught in object, equipment, material	4,235	260
Fall to lower level	13,105	296
Fall on same level	17,405	35
Slips, trips	6,426	—
Overexertion	46,231	—
Overexertion in lifting	23,258	—
Repetitive motion	5,030	—
Exposed to harmful substance	4,876	534
Transportation accidents	16,201	6,592
Fires, explosions	210	150
Assault, violent act	1,775	995
by person	730	833
by other	1,045	162
All other	21,679	40

Source: National Safety Council tabulations of Bureau of Labor Statistics data.
Note: Because of rounding and data exclusion of nonclassifiable responses, data may not sum to the totals. Dashes (—) indicate data that do not meet publication guidelines.
[a] Days away from work include those that result in days away from work with or without restricted work activity.

[b] Data conforming to OSHA definitions for employees in railroad transportation are provided to BLS by the Federal Railroad Administration, U.S. Department of Transportation.
[c] In the fatalities column, non-Hispanic categories include cases with Hispanic origin not reported.

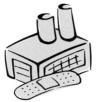

Establishments in Wholesale Trade generally sell merchandise to retailers; to industrial, commercial, institutional, farm construction contractors, or professional business users; to other wholesalers; or to agents or brokers.

Wholesale Trade employed 5,066,000 people in 2002 and an average of 4,992,000 people annually from 1993 through 2002.

NUMBER OF NONFATAL OCCUPATIONAL INJURIES AND ILLNESS INVOLVING DAYS AWAY FROM WORK[a] AND FATAL OCCUPATIONAL INJURIES BY SELECTED WORKER AND CASE CHARACTERISTICS, UNITED STATES, WHOLESALE TRADE

Characteristic	Nonfatal Cases, 2002	Fatalities, 1993–2002
Total	**108,791**	**2,412**
Sex		
Men	92,259	2,287
Women	16,532	125
Age		
Under 16	—	—
16 to 19	1,980	47
20 to 24	10,760	183
25 to 34	29,837	483
35 to 44	31,577	603
45 to 54	23,214	526
55 to 64	9,219	364
65 and over	1,869	199
Occupation		
Managerial and professional	3,842	191
Technical, sales, and administrative support	17,812	625
Service	1,572	34
Farming, forestry, and fishing	1,326	49
Precision production, craft, and repair	13,049	247
Operators, fabricators, and laborers	71,058	1,251
Race or ethnic origin[b]		
White, non-Hispanic	58,935	1,669
Black, non-Hispanic	9,253	182
Hispanic	15,505	266
Asian or Pacific Islander	1,560	65
American Indian or Alaskan Native	575	6
Not reported	22,962	224
Nature of injury, illness		
Sprains, strains	51,385	9
Fractures	7,694	14
Cuts, lacerations, punctures	9,040	246
Bruises, contusions	10,196	—
Heat burns	673	80
Chemical burns	468	—
Amputations	701	10
Carpal tunnel syndrome	1,188	—
Tendonitis	540	—
Multiple injuries	4,346	773
Soreness, pain	7,325	—
Back pain	2,873	—
All other	15,234	1,278

Characteristic	Nonfatal Cases, 2002	Fatalities, 1993–2002
Part of body affected		
Head	6,044	586
Eye	2,554	—
Neck	2,438	47
Trunk	42,211	477
Back	28,302	24
Shoulder	6,443	—
Upper extremities	21,143	6
Finger	8,296	—
Hand, except finger	3,600	—
Wrist	3,989	—
Lower extremities	25,174	33
Knee	8,308	5
Foot, toe	5,469	—
Body systems	727	306
Multiple	10,300	942
All other	754	15
Source of injury, illness		
Chemicals, chemical products	1,121	55
Containers	24,863	66
Furniture, fixtures	2,968	—
Machinery	6,719	171
Parts and materials	12,420	135
Worker motion or position	14,373	—
Floor, ground surfaces	17,399	169
Handtools	3,638	28
Vehicles	15,475	1,389
Health care patient	86	—
All other	9,728	396
Event or exposure		
Contact with object, equipment	29,379	425
Struck by object	14,570	236
Struck against object	7,580	—
Caught in object, equipment, material	5,537	185
Fall to lower level	6,750	149
Fall on same level	10,888	24
Slips, trips	3,184	—
Overexertion	32,486	—
Overexertion in lifting	19,807	—
Repetitive motion	2,620	—
Exposed to harmful substance	2,378	130
Transportation accidents	8,682	1,279
Fires, explosions	241	91
Assault, violent act	641	298
by person	348	202
by other	293	96
All other	11,544	12

Source: National Safety Council tabulations of Bureau of Labor Statistics data.
Note: Because of rounding and data exclusion of nonclassifiable responses, data may not sum to the totals. Dashes (—) indicate data that do not meet publication guidelines.

[a]Days away from work include those that result in days away from work with or without restricted work activity.
[b]In the fatalities column, non-Hispanic categories include cases with Hispanic origin not reported.

RETAIL TRADE

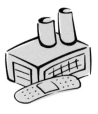

Establishments in Retail Trade generally sell merchandise for personal or household consumption. Retail Trade is the second largest industry division after Services.

Retail Trade employed 22,900,000 people in 2002 and an average of 21,721,000 people annually from 1993 through 2002.

NUMBER OF NONFATAL OCCUPATIONAL INJURIES AND ILLNESS INVOLVING DAYS AWAY FROM WORK[a] AND FATAL OCCUPATIONAL INJURIES BY SELECTED WORKER AND CASE CHARACTERISTICS, UNITED STATES, RETAIL TRADE

Characteristic	Nonfatal Cases, 2002	Fatalities, 1993–2002
Total	**263,401**	**6,343**
Sex		
Men	144,757	5,223
Women	118,631	1,120
Age		
Under 16	121	21
16 to 19	16,366	298
20 to 24	43,408	595
25 to 34	64,011	1,352
35 to 44	63,193	1,453
45 to 54	46,181	1,268
55 to 64	22,342	814
65 and over	6,901	532
Occupation		
Managerial and professional	9,259	831
Technical, sales, and administrative support	92,140	3,229
Service	67,892	740
Farming, forestry, and fishing	1,159	16
Precision production, craft, and repair	24,716	297
Operators, fabricators, and laborers	67,782	1,185
Race or ethnic origin[b]		
White, non-Hispanic	125,062	3,614
Black, non-Hispanic	16,245	681
Hispanic	28,835	783
Asian or Pacific Islander	3,167	703
American Indian or Alaskan Native	2,122	31
Not reported	87,971	531
Nature of injury, illness		
Sprains, strains	108,397	8
Fractures	16,494	43
Cuts, lacerations, punctures	32,985	3,634
Bruises, contusions	27,428	—
Heat burns	8,184	95
Chemical burns	1,199	—
Amputations	714	6
Carpal tunnel syndrome	3,007	—
Tendonitis	1,228	—
Multiple injuries	7,369	900
Soreness, pain	21,049	—
Back pain	*8,410*	—
All other	35,347	1,652

Characteristic	Nonfatal Cases, 2002	Fatalities, 1993–2002
Part of body affected		
Head	16,285	1,953
Eye	*6,799*	—
Neck	3,680	194
Trunk	93,833	1,757
Back	*64,056*	*150*
Shoulder	*13,307*	*9*
Upper extremities	65,987	11
Finger	*26,908*	—
Hand, except finger	*11,352*	—
Wrist	*12,003*	—
Lower extremities	55,649	56
Knee	*18,775*	*8*
Foot, toe	*13,511*	—
Body systems	2,823	425
Multiple	23,458	1,905
All other	1,687	42
Source of injury, illness		
Chemicals, chemical products	3,324	104
Containers	59,478	43
Furniture, fixtures	15,006	20
Machinery	17,435	78
Parts and materials	15,401	205
Worker motion or position	35,687	—
Floor, ground surfaces	51,361	288
Handtools	15,540	342
Vehicles	16,635	1,515
Health care patient	—	—
All other	33,524	3,745
Event or exposure		
Contact with object, equipment	74,643	267
Struck by object	*41,520*	*162*
Struck against object	*20,615*	*8*
Caught in object, equipment, material	*8,808*	*94*
Fall to lower level	11,827	177
Fall on same level	42,467	87
Slips, trips	9,927	—
Overexertion	69,653	—
Overexertion in lifting	*45,817*	—
Repetitive motion	8,367	—
Exposed to harmful substance	12,996	198
Transportation accidents	6,624	1,423
Fires, explosions	768	112
Assault, violent act	2,851	4,035
by person	*2,416*	*3,714*
by other	*435*	*321*
All other	23,278	37

Source: National Safety Council tabulations of Bureau of Labor Statistics data.
Note: Because of rounding and data exclusion of nonclassifiable responses, data may not sum to the totals. Dashes (—) indicate data that do not meet publication guidelines.

[a] Days away from work include those that result in days away from work with or without restricted work activity.
[b] In the fatalities column, non-Hispanic categories include cases with Hispanic origin not reported.

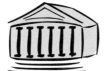

Establishments in the Finance, Insurance, and Real Estate industry division include banks and other savings institutions; securities and commodities brokers, dealers, exchanges, and services; insurance carriers, brokers, and agents; real estate operators, developers, agents, and brokers; and holding and other investment offices.

Finance, Insurance, and Real Estate had 8,939,000 workers in 2002 and an annual average of 8,243,000 from 1993 through 2002.

NUMBER OF NONFATAL OCCUPATIONAL INJURIES AND ILLNESS INVOLVING DAYS AWAY FROM WORK[a] AND FATAL OCCUPATIONAL INJURIES BY SELECTED WORKER AND CASE CHARACTERISTICS, UNITED STATES, FINANCE, INSURANCE, AND REAL ESTATE

Characteristic	Nonfatal Cases, 2002	Fatalities, 1993–2002
Total	**36,689**	**1,020**
Sex		
Men	17,874	789
Women	18,814	231
Age		
Under 16	—	—
16 to 19	432	—
20 to 24	2,820	40
25 to 34	8,125	163
35 to 44	10,481	235
45 to 54	8,841	266
55 to 64	5,056	170
65 and over	897	141
Occupation		
Managerial and professional	5,668	374
Technical, sales, and administrative support	15,883	376
Service	8,206	121
Farming, forestry, and fishing	1,693	42
Precision production, craft, and repair	3,739	53
Operators, fabricators, and laborers	1,483	46
Race or ethnic origin[b]		
White, non-Hispanic	15,119	714
Black, non-Hispanic	2,991	75
Hispanic	4,635	105
Asian or Pacific Islander	983	30
American Indian or Alaskan Native	390	—
Not reported	12,571	95
Nature of injury, illness		
Sprains, strains	13,327	—
Fractures	2,969	10
Cuts, lacerations, punctures	2,400	311
Bruises, contusions	2,793	—
Heat burns	222	10
Chemical burns	150	—
Amputations	67	—
Carpal tunnel syndrome	1,904	—
Tendonitis	476	—
Multiple injuries	1,430	281
Soreness, pain	3,693	—
Back pain	1,571	—
All other	7,259	400

Characteristic	Nonfatal Cases, 2002	Fatalities, 1993–2002
Part of body affected		
Head	1,601	264
Eye	465	—
Neck	433	20
Trunk	11,119	203
Back	7,672	20
Shoulder	1,517	—
Upper extremities	8,642	—
Finger	2,146	—
Hand, except finger	1,114	—
Wrist	3,279	—
Lower extremities	8,063	13
Knee	2,957	—
Foot, toe	1,490	—
Body systems	1,680	139
Multiple	5,026	369
All other	125	10
Source of injury, illness		
Chemicals, chemical products	523	27
Containers	3,313	—
Furniture, fixtures	2,002	—
Machinery	1,816	36
Parts and materials	1,678	43
Worker motion or position	8,417	—
Floor, ground surfaces	9,049	120
Handtools	1,398	35
Vehicles	2,821	360
Health care patient	213	—
All other	5,461	392
Event or exposure		
Contact with object, equipment	6,345	45
Struck by object	3,033	26
Struck against object	2,568	—
Caught in object, equipment, material	497	18
Fall to lower level	2,763	100
Fall on same level	6,265	20
Slips, trips	1,315	—
Overexertion	7,258	—
Overexertion in lifting	4,207	—
Repetitive motion	3,566	—
Exposed to harmful substance	1,358	74
Transportation accidents	2,047	360
Fires, explosions	—	8
Assault, violent act	459	406
by person	350	313
by other	108	93
All other	5,292	7

Source: National Safety Council tabulations of Bureau of Labor Statistics data.
Note: Because of rounding and data exclusion of nonclassifiable responses, data may not sum to the totals. Dashes (—) indicate data that do not meet publication guidelines.

[a]Days away from work include those that result in days away from work with or without restricted work activity.
[b]In the fatalities column, non-Hispanic categories include cases with Hispanic origin not reported.

SERVICES

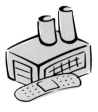

Establishments in the Services industry division provide services, rather than merchandise, for individuals, businesses, government agencies, and other organizations. Broad categories in this industry division include lodging places, personal and business services, automobile services, repair services, motion pictures, amusement and recreation services, health, legal, education, social services, etc.

Services is the largest industry division with 40,729,000 workers in 2002 and an annual average of 36,491,000 from 1993 through 2002.

NUMBER OF NONFATAL OCCUPATIONAL INJURIES AND ILLNESS INVOLVING DAYS AWAY FROM WORK[a] AND FATAL OCCUPATIONAL INJURIES BY SELECTED WORKER AND CASE CHARACTERISTICS, UNITED STATES, SERVICES

Characteristic	Nonfatal Cases, 2002	Fatalities, 1993–2002
Total	**372,159**	**7,599**
Sex		
Men	135,484	6,314
Women	236,651	1,285
Age		
Under 16	—	22
16 to 19	9,500	193
20 to 24	37,625	621
25 to 34	86,899	1,639
35 to 44	101,238	1,893
45 to 54	83,711	1,543
55 to 64	43,538	1,021
65 and over	8,524	657
Occupation		
Managerial and professional	62,599	2,338
Technical, sales, and administrative support	63,115	889
Service	175,604	1,585
Farming, forestry, and fishing	5,474	174
Precision production, craft, and repair	22,749	1,183
Operators, fabricators, and laborers	41,983	1,375
Race or ethnic origin[b]		
White, non-Hispanic	171,470	5,055
Black, non-Hispanic	45,861	805
Hispanic	39,909	817
Asian or Pacific Islander	8,257	259
American Indian or Alaskan Native	2,266	44
Not reported	104,397	618
Nature of injury, illness		
Sprains, strains	181,341	13
Fractures	19,930	80
Cuts, lacerations, punctures	18,984	1,546
Bruises, contusions	32,369	5
Heat burns	4,912	152
Chemical burns	2,165	5
Amputations	745	16
Carpal tunnel syndrome	4,560	—
Tendonitis	2,089	—
Multiple injuries	13,470	2,226
Soreness, pain	36,475	—
Back pain	14,125	—
All other	55,118	3,553

Characteristic	Nonfatal Cases, 2002	Fatalities, 1993–2002
Part of body affected		
Head	21,970	1,885
Eye	8,401	—
Neck	6,423	152
Trunk	144,724	1,341
Back	103,584	92
Shoulder	21,474	—
Upper extremities	67,023	25
Finger	19,162	—
Hand, except finger	10,869	—
Wrist	17,112	—
Lower extremities	77,155	85
Knee	31,445	13
Foot, toe	11,762	7
Body systems	7,279	1,232
Multiple	45,561	2,824
All other	2,024	55
Source of injury, illness		
Chemicals, chemical products	5,782	343
Containers	28,038	72
Furniture, fixtures	18,324	40
Machinery	14,917	306
Parts and materials	12,352	390
Worker motion or position	55,719	5
Floor, ground surfaces	74,885	747
Handtools	9,443	200
Vehicles	25,223	3,288
Health care patient	68,240	13
All other	59,237	2,195
Event or exposure		
Contact with object, equipment	67,301	734
Struck by object	33,962	459
Struck against object	21,900	35
Caught in object, equipment, material	7,728	235
Fall to lower level	16,815	563
Fall on same level	58,895	155
Slips, trips	13,891	—
Overexertion	114,747	12
Overexertion in lifting	57,831	8
Repetitive motion	11,803	—
Exposed to harmful substance	17,743	724
Transportation accidents	14,850	3,053
Fires, explosions	319	253
Assault, violent act	14,877	2,027
by person	13,587	1,443
by other	1,291	584
All other	40,920	78

Source: National Safety Council tabulations of Bureau of Labor Statistics data.
Note: Because of rounding and data exclusion of nonclassifiable responses, data may not sum to the totals. Dashes (—) indicate data that do not meet publication guidelines.

[a] Days away from work include those that result in days away from work with or without restricted work activity.
[b] In the fatalities column, non-Hispanic categories include cases with Hispanic origin not reported.

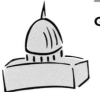

GOVERNMENT

Government includes workers at all levels from federal civilian and military to state, county, and municipal.

Government employment totaled 20,870,000 in 2002. From 1993 through 2002, Government employment averaged 19,953,000 per year.

NUMBER OF NONFATAL OCCUPATIONAL INJURIES AND ILLNESS INVOLVING DAYS AWAY FROM WORK[a] AND FATAL OCCUPATIONAL INJURIES BY SELECTED WORKER AND CASE CHARACTERISTICS, UNITED STATES, GOVERNMENT

Characteristic	Nonfatal Cases, 2002	Fatalities, 1993–2002
Total	(b)	6,295
Sex		
Men		5,526
Women		769
Age		
Under 16		9
16 to 19		158
20 to 24		565
25 to 34		1,588
35 to 44		1,514
45 to 54		1,370
55 to 64		783
65 and over		286
Occupation		
Managerial and professional		965
Technical, sales, and administrative support		659
Service		2,246
Farming, forestry, and fishing		120
Precision production, craft, and repair		567
Operators, fabricators, and laborers		866
Military occupations		831
Race or ethnic origin[c]		
White, non-Hispanic		4,457
Black, non-Hispanic		697
Hispanic		397
Asian or Pacific Islander		96
American Indian or Alaskan Native		55
Not reported		593
Nature of injury, illness		
Sprains, strains		20
Fractures		51
Cuts, lacerations, punctures		1,147
Bruises, contusions		—
Heat burns		126
Chemical burns		—
Amputations		14
Carpal tunnel syndrome		—
Tendonitis		—
Multiple injuries		2,221
Soreness, pain		—
Back pain		—
All other		2,708

Characteristic	Nonfatal Cases, 2002	Fatalities, 1993–2002
Part of body affected	(b)	
Head		1,490
Eye		—
Neck		138
Trunk		993
Back		96
Shoulder		—
Upper extremities		11
Finger		—
Hand, except finger		—
Wrist		—
Lower extremities		68
Knee		13
Foot, toe		5
Body systems		848
Multiple		2,689
All other		58
Source of injury, illness		
Chemicals, chemical products		91
Containers		50
Furniture, fixtures		17
Machinery		218
Parts and materials		208
Worker motion or position		5
Floor, ground surfaces		343
Handtools		62
Vehicles		3,382
Health care patient		8
All other		1,911
Event or exposure		
Contact with object, equipment		396
Struck by object		245
Struck against object		12
Caught in object, equipment, material		136
Fall to lower level		242
Fall on same level		82
Slips, trips		—
Overexertion		13
Overexertion in lifting		8
Repetitive motion		—
Exposed to harmful substance		405
Transportation accidents		3,402
Fires, explosions		293
Assault, violent act		1,414
by person		1,039
by other		375
All other		45

Source: National Safety Council tabulations of Bureau of Labor Statistics data.
Note: Because of rounding and data exclusion of nonclassifiable responses, data may not sum to the totals. Dashes (—) indicate data that do not meet publication guidelines.
[a]Days away from work include those that result in days away from work with or without restricted work activity.

[b]Data for government entities not collected in the national BLS Survey of Occupational Injuries and Illnesses.
[c]In the fatalities column, non-Hispanic categories include cases with Hispanic origin not reported.

MINING

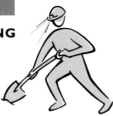

The federal Mine Safety and Health Administration (MSHA), part of the U.S. Department of Labor, collects and compiles data on mining accidents, injuries, employment, and coal production. Federal regulations require that operators of coal, metal, or nonmetallic mines and certain independent contractors working on mine property report accidents, occupational injuries, and illnesses to MSHA. From this collection of information MSHA develops and publishes statistical data that mine operators, labor organizations, academia, and state and federal agencies use to help identify potential health and safety improvements.

The statistics on pages 78-81 are derived from information the mining industry reports to MSHA and differs from the Bureau of Labor Statistics' (BLS) Census of Fatal Occupational Injuries and Survey of Occupational Injuries and Illnesses. In general, MSHA statistics include all injuries that occur on mine property. The BLS mining statistics exclude data on contract workers and classify certain types of injuries that occur on mine property in industries other than mining. The BLS mining statistics also include information on oil and gas extraction industries, which are not included here.

The table below presents the average industry employment, number of fatal occupational injuries, nonfatal injuries involving time away from work, total mining injuries, and the associated incidence rates from 1994 through 2003. As the data indicate, underground miners experience much higher injury rates than surface miners. Most underground mining occurs in the coal mining sector.

MINING INJURY STATISTICS, 1994-2003

Year	Avg. Employment (000's)	Fatal Injuries	Fatal Injury Incidence Rate[a]	Lost Time Injuries	Lost Time Injury Incidence Rate[a]	All Injuries	All-Injury Incidence Rate[a]
Underground Mining							
1994	76.6	32	.044	6,710	9.3	8,824	12.2
1995	73.0	34	.048	5,976	8.5	8,014	11.4
1996	70.4	39	.056	5,222	7.5	7,167	10.3
1997	70.5	31	.044	5,030	7.2	6,984	9.9
1998	68.6	30	.044	5,276	7.8	7,132	10.5
1999	63.2	31	.050	4,476	7.2	5,976	9.6
2000	59.7	31	.053	4,279	7.3	5,744	9.9
2001	61.8	43	.070	3,929	6.4	5,409	8.8
2002	58.5	22	.039	3,695	6.5	4,963	8.7
2003	55.4	19	.034	3,168	5.7	4,272	7.6
Surface Mining							
1994	292.5	53	.020	9,199	3.5	14,326	5.5
1995	288.7	66	.025	7,968	3.1	12,793	4.9
1996	285.1	47	.018	7,368	2.8	11,724	4.5
1997	291.8	60	.023	7,113	2.7	11,312	4.3
1998	288.7	50	.019	6,987	2.7	10,915	4.2
1999	290.1	59	.023	6,632	2.6	10,230	4.0
2000	288.9	54	.021	6,698	2.6	10,281	4.0
2001	285.4	29	.012	6,120	2.5	9,328	3.7
2002	270.6	46	.020	5,758	2.5	8,445	3.6
2003	264.5	37	.016	5,138	2.3	7,494	3.3

Source: MSHA.
[a] Incidence rate = (number of injuries x 200,000)/hours of employee exposure
Notes:
The term "injury," includes all reportable occupational injuries that result from a work accident involving a single incident in the work environment. A "reportable" injury is an injury to an individual, occurring at a mining operation that requires medical treatment or results in death or loss of consciousness or inability to perform all job duties on any workday after the injury or temporary assignment to other duties or transfer to another job. Lost time injuries are those that result in days away from work or days of restricted activity. The "All Injuries" category includes injuries reported to MSHA that resulted in no time away from work or restricted work activity.
The mining data compiled by MSHA include establishments in Standard Industrial Classification codes 10, 12, and 14 (except 1081, 1241, 1481), codes 1311, 3241, 3274, and parts of codes 2819 and 2899.

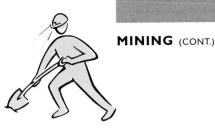

The United States has over 14,000 mines, employing more than 300,000 workers. The nation's 2,000 coal mines produce over one billion tons of coal per year. Metal and nonmetal mines extract close to 100 different mineral classifications with some type of mining occurring in every state. Safety and health in America's mining industry has improved dramatically. In the early part of the twentieth century, annual mining fatalities sometimes exceeded 3,500. For the last three years, mining fatalities have been at record low levels. In 2003, there were 56 mining fatalities — the lowest number ever recorded.

MINING DEATHS AND DEATH RATES, UNITED STATES, 1910–2003

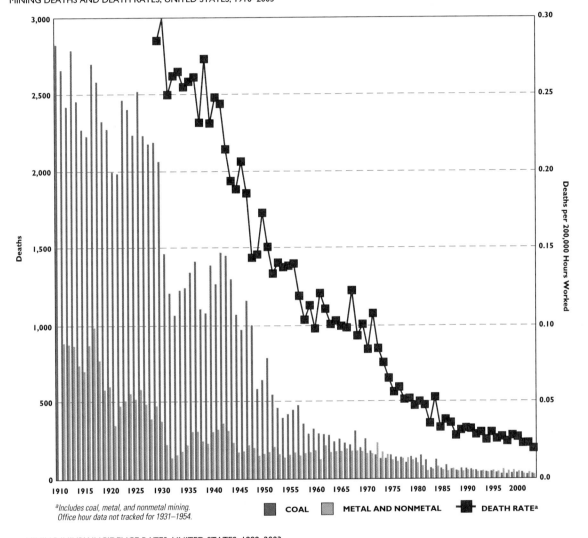

aIncludes coal, metal, and nonmetal mining.
Office hour data not tracked for 1931–1954.

COAL   METAL AND NONMETAL   DEATH RATEa

MINING INJURY INCIDENCE RATES, UNITED STATES, 1989–2003

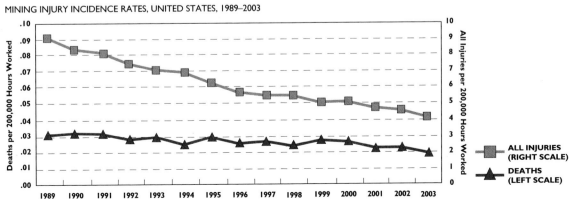

ALL INJURIES (RIGHT SCALE)

DEATHS (LEFT SCALE)

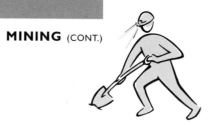

MINING (CONT.)

Explosions, ignitions, and roof falls, once the cause of the majority of mining fatalities, are increasingly rare. Today, powered haulage (the transport of ore, coal, supplies, and waste) and machinery (accidents related to the motion of machinery) represent more than half of the fatalities occurring in the industry. Over half of non-fatal mining injuries are classified as handling materials (lifting, pulling, and shoveling) and slips or falls.

MINING FATALITIES BY ACCIDENT CLASSIFICATION, UNITED STATES, 2003

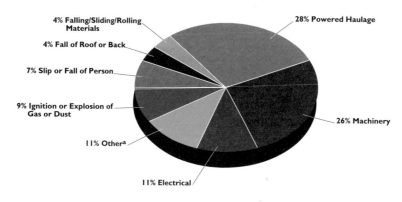

4% Falling/Sliding/Rolling Materials
4% Fall of Roof or Back
7% Slip or Fall of Person
9% Ignition or Explosion of Gas or Dust
11% Other[a]
11% Electrical
28% Powered Haulage
26% Machinery

[a] *"Other" includes 5 other accidental classifications*

MINING INJURIES BY ACCIDENT CLASSIFICATION, UNITED STATES, 2003

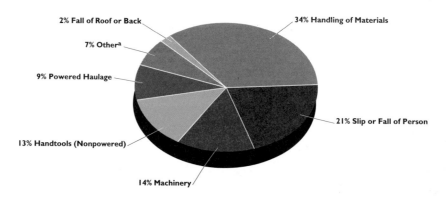

2% Fall of Roof or Back
7% Other[a]
9% Powered Haulage
13% Handtools (Nonpowered)
14% Machinery
34% Handling of Materials
21% Slip or Fall of Person

[a] *"Other" includes 13 other accidental classifications.*

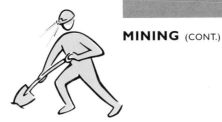

The activities miners are performing when they incur fatal injuries are diverse. In 2003, miners performing machine maintenance and repair activities accounted for the single largest portion of mining fatalities, with truck drivers representing the second largest portion.

Nonfatal injuries followed a similar pattern in 2003, with equipment operation and maintenance and repair activities accounting for over 60% of all reported mining injuries.

MINING FATALITIES BY ACTIVITY, UNITED STATES, 2003

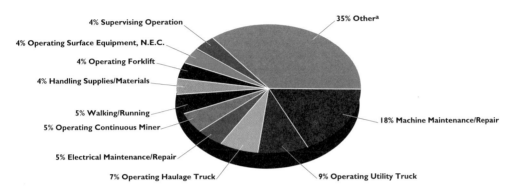

4% Supervising Operation

4% Operating Surface Equipment, N.E.C.

4% Operating Forklift

4% Handling Supplies/Materials

5% Walking/Running

5% Operating Continuous Miner

5% Electrical Maintenance/Repair

7% Operating Haulage Truck

35% Other[a]

18% Machine Maintenance/Repair

9% Operating Utility Truck

[a] "Other" includes 17 other activities (1 incident each).
N.E.C. means not elsewhere classified.

MINING INJURIES BY ACTIVITY, UNITED STATES, 2003

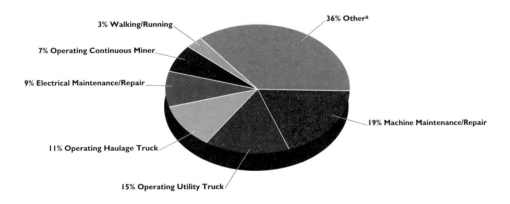

3% Walking/Running

7% Operating Continuous Miner

9% Electrical Maintenance/Repair

11% Operating Haulage Truck

15% Operating Utility Truck

36% Other[a]

19% Machine Maintenance/Repair

[a] "Other" includes 87 other activities.

OCCUPATIONAL HEALTH

Skin diseases or disorders were the most common illness, with nearly 45,000 new cases in 2002.

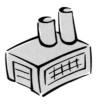

Approximately 294,500 occupational illnesses were recognized or diagnosed by employers in 2002 according to the Bureau of Labor Statistics (BLS). Manufacturing accounted for nearly 45% of these cases. Skin diseases or disorders were the most common illness with 44,900 new cases, followed by respiratory conditions with 22,000, and poisonings with 4,700. Since the revised recordkeeping guidelines that became effective January 1, 2002 no longer provide categories to separately record cases such as disorders associated with repeated trauma or disorders due to physical agents, these cases are now being captured in the "all other illnesses" category, which accounted for 222,900 illnesses, or nearly 76% of all new illness cases in 2002.

The overall incidence rate of occupational illness for all workers was 33.3 per 10,000 full-time workers. Of the major industry divisions, manufacturing had the highest rate in 2002, 81.7 per 10,000 full-time workers. Workers in manufacturing also had the highest rates in the "all other illnesses" category. Agriculture had the second highest incidence rate, 40.7, although agricultural workers had the highest rate of all the industry divisions for skin diseases or disorders, respiratory conditions, and poisonings.

The table below shows the number of occupational illnesses and the incidence rate per 10,000 full-time workers as measured by the 2002 BLS survey. To convert these to incidence rates per 100 full-time workers, which are comparable to other published BLS rates, divide the rates in the table by 100. The BLS survey records illnesses only for the year in which they are recognized or diagnosed as work-related. Since only recognized cases are included, the figures underestimate the incidence of occupational illness.

NUMBER OF OCCUPATIONAL ILLNESSES AND INCIDENCE RATES BY INDUSTRY AND TYPE OF ILLNESS, UNITED STATES, 2002

Occupational Illness	Private Sector[a]	Agriculture[a,b]	Mining[b]	Construction	Manufacturing	Trans. & Pub. Util.[c]	Trade[b]	Finance[b]	Services
Number of Illnesses (in thousands)									
All Illnesses	**294.5**	**6.2**	**1.0**	**9.3**	**131.0**	**20.4**	**37.4**	**12.8**	**76.4**
Skin diseases, disorders	44.9	2.8	0.1	2.3	13.5	2.3	6.0	1.3	16.6
Respiratory conditions	22.0	0.6	0.1	0.9	4.4	1.4	4.2	0.7	9.8
Poisoning	4.7	0.2	(d)	0.5	1.1	0.3	1.1	0.1	1.2
All other occupational illnesses	222.9	2.5	0.8	5.6	112.0	16.4	26.1	10.6	48.8
Incidence Rate per 10,000 Full-Time Workers									
All Illnesses	**33.3**	**40.7**	**17.7**	**15.8**	**81.7**	**32.8**	**16.0**	**18.6**	**27.5**
Skin diseases, disorders	5.1	18.8	1.5	3.9	8.4	3.8	2.5	1.8	6.0
Respiratory conditions	2.5	3.9	2.4	1.5	2.7	2.2	1.8	1.1	3.5
Poisoning	0.5	1.6	0.5	0.9	0.7	0.5	0.5	0.2	0.4
All other occupational illnesses	25.2	16.5	13.4	9.5	69.8	26.4	11.2	15.5	17.5

Source: Bureau of Labor Statistics, U.S. Department of Labor. Components may not add to totals due to rounding.
[a] Private sector includes all industries except government, but excludes farms with less than 11 employees.
[b] Agriculture includes forestry and fishing; mining includes quarrying and oil and gas extraction; trade includes wholesale and retail; finance includes insurance and real estate.
[c] Data for transportation and public utilities do not reflect the changes OSHA made to its recordkeeping requirements effective January 1, 2002; therefore, estimates for these industries are not comparable with estimates for other industries.
[d] Fewer than 50 cases.

NONFATAL OCCUPATIONAL ILLNESS INCIDENCE RATES, U.S. INDUSTRY, 1996–2002

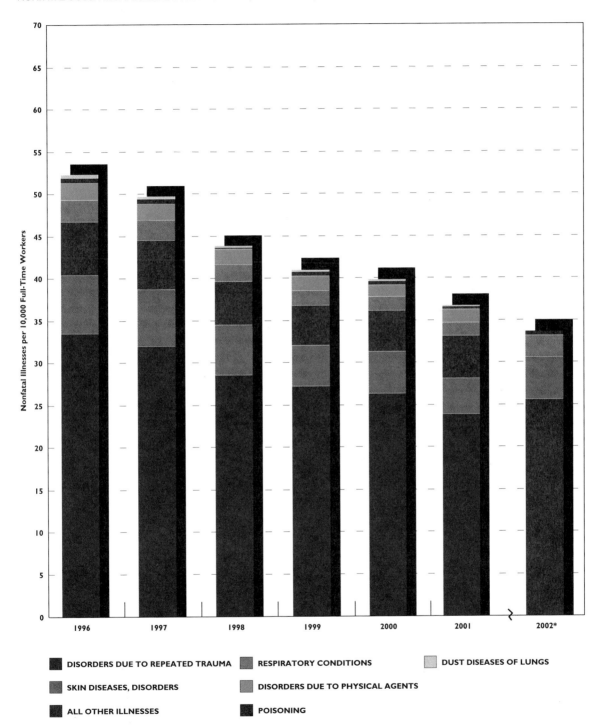

DISORDERS DUE TO REPEATED TRAUMA   RESPIRATORY CONDITIONS   DUST DISEASES OF LUNGS

SKIN DISEASES, DISORDERS   DISORDERS DUE TO PHYSICAL AGENTS

ALL OTHER ILLNESSES   POISONING

*Due to revised requirements for recording occupational injuries and illnesses,
the data for 2002 are not comparable to those from previous years.*

84

INJURY FACTS®

NATIONAL SAFETY COUNCIL

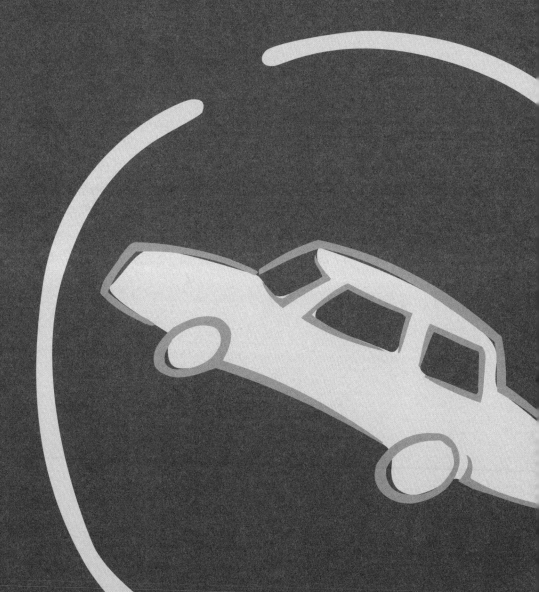

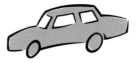

Between 1912 and 2003, motor-vehicle deaths per 10,000 registered vehicles were reduced 94%, from 33 to about 2. In 1912, there were 3,100 fatalities when the number of registered vehicles totaled only 950,000. In 2003, there were 44,800 fatalities, but registrations soared to 240 million.

While mileage data were not available in 1912, the 2003 mileage death rate of 1.56 per 100,000,000 vehicle miles was up 1% from the revised 2002 rate of 1.54, which is the lowest on record. Disabling injuries in motor-vehicle accidents totaled 2,400,000 in 2003, and total motor-vehicle costs were estimated at $240.7 billion. Costs include wage and productivity losses, medical expenses, administrative expenses, motor-vehicle property damage, and employer costs.

Motor-vehicle deaths increased 2% from 2002 to 2003 and also increased 2% from 2001. Miles traveled was up about 1%, the number of registered vehicles increased 2%, and the population increased 1%. As a result, the mileage death rate was up 1%, the registration death rate was down 1%, and the population death rate was up 1% from 2002 to 2003.

Compared with 1993, 2003 motor-vehicle deaths increased by about 7%. However, mileage, registration, and population death rates were all sharply lower in 2003 compared to 1993 (see chart on next page).

The word "accident" may be used in this section as well as the word "crash." When used, "accident" has a specific meaning as defined in the *Manual on Classification of Motor Vehicle Traffic Accidents, ANSI D16.1-1996.* "Crash" is generally used by the National Highway Traffic Safety Administration to mean the same as accident, but it is not formally defined.

Deaths **44,800**
Disabling Injuries **2,400,000**
Cost . . . . **$240.7 billion**
Motor-Vehicle Mileage . . . . **2,880 billion**
Registered Vehicles in the United States **239,600,000**
Licensed Drivers in the United States **196,700,000**
Death Rate per 100,000,000 Vehicle Miles **1.56**
Death Rate per 10,000 Registered Vehicles **1.87**
Death Rate per 100,000 Population **15.4**

ACCIDENT AND VEHICLE TOTALS, 2003

Severity of Accident	Number of Accidents	Drivers (Vehicles) Involved
Fatal	41,600	54,000
Disabling injury	1,800,000	2,600,000
Property damage and nondisabling injury[a]	10,000,000	17,300,000
Total (rounded)	11,800,000	20,000,000

[a]*Estimating procedures for these figures were revised beginning with the 1990 edition.*

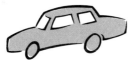

TRAVEL, DEATHS, AND DEATH RATES, UNITED STATES, 1925–2003

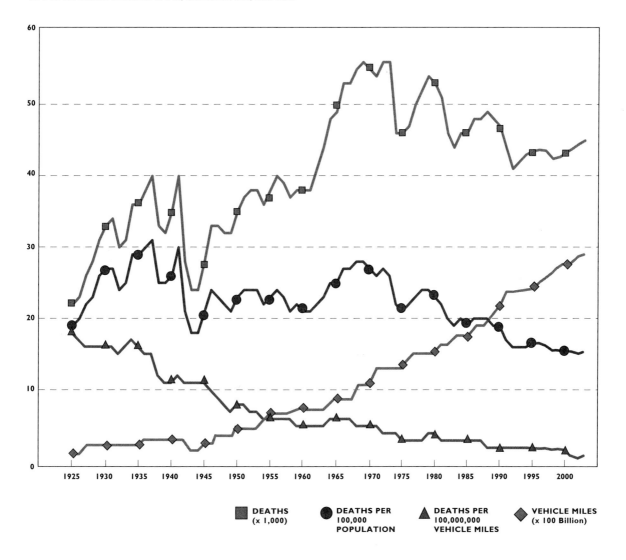

■ DEATHS (x 1,000)	● DEATHS PER 100,000 POPULATION	▲ DEATHS PER 100,000,000 VEHICLE MILES	◆ VEHICLE MILES (x 100 Billion)

DEATHS DUE TO MOTOR-VEHICLE ACCIDENTS, 2003

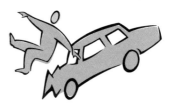

TYPE OF EVENT AND AGE OF VICTIM

All Motor-Vehicle Accidents

Includes deaths involving mechanically or electrically powered highway-transport vehicles in motion (except those on rails), both on and off the highway or street.

	Total	Change from 2002	Death Rate[a]
Deaths	44,800	+2%	15.4
Nonfatal injuries	2,400,000		

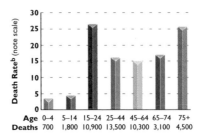

Age	0–4	5–14	15–24	25–44	45–64	65–74	75+
Deaths	700	1,800	10,900	13,500	10,300	3,100	4,500

Collision Between Motor Vehicles

Includes deaths from collisions of two or more motor vehicles. Motorized bicycles and scooters, trolley buses, and farm tractors or road machinery traveling on highways are motor vehicles.

	Total	Change from 2002	Death Rate[a]
Deaths	19,900	+6%	6.8
Nonfatal injuries	1,780,000		

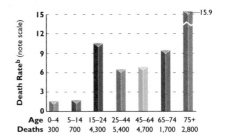

Age	0–4	5–14	15–24	25–44	45–64	65–74	75+
Deaths	300	700	4,300	5,400	4,700	1,700	2,800

Collision with Fixed Object

Includes deaths from collisions in which the first harmful event is the striking of a fixed object such as a guardrail, abutment, impact attenuator, etc.

	Total	Change from 2002	Death Rate[a]
Deaths	13,000	–3%	4.5
Nonfatal injuries	400,000		

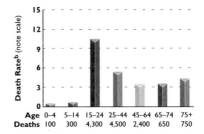

Age	0–4	5–14	15–24	25–44	45–64	65–74	75+
Deaths	100	300	4,300	4,500	2,400	650	750

Pedestrian Accidents

Includes all deaths of persons struck by motor vehicles, either on or off a street or highway, regardless of the circumstances of the accident.

	Total	Change from 2002	Death Rate[a]
Deaths	5,600	–2%	1.9
Nonfatal injuries	80,000		

See footnotes on page 89.

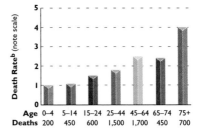

Age	0–4	5–14	15–24	25–44	45–64	65–74	75+
Deaths	200	450	600	1,500	1,700	450	700

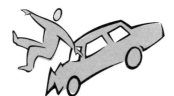

Noncollision Accidents

Includes deaths from accidents in which the first injury or damage-producing event was an overturn, jackknife, or other type of noncollision.

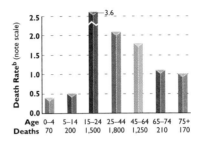

	Total	Change from 2002	Death Rate[a]
Deaths	5,200	0%	1.8
Nonfatal injuries	100,000		

Collision with Pedalcycle

Includes deaths of pedalcyclists and motor-vehicle occupants from collisions between pedalcycles and motor vehicles on streets, highways, private driveways, parking lots, etc.

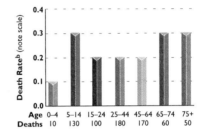

	Total	Change from 2002	Death Rate[a]
Deaths	700	0%	0.2
Nonfatal injuries	28,000		

Collision with Railroad Train

Includes deaths from collisions of motor vehicles (moving or stalled) and railroad vehicles at public or private grade crossings. In other types of accidents, classification requires motor vehicle to be in motion.

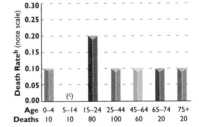

	Total	Change from 2002	Death Rate[a]
Deaths	300	0%	0.1
Nonfatal injuries	2,000		

Other Collision

Includes deaths from motor-vehicle collisions not specified in other categories above. Most of the deaths arose out of accidents involving animals or animal-drawn vehicles.

	Total	Change from 2002	Death Rate[a]
Deaths	100	0%	[c]
Nonfatal Injuries	10,000		

Note: Procedures and benchmarks for estimating deaths by type of accident and age were changed in 1990. Estimates for 1987 and later years are not comparable to earlier years. The noncollision and fixed object categories were most affected by the changes.
[a]*Deaths per 100,000 population.*
[b]*Deaths per 100,000 population in each age group.*
[c]*Death rate was less than 0.05.*

TYPE OF MOTOR-VEHICLE ACCIDENT

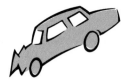

Although motor-vehicle deaths occur more often in collisions between motor vehicles than any other type of accident, this type represents only about 44% of the total. Collisions between a motor vehicle and a fixed object were the next most common type, with about 29% of the deaths, followed by pedestrian accidents and noncollisions (rollovers, etc.).

While collisions between motor vehicles accounted for less than half of motor-vehicle fatalities, this accident type represented 74% of injuries, 70% of injury accidents, and 68% of all accidents. Single-vehicle accidents involving collisions with fixed objects, pedestrians, and noncollisions, on the other hand,

accounted for a greater proportion of fatalities and fatal accidents compared to less serious accidents. These three accident types made up 53% of fatalities and 54% of fatal accidents, but 28% or less of injuries, injury accidents, or all accidents.

Of collisions between motor vehicles, angle collisions cause the greatest number of deaths, about 10,500 in 2003, and the greatest number of nonfatal injuries as well as fatal and injury accidents. The table below shows the estimated number of motor-vehicle deaths, injuries, fatal accidents, injury accidents, and all accidents, for various types of accidents.

MOTOR-VEHICLE DEATHS AND INJURIES AND NUMBER OF ACCIDENTS BY TYPE OF ACCIDENT, 2003

Type of Accident	Deaths	Nonfatal Injuries	Fatal Accidents	Injury Accidents	All Accidents
Total	**44,800**	**2,400,000**	**41,600**	**1,800,000**	**11,800,000**
Collision with —					
Pedestrian	5,600	80,000	5,100	70,000	130,000
Other motor vehicle	19,900	1,780,000	17,900	1,260,000	7,980,000
Angle collision	*10,500*	*916,000*	*10,000*	*634,000*	*3,740,000*
Head-on collision	*5,300*	*146,000*	*5,100*	*84,000*	*300,000*
Rear-end collision	*2,400*	*657,000*	*1,700*	*497,000*	*3,360,000*
Sideswipe and other two-vehicle collisions	*1,700*	*61,000*	*1,100*	*45,000*	*580,000*
Railroad train	300	2,000	300	2,000	5,000
Pedalcycle	700	28,000	700	28,000	100,000
Animal, animal-drawn vehicle	100	10,000	100	10,000	530,000
Fixed object	13,000	400,000	12,300	330,000	2,685,000
Noncollision	**5,200**	**100,000**	**5,200**	**100,000**	**370,000**

Source: National Safety Council estimates, based on reports from state traffic authorities. Procedures for estimating the number of accidents by type were changed for the 1998 edition and are not comparable to estimates in previous editions (see Technical Appendix).

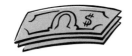

ESTIMATING MOTOR-VEHICLE CRASH COSTS

There are two methods commonly used to measure the costs of motor-vehicle crashes. One is the *economic cost* framework and the other is the *comprehensive cost* framework.

Economic costs may be used by a community or state to estimate the economic impact of motor-vehicle crashes that occurred within its jurisdiction in a given time period. It is a measure of the productivity lost and expenses incurred because of the crashes. Economic costs, however, should not be used for cost-benefit analysis because they do not reflect what society is willing to pay to prevent a statistical fatality or injury.

There are five economic cost components: (a) wage and productivity losses, which include wages, fringe benefits, household production, and travel delay; (b) medical expenses, including emergency service costs; (c) administrative expenses, which include the administrative cost of private and public insurance plus police and legal costs; (d) motor-vehicle damage, including the value of damage to property; and (e) uninsured employer costs for crashes involving workers.

The information below shows the average economic costs in 2003 per death (*not* per fatal crash), per injury (*not* per injury crash), and per property damage crash.

ECONOMIC COSTS, 2003

Death	**$1,120,000**
Nonfatal Disabling Injury	**$45,500**
Incapacitating injury[a]	*$55,500*
Nonincapacitating evident injury[a]	*$18,200*
Possible injury[a]	*$10,300*
Property Damage Crash (including minor injuries)	**$8,200**

Comprehensive costs include not only the economic cost components, but also a measure of the value of lost quality of life associated with the deaths and injuries, that is, what society is willing to pay to prevent them. The values of lost quality of life were obtained through empirical studies of what people actually pay to reduce their safety and health risks, such as through the purchase of air bags or smoke detectors. Comprehensive costs should be used for cost-benefit analysis, but because the lost quality of life represents only a dollar equivalence of intangible qualities, they do not represent real economic losses and should not be used to determine the economic impact of past crashes.

The information below shows the average comprehensive costs in 2003 on a per person basis.

COMPREHENSIVE COSTS, 2003

Death	**$3,610,000**
Incapacitating injury[a]	*$181,000*
Nonincapacitating evident injury[a]	*$46,200*
Possible injury[a]	*$22,000*
No Injury	**$2,000**

Source: National Safety Council estimates (see the Technical Appendix) and Children's Safety Network Economics and Insurance Resource Center, Pacific Institute for Research and Evaluation.
[a] Committee on Motor Vehicle Traffic Accident Classification. (1997). Manual on Classification of Motor Vehicle Traffic Accidents, ANSI D16.1-1996 (6th ed.). Itasca, IL: National Safety Council.
Note: The National Safety Council's cost estimating procedures were extensively revised for the 1993 edition. New components were added, new benchmarks adopted, and a new discount rate assumed. The costs are not comparable to those of prior years.

STATE LAWS

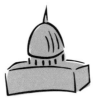

All states and the District of Columbia have 21-year-old drinking age and child safety seat laws. Breath alcohol ignition interlock device laws are in effect in 42 states. Mandatory belt use laws are in effect in 49 states plus the District of Columbia, of which 20 states and D.C. are standard enforcement. Graduated licensing is in effect in some form in 45 states and the District of Columbia.

STATE LAWS

State	Alcohol Laws Administrative License Revocation[a]	BAC Limit[b]	Zero Tolerance Limit[c] for Minors	Alcohol Ignition Interlock Device[d]	Mandatory Belt Use Law Enforcement	Seating Positions Covered by Law	Minimum Instructional Permit Period[e]	Minimum Hours of Supervised Driving[f]	Passenger Restrictions	Nighttime Driving Restrictions	Unrestricted License Minimum Age[g]
Alabama	1996	0.08	0.02	no	standard	front	6 mo.	30/–	yes	yes	16yrs.
Alaska	1983	0.08	0.00	yes	secondary	all	6 mo.	none	no	no	16yrs.
Arizona	1992	0.08	0.00	yes[h]	secondary	front	6 mo.	25/5	no	no	16yrs.
Arkansas	1995	0.08	0.02	yes	secondary	front	until 16 yrs.	none	no	no	18yrs.
California	1989	0.08	0.01	yes[h]	standard	all	6 mo.	50/10	yes	yes	16yrs.
Colorado	1983	0.10	0.02	yes[h]	secondary	front	6 mo.	50/10	yes	yes	17yrs.
Connecticut	1990	0.08	0.02	yes[h]	standard	front[i]	6 mo.	none	yes	no	16yrs., 4 mo.
Delaware	yes	0.10	0.02	yes[h]	standard	all	12 mo.	none[j]	yes	yes	16yrs., 10 mo.
Dist. of Columbia	yes	0.08	0.00	no	standard	all	6 mo.	40+10[k]	yes	yes	18yrs.
Florida	1990	0.08	0.02	yes[h]	secondary	front	12 mo.	50/10	no	yes	18yrs.
Georgia	1995	0.08	0.02	yes[h]	standard	front[i]	12 mo.	40/6	yes	yes	18yrs.
Hawaii	1990	0.08	0.02	no	standard	front[i]	3 mo.	none	no	no	16yrs.
Idaho	1994	0.08	0.02	yes	secondary	all	4 mo.	50/10	no	yes	16yrs.
Illinois	1986	0.08	0.00	yes[h]	standard	front	3 mo.	25/–	yes	yes	18yrs.
Indiana	yes	0.08	0.02	yes[h]	standard	front	2 mo.	none	yes	yes	18yrs.
Iowa	1982	0.08	0.02	yes	standard	front	6 mo.	20/2	no	yes	17yrs.
Kansas	1988	0.08	0.02	yes[h]	secondary	front	6 mo.	50/10	no	no	16yrs.
Kentucky	no	0.08	0.02	yes[h]	secondary	all	6 mo.	none	no	yes[n]	16yrs., 6 mo.
Louisiana	1984	0.08	0.02	yes	standard	front[i]	3 mo.	none	yes	yes	17yrs.
Maine	1984	0.08	0.00	no	secondary	all	6 mo.	35/5	yes	yes	16yrs., 6 mo.
Maryland	1989	0.08[m]	0.00	yes[h]	standard	front[i]	4 mo.	40/–	no	yes	17yrs., 7 mo.
Massachusetts	1994	0.08	0.02	yes[h]	secondary	all	6 mo.	12/–	yes	yes	18yrs.
Michigan	no	0.08	0.02	yes[h]	standard	front[i]	6 mo.	50/10	no	yes	17yrs.
Minnesota	1976	0.10	0.01	no	secondary	front[i]	6 mo.	30/10	no	no	17yrs.
Mississippi	1983	0.08	0.02	yes[h]	secondary	front	6 mo.	none	no	yes	16yrs.
Missouri	1987	0.08	0.02	yes[h]	secondary	front[i]	6 mo.	20/–	no	yes	18yrs.
Montana	no	0.08	0.02	yes	secondary	all	none	none	no	no	15yrs.
Nebraska	1993	0.08	0.02	yes	secondary	front[i]	none	50/–	no	yes	17yrs.
Nevada	1983	0.08	0.02	yes[h]	secondary	all	30–90 days	50/–	yes	no	18yrs.
New Hampshire	1993	0.08	0.02	yes[h]	(l)	(l)	6 mo.	20/–	yes	yes	18yrs.
New Jersey	no	0.08	0.01	yes[h]	standard	front	12 mo.	1 year	yes	yes	18yrs.
New Mexico	1984	0.08	0.02	yes	standard	all	6 mo.	50/10	yes	yes	16yrs., 6 mo.
New York	1994[o]	0.08[m]	0.02	yes[h]	standard	front[i]	6 mo.	20/–	no	yes	18yrs.
North Carolina	1983	0.08	0.00	yes[h]	standard	all	12 mo.	none	yes	yes	16yrs., 6 mo.
North Dakota	1983	0.08	0.02	yes[h]	secondary	front	6 mo.	none	no	no	16yrs.
Ohio	1993	0.08	0.02	yes	secondary	front	6 mo.	50/10	no	yes	17yrs.
Oklahoma	1983	0.08	0.00	yes	standard	front	none	none	no	no	16yrs.
Oregon	1983	0.08	0.00	yes	standard	all	6 mo.	100/–	yes	yes	18yrs.
Pennsylvania	no	0.08	0.02	yes[h]	secondary	front[i]	6 mo.	50/–	yes	yes	17yrs., 6 mo.
Rhode Island	no	0.08	0.02	yes[h]	secondary	all	6 mo.	none	no	yes	17yrs.
South Carolina	1998	0.08	0.02	yes	secondary	front[p]	180 days	40/10	yes	yes	17yrs.
South Dakota	no	0.08	0.02	no	secondary	front	6 mo.	none	no	yes	16yrs.
Tennessee	no	0.08	0.02	yes	secondary	front[i]	180 days	50/10	yes	yes	18yrs.
Texas	1995	0.08	0.00	yes[h]	standard	front[i]	6 mo.	none	yes	yes	18yrs.
Utah	1983	0.08	0.00	yes	secondary[q]	all	none	40/10	yes	yes	17yrs.
Vermont	1969[o]	0.08	0.02	no	secondary	all	12 mo.	40/10	yes	no	16yrs., 6 mo.
Virginia	1995	0.08	0.02	yes	secondary	front[i]	9 mo.	40/10	yes	yes	18yrs.
Washington	1998	0.08	0.02	yes	standard	all	6 mo.	50/10	yes	yes	18yrs.
West Virginia	1981	0.08	0.02	yes	secondary	front[i]	6 mo.	30/–	yes	yes	18yrs.
Wisconsin	1988	0.08	0.00	yes[h]	secondary	front[p]	12 mo.	30/10	yes	yes	18yrs.
Wyoming	1973	0.08	0.02	no	secondary	all	10 days	none	no	no	16yrs.

Source: Survey of state officials. Laws as of April 2004. Virginia did not respond to the 2004 survey.

a Year original law became effective, not when grandfather clauses expired.
b Blood alcohol concentration that constitutes the threshold of legal intoxication.
c Blood alcohol concentration that constitutes "zero tolerance" threshold for minors (<21 years of age unless otherwise noted).
d Instruments designed to prevent drivers from starting their cars when breath alcohol content is at or above a set point.
e Minimum instructional periods often include time spent in driver's education classes.
f Figures shown as follows: Total hours/Nighttime hours. For example, 25/5 means 25 hours of supervised driving, 5 of which must be at night. Some states (GA, MD, OR, WV) have lower requirements if driver ed is taken.
g Minimum age to obtain unrestricted license provided driver is crash and violation free. Alcohol restrictions still apply at least until 21.
h Primarily for repeat offenders.

i Required for certain ages at all seating positions.
j No minimum amount of supervised driving, but with level 1 permit driving has to be supervised at all times for the first 6 months.
k 40 hours of supervised driving during learner's stage; 10 hours at night during intermediate stage.
l Standard enforcement law in effect for ages under 18 only.
m BAC of 0.07 is prima facia evidence of DUI (MD). BAC of 0.05–0.07 constitutes driving while ability impaired (NY).
n During permit period only.
o Revocation by judicial action (NY) or Department of Motor Vehicles (VT).
p Belt use required in rear seat if lap/shoulder belt is available.
q Secondary for 19 and older, standard for under 19.

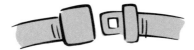

Safety belts are considered the most effective means of reducing deaths and injuries due to motor-vehicle crashes. The National Occupant Protection Use Survey (NOPUS) conducted by the National Highway Traffic Safety Administration (NHTSA) provides estimates of safety belt use and helps to evaluate the impact of specific transportation improvement initiatives on public safety. From 2000 to 2003, NHTSA implemented state-based Selective Traffic Enforcement Programs, including the *Click It or Ticket* program, that combined elements of high-visibility safety belt use enforcement and extensive media coverage.

In June 2003, safety belt use was estimated at a record high of 79%, up by 4 percentage points from June 2002 and 8 percentage points from June 2000. Between 2000 and 2003, the rate of nonuse of safety belts decreased by 28%.

The District of Columbia and all U.S. states, except New Hampshire, have enacted either a primary or a secondary safety belt use law. In June 2003, the use of safety belts in states with primary enforcement laws was 83%, 8 percentage points higher than in states with secondary enforcement laws. The gap between secondary and primary law states narrowed from 14 percentage points in 2000 to 8 percentage points

in 2003, but the difference remained significant.

Regional trends indicate that Western states typically have higher safety belt usage rates. Between 2002 and 2003, the West also showed the highest decline (24%) in nonuse rates compared to other regions.

The rate of safety belt use was 77% among passengers and 80% among drivers in 2003, up from 71% and 74%, respectively, in 2000. During the same time period, the rate of nonuse declined by 21% among passengers and by 23% among drivers.

In 2003, safety belt use among occupants of passenger cars was 81%, compared with 69% in pickup trucks and 83% in vans and SUVs.

NOPUS data also indicate that (a) women tend to have higher use rates, (b) recent enforcement programs led to substantial gains in safety belt use among black and other nonwhite occupants, and (c) children are at least three times more likely to be unrestrained when riding with an unrestrained driver than with a restrained driver.

These and other statistics can be found in a special section of the *Journal of Safety Research* (Vol. 35, No. 2, 2004) dedicated to issues of high-visibility safety belt use enforcement in the United States and Canada.

SAFETY BELT USE BY GEOGRAPHICAL REGION, UNITED STATES, 2000–2003

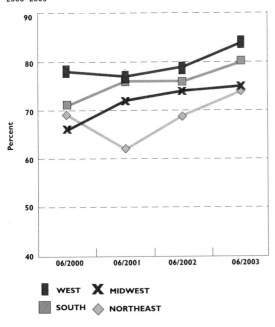

■ WEST   ✕ MIDWEST
■ SOUTH   ◆ NORTHEAST

SAFETY BELT USE BY TYPE OF STATE LAW ENFORCEMENT, UNITED STATES, 2000–2003

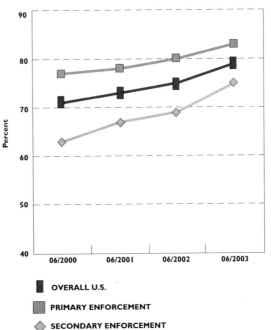

■ OVERALL U.S.

■ PRIMARY ENFORCEMENT

◆ SECONDARY ENFORCEMENT

ALCOHOL

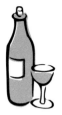

According to studies conducted by the National Highway Traffic Safety Administration (NHTSA), about 41% of all traffic fatalities in 2002 involved an intoxicated or alcohol-impaired driver or nonmotorist. In 2002, 35% of all traffic fatalities occurred in crashes where at least one driver or nonoccupant was intoxicated (blood alcohol concentration [BAC] of 0.08 grams per deciliter [g/dl] or greater). Of the 15,019 people killed in such crashes, 68% were themselves intoxicated. The other 32% were passengers, nonintoxicated drivers, or nonintoxicated nonoccupants. The following data summarize the extent of alcohol involvement in motor-vehicle crashes:

• Traffic fatalities in alcohol-related crashes rose by 0.1% from 2001 to 2002 and declined by 5% from 1992 to 2002. (See corresponding chart.) In 1992, alcohol-related fatalities accounted for 47% of all traffic deaths.

• According to NHTSA, alcohol was involved in 41% of fatal crashes and 6% of all crashes, both fatal and nonfatal, in 2002.

• Approximately 1.4 million drivers were arrested in 2001 for driving under the influence of alcohol or narcotics.

• There were 17,419 alcohol-related traffic fatalities in 2002, an average of one alcohol-related fatality every 30 minutes. An average of one person every 2 minutes is injured in a crash where alcohol is present.

• In 2002, alcohol was present in 31% of all fatal crashes on weekdays, compared to 54% on weekends. The rate of alcohol involvement in fatal crashes during the day is 19%, compared to 63% at night.

PERCENT OF TOTAL TRAFFIC FATALITIES WITH ALCOHOL PRESENT, BY STATE, 2002

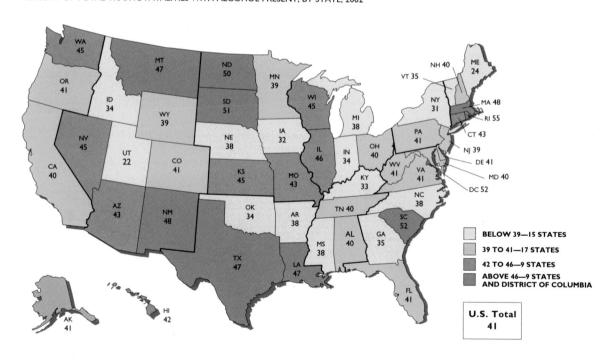

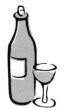

ALCOHOL (CONT.)

- From 1992 to 2002, intoxication rates decreased for drivers of all age groups involved in fatal crashes, except for the group of drivers 45 to 64 years old, which had the same rate in 1992 and 2002. The greatest decrease was for drivers over 64 years old (29%), followed by drivers 25 to 34 years old (20%). NHTSA estimates that 21,887 lives have been saved by 21-year-old minimum drinking age laws since 1975. All states and the District of Columbia now have such laws.

- Safety belts were used by only 23% of fatally injured intoxicated drivers, compared to 36% of fatally injured alcohol-impaired drivers (BAC of 0.01 to 0.07 g/dl) and 53% of fatally injured sober drivers (BAC of 0.00 g/dl).

- The driver, pedestrian, or both were intoxicated in 41% of all fatal pedestrian crashes in 2002. In these crashes, the intoxication rate for pedestrians was nearly triple the rate for drivers.

- The cost of alcohol-related motor-vehicle crashes is estimated by the National Safety Council at $34.5 billion in 2003.

Source: National Center for Statistics and Analysis. (2003). Traffic Safety Facts 2002 — Alcohol. Washington, DC: National Highway Traffic Safety Administration.

PERCENT OF ALL TRAFFIC FATALITIES THAT OCCURRED IN ALCOHOL-RELATED CRASHES, 1992–2002

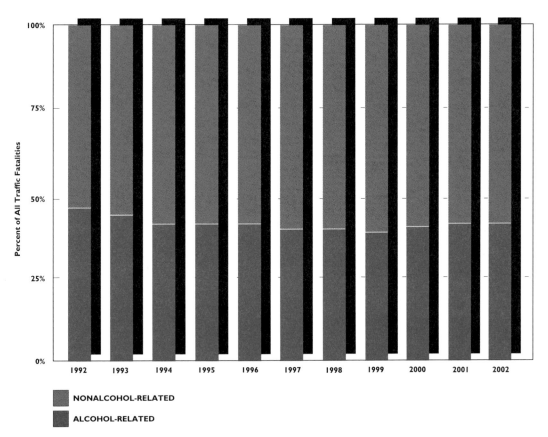

- NONALCOHOL-RELATED
- ALCOHOL-RELATED

OCCUPANT PROTECTION

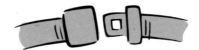

Safety Belts

- When used, lap/shoulder safety belts reduce the risk of fatal injury to front seat passenger car occupants by 45% and reduce the risk of moderate-to-critical injury by 50%.

- For light truck occupants, safety belts reduce the risk of fatal injury by 60% and moderate-to-critical injury by 65%.

- Forty-nine states and the District of Columbia have mandatory belt use laws in effect, the only exception being New Hampshire. Thirty-two of the states with belt use laws in effect in 2002 specified secondary enforcement (i.e., police officers are permitted to write a citation only after a vehicle is stopped for some other traffic infraction). Seventeen states and the District of Columbia had laws that allowed primary enforcement, enabling officers to stop vehicles and write citations whenever they observe violations of the belt law.

- Safety belts saved an estimated 14,164 lives in 2002 among passenger vehicle occupants over 4 years old. An *additional* 7,153 lives could have been saved in 2002 if all passenger vehicle occupants over age 4 wore safety belts. From 1975 through 2002, an estimated 164,753 lives were saved by safety belts.

- Safety belts provide the greatest protection against occupant ejection. Among crashes in which a fatality occurred in 2002, only 1% of restrained passenger car occupants were ejected, compared to 30% of unrestrained occupants.

- The results of a 1995 study by the National Highway Traffic Safety Administration (NHTSA) suggest that belt use among fatally injured occupants was at least 15% higher in states with primary enforcement laws.

Air Bags

- Air bags, combined with lap/shoulder belts, offer the best available protection for passenger vehicle occupants. The overall fatality-reducing effectiveness

for air bags is estimated at 12% over and above the benefits from using safety belts alone.

- Lap/shoulder belts should always be used, even in a vehicle with an air bag. Air bags are a supplemental form of protection, and most are designed to deploy only in moderate-to-severe *frontal* crashes.

- Children in rear-facing child seats should not be placed in the front seat of vehicles equipped with passenger-side air bags. The impact of the deploying air bag could result in injury to the child.

- An estimated 2,248 lives were saved by air bags in 2002, and a total of 11,663 lives were saved from 1987 through 2002.

- Beginning September 1997, all new passenger cars were required to have driver and passenger side air bags. In 1998, the same requirement went into effect for light trucks.

Child Restraints

- Child restraints saved an estimated 376 lives in 2002 among children under the age of 5. Of the 376 lives saved, 329 were attributed to the use of child safety seats while 47 lives were spared with the use of adult belts.

- At 100% child safety seat use for children under the age of 5, an estimated 109 *additional* lives could have been saved in 2002.

- All states and the District of Columbia have had child restraint use laws in effect since 1985.

- Research has shown that child safety seats reduce fatal injury in passenger cars by 71% for infants (less than 1 year old), and by 54% for toddlers (1-4 years old). For infants and toddlers in light trucks, the corresponding reductions are 58% and 59%, respectively.

- In 2002, there were 459 occupant fatalities among children less than 5 years of age. Of these, an estimated 40% were totally unrestrained.

- An estimated 6,567 lives have been saved by child restraints from 1975 through 2002.

ESTIMATED NUMBER OF LIVES SAVED BY RESTRAINT SYSTEMS, 1975–2002

Restraint Type	1975–94	1995	1996	1997	1998	1999	2000	2001	2002
Seat Belts	68,940	9,882	10,710	11,259	11,680	11,941	12,882	13,295	14,164
Air Bags	730	536	783	973	1,208	1,491	1,716	1,978	2,248
Child Restraints	3,107	408	480	444	438	447	479	388	376

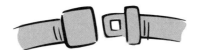

Motorcycle Helmets

- Technological changes over the past 15 years have led to improvements in helmet design and materials that have resulted in an increase in the effectiveness of helmets in preventing fatalities. The effectiveness of motorcycle helmets has increased from 29% in 1982 through 1987 to 37% over the years 1993 through 2002.

- Based on this new effectiveness data, it was estimated that motorcycle helmets saved the lives of 1,005 motorcyclists in 2002 (up from 692 using the old effectiveness data). An *additional* 579 lives could have been saved if all motorcyclists had worn helmets.

- Reported helmet use rates for fatally injured motorcyclists in 2002 were 53% for operators and 41% for passengers, the same as the corresponding rates of 53% and 41%, respectively, in 2001.

- In 2002, 20 states, the District of Columbia, and Puerto Rico required helmet use by all motorcycle operators and passengers. In another 27 states, only persons under 18 were required to wear helmets. Three states had no laws requiring helmet use.

Safety Belt and Helmet Use

- According to the latest observational survey by the National Highway Traffic Safety Administration, the national safety belt use rate was 79% in 2003, the highest rate yet observed and a continuation of the relatively steady pattern of increased use since belt use was first measured by a national survey at 58% in 1994.

- States with primary enforcement of belt laws reached a milestone of 83% belt use in 2003, while use in states with secondary enforcement was significantly lower at 75%.

- From 2002 to 2003, all regions of the nation experienced a significant 4–5 percentage point increase in belt use except for the Midwest, which experienced an increase of only 1 percentage point, leaving it nearly tied with the Northeast with the lowest rate of safety belt use. In 2003, the use rates for the four regions were 84% for the West, 80% for the South, 75% for the Midwest, and 74% for the Northeast.

- Belt use increased significantly among occupants of all types of vehicles from 2002 to 2003. Belt use increased 5 percentage points among occupants of vans and SUVs to reach 83%, while usage rates for occupants of passenger cars increased 4 percentage points to achieve a level of 81%. The use rate for pickups also increased 5 percentage points during this period to reach 69%, but continues to lag significantly behind the use rates for other passenger vehicles.

- Helmet use declined by 13 percentage points over 2 years, from 71% in 2000 to 58% in 2002. This drop is statistically significant and corresponds to a 45% increase in nonuse.

See page 93 for additional information on safety belt use.
Source: Deutermann, W. (2004). Motorcycle Helmet Effectiveness Revisited (DOT HS 809-715, March). Washington, DC: National Center for Statistics and Analysis. Glassbrenner, D. (2003). Safety Belt Use in 2003 (DOT HS 809 646, September). Washington, DC: National Center for Statistics and Analysis. National Center for Statistics and Analysis. (2003). Traffic Safety Facts 2002 — Occupant Protection; Traffic Safety Facts 2002 — Motorcycles. Washington, DC: Author.

BELT USE BY VEHICLE TYPE AND DAY OF WEEK

	Belt Use						
	Use in June 2003		Use in June 2002		2002–2003 Change		
Category	Estimate (%)	Std. Error (%)	Estimate (%)	Std. Error (%)	Estimate (%)	Std. Error (%)	Conversion Rate[a] (%)
Vehicle Type							
Passenger Cars	81	1.0	77	1.0	4[b]	1.0	17
SUVs and Vans	83	1.0	78	1.1	5[b]	1.3	23
Pickup Trucks	69[c]	2.2	64[c]	1.6	5[b]	2.4	14
Day of Week							
Weekday	78	1.3	75	1.0	3[b]	1.6	12
Rush Hour	79	1.6	76	1.2	3[b]	1.5	13
Non-Rush Hour	79	1.2	75	1.2	4[b]	1.4	16
Weekend	81	1.7	76	1.9	5[b]	1.6	21

[a] The rate of decrease of belt nonuse from one year to the next.
[b] Significant at the 95% confidence level.
[c] Significantly low in category at the 95% confidence level.

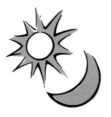

DEATHS AND DEATH RATES
BY DAY AND NIGHT

About 57% of all motor-vehicle deaths in 2003 occurred during the day, while the remainder occurred at night. Death rates based on mileage, however, were over two times higher at night than during the day with vehicle miles traveled by night representing only 25% of the total.

Source: State traffic authorities and the Federal Highway Administration.

DEATH RATES BY DAY AND NIGHT, 2003

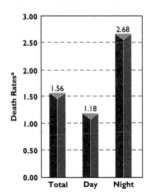

a Per 100,000,000 vehicle miles.

DEATHS AND MILEAGE DEATH RATES
BY MONTH

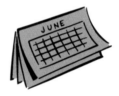

Motor-vehicle deaths in 2003 were at their lowest level in February and increased to their highest level in August. In 2003, the highest monthly mileage death rate of 1.69 deaths per 100,000,000 vehicle miles occurred in November. The overall rate for the year was 1.56.

Source: Deaths — National Safety Council estimates. Mileage — Federal Highway Administration, Traffic Volume Trends.

MOTOR-VEHICLE DEATHS AND MILEAGE DEATH RATES BY MONTH, 2003

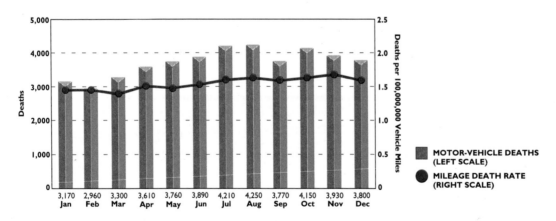

98

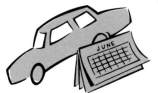

MOTOR-VEHICLE ACCIDENTS
BY TIME OF DAY AND DAY OF WEEK

More fatal accidents occurred on Saturday than any other day of the week in 2003, according to reports from state traffic authorities. About 18% of fatal accidents occurred on Saturday, compared to about 16% on Sundays and 15% on Fridays. For all accidents, Friday had the highest percentage with over 17%.

Patterns by hour of day for fatal accidents show peaks during afternoon rush hour for weekdays and, especially, late night for weekends. For all accidents, peaks occur during both morning and afternoon rush hour.

PERCENT OF WEEKLY ACCIDENTS BY HOUR OF DAY AND DAY OF WEEK, UNITED STATES, 2003

Time of Day	Fatal Accidents								All Accidents							
	Total	Mon.	Tues.	Wed.	Thurs.	Fri.	Sat.	Sun.	Total	Mon.	Tues.	Wed.	Thurs.	Fri.	Sat.	Sun.
All Hours	100.0%	12.6%	12.5%	12.3%	13.4%	15.0%	18.0%	16.2%	100.0%	14.4%	14.4%	15.1%	15.0%	17.3%	13.4%	10.5%
Midnight–3:59 am	13.5%	1.4%	1.0%	1.1%	1.5%	1.6%	3.1%	3.7%	6.0%	0.6%	0.5%	0.6%	0.6%	0.8%	1.5%	1.5%
4:00–7:59 am	12.2%	1.5%	1.5%	1.9%	1.7%	1.9%	2.1%	1.8%	10.5%	1.7%	1.8%	1.8%	1.7%	1.7%	1.0%	0.8%
8:00–11:59am	13.9%	2.0%	2.2%	1.8%	2.0%	2.0%	2.3%	1.8%	17.9%	2.9%	2.8%	2.8%	2.7%	2.9%	2.3%	1.5%
Noon–3:59 pm	19.3%	3.0%	2.7%	2.4%	2.7%	2.4%	3.1%	3.0%	26.2%	3.9%	3.8%	4.0%	3.8%	4.6%	3.4%	2.6%
4:00–7:59 pm	21.8%	2.6%	2.9%	2.7%	2.7%	3.6%	3.7%	3.6%	26.9%	3.9%	4.0%	4.3%	4.3%	4.8%	3.0%	2.6%
8:00–11:59pm	19.3%	2.2%	2.3%	2.5%	2.8%	3.6%	3.8%	2.3%	12.5%	1.4%	1.5%	1.6%	1.9%	2.4%	2.2%	1.5%

Source: Based on reports from 7 state traffic authorities.
Note: Column and row totals may not equal sum of parts due to rounding.

PERCENT OF ACCIDENTS BY TIME OF DAY AND DAY OF WEEK, 2003

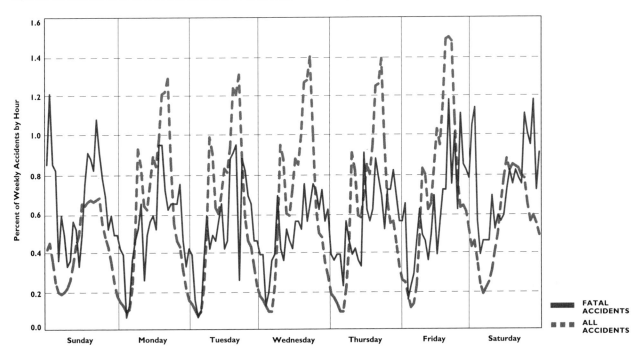

TYPE OF MOTOR VEHICLE

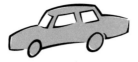

The types of vehicles listed in the table below are classified by body style, not by vehicle use. The light truck category includes both commercial and noncommercial trucks under 10,000 pounds gross vehicle weight. It also includes minivans and sport-utility vehicles. The medium/heavy truck category includes truck tractors with or without semi-trailers.

Passenger Cars

In 2003, passenger cars comprised about 58% of the registered vehicles and were involved in about an identical share of motor-vehicle accidents. Approximately 53% of all motor-vehicle occupant fatalities are passenger car occupants. (see corresponding chart.)

Trucks

Light trucks represent about 36% of all motor-vehicle registrations and an equivalent percentage of vehicles involved in fatal accidents. Medium and heavy trucks account for nearly 4% of registered vehicles and about 9% of vehicles involved in fatal accidents. Medium and heavy truck occupants as well as light truck occupants are slightly under-represented in motor-vehicle occupant fatalities compared to their proportion of registrations. Medium and heavy truck occupants

account for only about 2% of all motor-vehicle occupant fatalities and light truck occupants account for 32%.

There were 879,000 light truck occupants and 26,000 large truck occupants injured in 2002, according to the National Highway Traffic Safety Administration.

Motorcycles

The number of registered motorcycles in the United States totaled about 5,004,000 in 2003, compared to approximately 4,001,000 a decade earlier. Although motorcycles accounted for about 2% of the total 239,600,000 vehicle registrations in 2003, they were over-represented in the distribution of fatalities by type of vehicle. Of the 38,400 occupant deaths in motor-vehicle accidents in 2003, about 3,300 (9%) were motorcycle riders. Approximately 65,000 riders and passengers were injured in 2002 according to the National Highway Traffic Safety Administration.

Motorcycles traveled an estimated 9.5 billion miles in 2003. The 2003 mileage death rate for motorcycle riders is estimated to be about 35 occupant deaths per 100,000,000 miles of motorcycle travel, about 29 times the mileage death rate for occupants of other types of vehicles (passenger autos, trucks, buses, etc.).

TYPES OF MOTOR VEHICLES INVOLVED IN ACCIDENTS, 2003

Type of Vehicle	In Fatal Accidents		In All Accidents		Percent of Total Vehicle Registrations[a]	No. of Occupant Fatalities
	Number	Percent	Number	Percent		
All Types	**54,000**	**100.0%**	**20,000,000**	**100.0%**	**100.0%**	**38,400[b]**
Passenger cars	24,500	45.4	11,520,000	57.6	57.9	20,500
Trucks	24,200	44.8	8,180,000	40.9	39.6	12,880
Light trucks	19,500	36.1	7,440,000	37.2	35.7	12,100
Medium/heavy trucks	4,700	8.7	740,000	3.7	3.9	780
Farm tractor, equipment	100	0.2	7,000	(c)	(d)	60
Buses, commercial	200	0.4	75,000	0.4	0.1	50
Buses, school	100	0.1	50,000	0.2	0.3	10
Motorcycles	3,300	6.1	150,000	0.8	} 2.1	3,300
Motor scooters, motor bikes	100	0.2	4,000	(c)		100
Other	1,500	2.8	14,000	0.1	(d)	1,500

Source: Based on reports from 9 state traffic authorities. Vehicle registrations based on data from Federal Highway Administration. Estimating procedures were changed for the 1998 edition and are not comparable to estimates in previous editions.
[a]Percentage figures are based on numbers of vehicles and do not reflect miles traveled or place of travel, both of which affect accident experience. Percents may not add due to rounding.
[b]In addition to these occupant fatalities, there were 5,600 pedestrian, 700 pedalcyclist, and 100 other deaths.
[c]Less than 0.05%.
[d]Data not available.

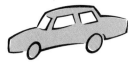

REGISTRATIONS, INVOLVEMENTS, AND OCCUPANT FATALITIES BY TYPE OF VEHICLE, 2003

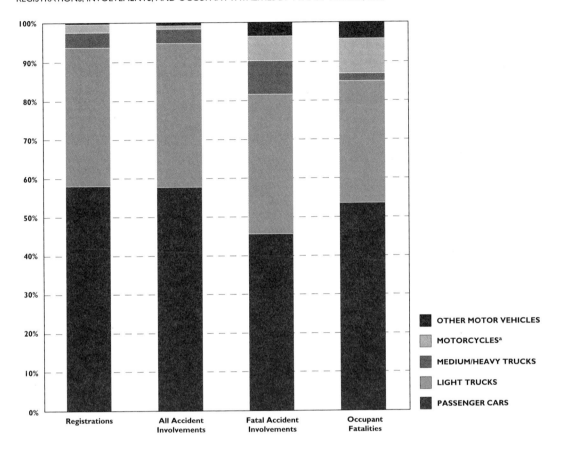

ᵃIncludes motor scooters and motorbikes.

SCHOOL BUS TRANSPORTATION

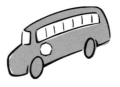

School bus–related crashes killed 127 persons and injured an estimated 18,000 persons nationwide in 2002, according to data from the National Highway Traffic Safety Administration's Fatality Analysis Reporting System (FARS) and General Estimates System (GES).

A school bus–related crash is defined by NHTSA to be any crash in which a vehicle, regardless of body design, used as a school bus is directly or indirectly involved, such as a crash involving school children alighting from a vehicle.

Over the period from 1997–2002, about 73% of the deaths in school bus–related crashes were occupants of vehicles other than the school bus, and 16% were pedestrians. About 5% were school bus passengers, and 4% were school bus drivers.

Of the pedestrians killed in school bus–related crashes over this period, approximately 79% were struck by the school bus.

Out of the people injured in school bus–related crashes from 1997 through 2002, about 45% were school bus

passengers, 9% were school bus drivers, and another 43% were occupants of other vehicles. The remainder were pedestrians, pedalcyclists, and other or unknown type persons.

Characteristics of school bus transportation

Forty-eight states reported that about 24.2 million public school pupils were transported at public expense and 33 states reported that public funds were used to transport another 1.0 million private school pupils. These data are prepared by *School Bus Fleet* (vol. 50, no. 1) for the latest year available with most states reporting for the 2001–02 school year, but in a few such as Maryland, New Mexico, and New York the latest year was 1998–99. This compares to estimates from the U.S. Department of Education of enrollments in fall 2001 in grades K–12 of about 47.6 million public school pupils and 5.9 million private school pupils nationwide. About 450,000 school buses were reported in use in 48 states, and the buses in 43 states traveled about 4.2 billion route miles.

FATALITIES IN SCHOOL BUS–RELATED CRASHES, U.S., 1993–2002

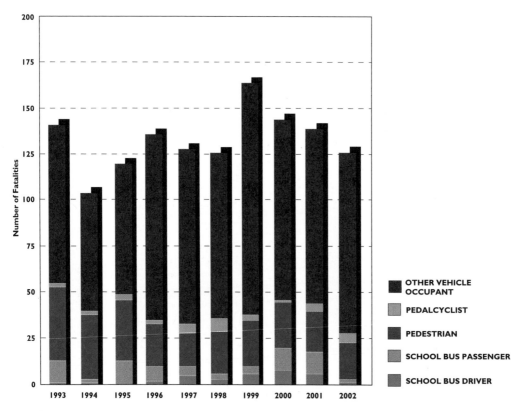

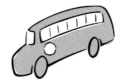

SCHOOL BUS TRANSPORTATION
(CONT.)

DEATHS AND INJURIES IN SCHOOL BUS–RELATED CRASHES, UNITED STATES, 1997–2002

	1997	1998	1999	2000	2001	2002
Deaths						
Total	128	126	164	144	141	127
School bus driver	5	3	6	8	6	1
School bus passenger	5	3	4	12	12	2
Pedestrian	18	23	25	25	22	20
Pedalcyclist	5	7	3	1	4	5
Occupant of other vehicle	95	90	126	98	95	98
Other or Unknown	0	0	0	0	2	1
Injuries						
Total	19,000	17,000	18,000	20,000	13,000	18,000
School bus driver	2,000	2,000	1,000	2,000	1,000	1,000
School bus passenger	10,000	6,000	8,000	8,000	6,000	9,000
Pedestrian	(a)	(a)	(a)	1,000	(a)	1,000
Pedalcyclist	(a)	(a)	(a)	(a)	(a)	(a)
Occupant of other vehicle	7,000	9,000	8,000	9,000	5,000	7,000
Other or Unknown	(a)	(a)	(a)	(a)	(a)	(a)

Source: National Highway Traffic Safety Administration. Traffic Safety Facts, *1997–2002 editions. Washington, DC: Author.*
[a] *Less than 500.*

PEDESTRIAN DEATHS IN SCHOOL BUS–RELATED CRASHES, UNITED STATES, 1997–2002

		Age Group			
Year	All Ages	Under 5	5–9	10–15	16 and older
1997	18	0	8	3	7
Struck by bus	*16*	*0*	*6*	*3*	*7*
1998	23	3	9	1	10
Struck by bus	*20*	*3*	*6*	*1*	*10*
1999	25	0	13	4	8
Struck by bus	*19*	*0*	*10*	*2*	*7*
2000	25	5	10	2	8
Struck by bus	*16*	*2*	*8*	*0*	*6*
2001	22	3	6	4	9
Struck by bus	*18*	*3*	*5*	*1*	*9*
2002	20	0	11	1	8
Struck by bus	*16*	*0*	*8*	*1*	*7*

Source: National Highway Traffic Safety Administration. Traffic Safety Facts, *1997-2002 editions. Washington, DC: Author.*

AGE OF DRIVER

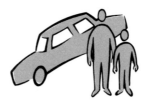

The table below shows the total number of licensed drivers and drivers involved in accidents by selected ages and age groups. The figures in the last two columns indicate the frequency of accident involvement on the basis of the number of drivers in each age group. The fatal accident involvement rates per 100,000 drivers in each age group ranged from a low of 16 for drivers 55 to 64 years of age to a high of 114 for drivers aged 16. The all accident involvement rates per 100 drivers in each age group ranged from 5 for drivers in the 55 to 64, 65 to 74, and 75 and over age groups to 63 for drivers aged 16.

On the basis of miles driven by each age group, however, involvement rates (not shown in the table) are highest for young and old drivers. For drivers aged 16 to 19, the fatal involvement rate per 100 million vehicle miles traveled was 9.2 in 1990, about three times the overall rate for all drivers in passenger vehicles, 3.0. The rate for drivers aged 75 and over was 11.5, the highest of all age groups. The same basic "U"-shaped curve is found for injury accident involvement rates.[a]

[a]Massie, D., Campbell, K., & Williams, A. (1995). Traffic accident involvement rates by driver age and gender. Accident Analysis and Prevention, 27 (1), 73–87.

AGE OF DRIVER — TOTAL NUMBER AND NUMBER IN ACCIDENTS, 2003

	Licensed Drivers		Drivers in Accidents					
			Fatal		All		Per No. of Drivers	
Age Group	Number	Percent	Number	Percent	Number	Percent	Fatal[a]	All[b]
Total	196,700,000	100.0%	54,000	100.0%	20,000,000	100.0%	27	10
Under 16	58,000	(c)	600	1.1	170,000	0.9	(d)	(d)
16	1,311,000	0.7	1,500	2.8	830,000	4.2	114	63
17	2,239,000	1.1	2,100	3.9	1,100,000	5.5	94	49
18	2,748,000	1.4	2,400	4.4	1,190,000	6.0	87	43
19	3,147,000	1.6	2,600	4.8	1,120,000	5.6	83	36
19 and under	9,503,000	4.8	9,200	17.0	4,410,000	22.1	97	46
20	3,322,000	1.7	2,400	4.4	1,050,000	5.3	72	32
21	3,294,000	1.7	2,000	3.7	720,000	3.6	61	22
22	3,221,000	1.6	2,000	3.7	680,000	3.4	62	21
23	3,342,000	1.7	1,700	3.1	630,000	3.2	51	19
24	3,317,000	1.7	1,800	3.3	580,000	2.9	54	17
20–24	16,496,000	8.4	9,900	18.3	3,660,000	18.3	60	22
25–34	34,021,000	17.3	7,600	14.1	3,580,000	17.9	22	11
35–44	40,876,000	20.8	9,100	16.9	3,150,000	15.8	22	8
45–54	40,740,000	20.7	8,200	15.2	2,490,000	12.5	20	6
55–64	26,168,000	13.3	4,300	8.0	1,400,000	7.0	16	5
65–74	16,165,000	8.2	2,800	5.2	730,000	3.6	17	5
75 and over	12,731,000	6.5	2,900	5.4	580,000	2.9	23	5

Source: National Safety Council estimates. Drivers in accidents based on reports from 9 state traffic authorities. Total licensed drivers from the Federal Highway Administration; age distribution by National Safety Council.
Note: Percents may not add to total due to rounding.
[a]Drivers in fatal accidents per 100,000 licensed drivers in each age group.
[b]Drivers in all accidents per 100 licensed drivers in each age group.
[c]Less than 0.05.
[d]Rates for drivers under age 16 are substantially overstated due to the high proportion of unlicensed drivers involved.

SEX OF DRIVER

Of the estimated 196,700,000 licensed drivers in 2003, about 98,600,000 (50.1%) were males and 98,100,000 (49.9%) were females. Males account for about 62% of the miles driven each year, according to the latest estimates, and females for 38%. At least part of the difference in involvement rates, cited below, may be due to differences in the time, place, and circumstances of driving.

For fatal accidents, males have higher involvement rates than females. About 40,000 male drivers and 14,000 female drivers were involved in fatal accidents in 2003. The involvement rate per one billion miles driven was 22 for males and 13 for females. For all accidents, females have higher involvement rates than males. About 11,600,000 male drivers and 8,400,000 female drivers were involved in all accidents in 2003. Their involvement rates per 10 million miles driven were 65 and 77, respectively.

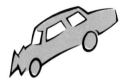

IMPROPER DRIVING

In most motor-vehicle accidents, factors are present relating to the driver, the vehicle and the road, and it is the interaction of these factors that often sets up the series of events that results in an accident. The table below relates only to the driver, and shows the principal kinds of improper driving in accidents in 2003 as reported by police.

Exceeding the posted speed limit or driving at an unsafe speed was the most common error in fatal and injury accidents. Right-of-way violations predominated in the all accidents category.

While some drivers were under the influence of alcohol or other drugs, this represents the driver's physical condition — not a driving error. See page 94 for a discussion of alcohol involvement in traffic accidents.

Correcting the improper practices listed below could reduce the number of accidents. This does not mean, however, that road and vehicle conditions can be disregarded.

IMPROPER DRIVING REPORTED IN ACCIDENTS, 2003

Kind of Improper Driving	Fatal Accidents	Injury Accidents	All Accidents
Total	100.0%	100.0%	100.0%
Improper driving	**57.0**	**50.3**	**49.9**
Speed too fast or unsafe	24.9	17.2	13.1
Right of way	16.3	16.5	18.1
Failed to yield	8.0	12.8	10.6
Disregarded signal	5.3	2.9	5.7
Passed stop sign	3.0	0.8	1.8
Drove left of center	5.9	0.8	0.8
Made improper turn	0.5	1.2	1.7
Improper overtaking	1.3	1.1	1.7
Followed too closely	0.4	3.4	6.3
Other improper driving	7.7	10.1	8.2
No improper driving stated	**43.0**	**49.7**	**50.1**

Source: Based on reports from 6 state traffic authorities. Percents may not add to totals due to rounding.

PEDESTRIANS

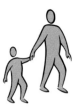

In 2003, there were an estimated 5,600 pedestrian deaths and 80,000 injuries in motor-vehicle accidents. About 45% of these deaths and injuries occur when pedestrians cross or enter streets. Walking in the roadway accounted for about 10% of pedestrian deaths and injuries, with more cases occurring while walking with traffic than against traffic.

The distribution of pedestrian deaths and injuries by action varies for persons of different ages. While crossing or entering at or between intersections was the leading type for each age group, this type varied from a low of 41.5% of the total for those aged 25 to 44 years to a high of 60.6% for those aged 5 to 9 years.

DEATHS AND INJURIES OF PEDESTRIANS BY AGE AND ACTION, 2003

Actions	Total[a]	Age of Persons Killed or Injured							
		0–4	5–9	10–14	15–19	20–24	25–44	45–64	65 & Over
All Actions	*100.0%*	2.2%	6.8%	9.8%	10.2%	9.6%	25.9%	18.3%	7.3%
Totals	**100.0%**	**100.0%**	**100.0%**	**100.0%**	**100.0%**	**100.0%**	**100.0%**	**100.0%**	**100.0%**
Crossing or entering at or between intersections	44.5%	52.7%	60.6%	55.9%	44.6%	42.3%	41.5%	52.6%	51.8%
Walking in the roadway	9.6%	0.9%	5.0%	10.7%	14.6%	11.9%	11.1%	10.5%	7.6%
with traffic	5.7%	0.9%	2.9%	6.4%	8.7%	7.8%	6.6%	5.9%	4.3%
against traffic	3.9%	0.0%	2.0%	4.2%	6.0%	4.1%	4.5%	4.5%	3.3%
Standing (or playing) in roadway	6.9%	5.4%	3.8%	5.0%	8.1%	9.9%	10.3%	5.3%	4.3%
Pushing/working on a vehicle in the roadway	0.7%	0.0%	0.3%	0.2%	0.2%	1.4%	1.4%	0.1%	0.3%
Other working in the roadway	1.6%	0.0%	0.0%	0.0%	0.8%	2.5%	3.0%	2.2%	0.8%
Not in the roadway	1.5%	0.0%	0.9%	0.2%	2.9%	2.1%	1.5%	1.5%	2.7%
Other	23.6%	32.1%	25.4%	23.7%	25.0%	25.9%	27.1%	24.0%	27.4%
Not stated	11.7%	8.9%	4.1%	4.2%	3.8%	4.1%	4.0%	3.9%	5.1%

Source: Based on reports from 6 state traffic authorities.
[a]Total includes "Age Unknown."

PEDESTRIAN DEATHS AND DEATH RATES BY SEX AND AGE GROUP, UNITED STATES, 2001

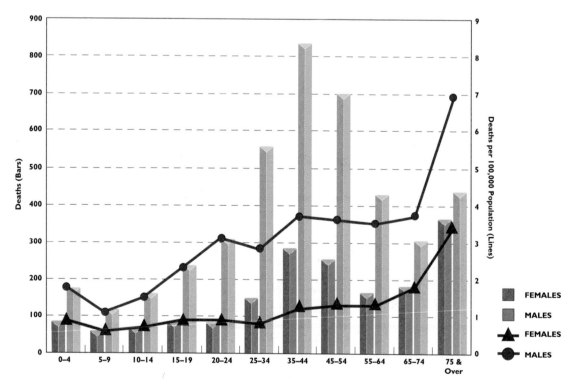

Source: National Safety Council based on National Center for Health Statistics data.

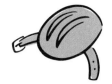

PEDALCYCLISTS

The estimated number of deaths from pedalcycle–motor-vehicle collisions increased from about 750 in 1940 to 1,200 in 1980, then declined to about 700 in 2003. Nonfatal disabling injuries were estimated to number 28,000 in 2003.

In 2001, 585 pedalcyclists died in motor-vehicle crashes and 207 in other accidents, according to National Center for Health Statistics mortality data. Males accounted for more than 90% of all pedalcycle deaths, nearly ten times the female fatalities.

Emergency-room–treated injuries associated with bicycles and bicycle accessories were estimated to total 521,328 in 2002, according to the U.S. Consumer

Product Safety Commission (see also page 126). The CPSC reported that bike helmet use was 50% in 1998. About 38% of adults and 69% of children under 16 reported wearing bike helmets regularly. The Bicycle Helmet Safety Institute estimates that helmets reduce the risk of all head injuries by up to 85% and reduce the risk of brain injuries by as much as 88%. In 2004, 19 states, the District of Columbia, and at least 134 localities had bicycle helmet laws, according to the Bicycle Helmet Safety Institute.

Source: National Safety Council estimates and tabulations of National Center for Health Statistics mortality data. Rodgers, G.B., & Tinsworth, D. (1999). Bike Helmets. Consumer Product Safety Review, (4), 2–4. Data from Bicycle Helmet Safety Institute retrieved 7/9/04 from www.bhsi.org.

PEDALCYCLE DEATHS AND DEATH RATES BY SEX AND AGE GROUP, UNITED STATES, 2001

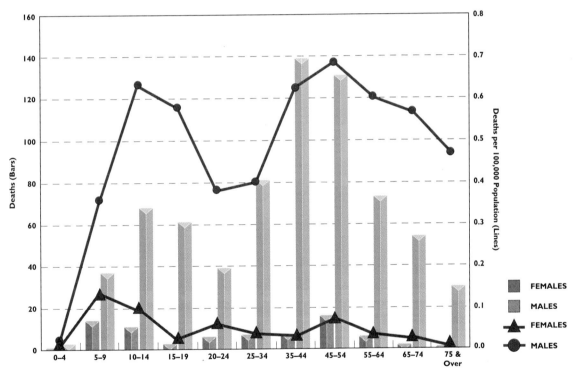

Source: National Safety Council based on National Center for Health Statistics data.

PEDALCYCLE FATALITIES BY MONTH, UNITED STATES, 2001

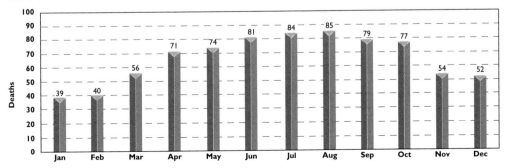

WORK ZONE DEATHS AND INJURIES

In 2002 there were 1,181 people killed and 51,988 people injured in work zone crashes (see table below). Compared to 2001, work zone fatalities and injuries increased 9% and 13%, respectively. Of the 1,181 people killed in work zones, 1,023 were in construction zones, 89 were in maintenance zones, 12 were in utility zones, and 57 were in an unknown type of work zone.

Over the ten years from 1993 through 2002, work zone deaths have ranged from 658 to 1,181 and averaged 875 per year.

Based on a National Safety Council survey in April 2004, 28 states reported having work zone speed laws and 49 states had special penalties for traffic violations in work zones, such as increased or doubled fines. Hawaii and District of Columbia were the only jurisdictions with neither.

PERSONS KILLED AND INJURED IN WORK ZONES, UNITED STATES, 2002

	Total	Vehicle Occupants	Pedestrians	Pedalcyclists	Other Nonmotorists
Killed	1,181	1,029	134	13	5
Injured	51,988	50,787	723	249	229

Source: National Safety Council tabulations of data from National Highway Traffic Safety Administration — 2002 Fatality Analysis Reporting System (FARS) and 2002 General Estimates Systems (GES).

EMERGENCY VEHICLES

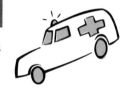

CRASHES INVOLVING EMERGENCY VEHICLES, UNITED STATES, 2002

	Ambulance		Fire Truck/Car		Police Car	
	Total	Emergency Use[a]	Total	Emergency Use[a]	Total	Emergency Use[a]
Emergency vehicles in fatal crashes	20	10	12	8	111	55
Emergency vehicles in injury crashes	2,064	1,396	822	589	10,652	3,876
Emergency vehicles in all crashes	**4,042**	**2,838**	**4,011**	**2,194**	**36,116**	**13,958**
Emergency vehicle drivers killed	0	0	3	2	25	12
Emergency vehicle passengers killed	3	1	2	2	3	2
Other vehicle occupants killed	17	9	6	3	76	41
Nonmotorists killed	2	0	1	1	18	7
Total killed in crashes	**22**	**10**	**12**	**8**	**122**	**62**
Total injured in crashes	**3,614**	**2,621**	**1,745**	**1,308**	**14,785**	**4,853**

Source: National Safety Council tabulations of data from National Highway Traffic Safety Administration — 2002 Fatality Analysis Reporting System (FARS) and 2002 General Estimates Systems (GES).
[a]Emergency lights and/or sirens in use.

The population of the United States is becoming increasingly older. The number and proportion of persons aged 65 years and over is expected to increase from 36 million, or 12.6%, in 2004 to 70.3 million, or 20%, in 2030. This demographic shift will lead to a substantial increase in the number and percent of older licensed drivers on the road.

Millions of older adults have to travel outside the home in order to maintain employment, interact with friends and family, buy groceries, access professional medical and social services, and just for pleasure. According to the 2001 National Household Travel Survey, American seniors (65+ years old) take approximately 42 billion short-distance trips (0–50 miles from home) and 220 million long-distance trips (50+ miles), representing 10.2% and 8.4%, respectively, of all travel by adults over 19. Seventy-five percent of older adults report taking short-distance trips (men — 81%, women — 72%), while their participation in long-distance travel is 35% (men — 40%, women — 31%).

Personal vehicles are the preferred mode of transportation for short-distance travel — older adults conduct 89% of all short trips in a personal automobile. With respect to the type of vehicle driven, 77% of the elderly use cars, 10% trucks, 8% vans, 4% sport utility vehicles, and less than 1% RVs or motorcycles. Women take a higher percentage of their short-distance trips as passengers than do men (38% vs. 12%).

Data collected on long-distance trips show that personal vehicles are used by older men in 91% of their travel, while older women rely on a personal vehicle in 87% of their travel. There is no difference in the frequency of personal vehicle use for long-distance travel between older and younger travelers. For older men, the average length of a long-distance trip made in a personal vehicle is 376 miles as compared to 364 miles for older women. Sixty-five percent of older adults take long-distance trips for pleasure purposes, as compared to 49% for younger people.

Many Americans will keep driving into old age. According to a survey conducted in Michigan, 43% of older drivers (ages 65+) do not plan to stop driving for at least 10 years; an additional 31% expect to continue driving for 5 to 10 years. About half of the older drivers, who feel that their ability to drive is likely to deteriorate within the next 5 years, still expect to keep driving for more than 5 years.

Use of public transportation services or other alternatives is relatively low among the elderly. The Michigan survey indicates that 60% of older adults have never used public transportation on a regular basis and some are not even aware of what public transportation services are available to them.

The automobile is also the principal mode of transportation for former drivers as they rely on getting rides from friends and relatives. In fact, most former drivers, who travel primarily as passengers in personal vehicles, report that they do not have a secondary mode of transportation.

The anticipated growth of the older population also represents an increase in the contribution of older adults to the total number of fatal and serious nonfatal injuries among vehicle occupants. Based on the occupant death rate per 100,000 population, the risk of adults aged 65–74 is similar to that of persons aged 35–44 and actually decreases with age. When the risk is described by death rates per vehicle miles traveled, which take exposure into account, the most elderly and teenage drivers appear to be the two most vulnerable groups. However, neither approach adequately captures the risk of motor-vehicle injury, as they disregard that (a) older adults (aged 65+) have a higher proportion of miles traveled per person as nondrivers compared to their younger counterparts; (b) older people are more likely to use passenger cars than younger people; and (c) in cases of serious injuries, older occupants are more likely to be involved in side-impact collisions than younger occupants.

The facts about transportation safety and mobility of the elderly were taken from 13 papers published in the *Journal of Safety Research* (Vol. 34, No. 4, November 2003) that summarized current research in that area.

MOTOR-VEHICLE DEATHS AND RATES

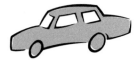

MOTOR-VEHICLE DEATHS AND RATES, UNITED STATES, 1913–2003

Year	No. of Deaths	Estimated No. of Vehicles (Millions)	Estimated Vehicle Miles (Billions)	Estimated No. of Drivers (Millions)	Death Rates		
					Per 10,000 Motor Vehicles	Per 100,000,000 Vehicle Miles	Per 100,000 Population
1913	4,200	1.3	(a)	2.0	33.38	(a)	4.4
1914	4,700	1.8	(a)	3.0	26.65	(a)	4.8
1915	6,600	2.5	(a)	3.0	26.49	(a)	6.6
1916	8,200	3.6	(a)	5.0	22.66	(a)	8.1
1917	10,200	5.1	(a)	7.0	19.93	(a)	10.0
1918	10,700	6.2	(a)	9.0	17.37	(a)	10.3
1919	11,200	7.6	(a)	12.0	14.78	(a)	10.7
1920	12,500	9.2	(a)	14.0	13.53	(a)	11.7
1921	13,900	10.5	(a)	16.0	13.25	(a)	12.9
1922	15,300	12.3	(a)	19.0	12.47	(a)	13.9
1923	18,400	15.1	85	22.0	12.18	21.65	16.5
1924	19,400	17.6	104	26.0	11.02	18.65	17.1
1925	21,900	20.1	122	30.0	10.89	17.95	19.1
1926	23,400	22.2	141	33.0	10.54	16.59	20.1
1927	25,800	23.3	158	34.0	11.07	16.33	21.8
1928	28,000	24.7	173	37.0	11.34	16.18	23.4
1929	31,200	26.7	197	40.0	11.69	15.84	25.7
1930	32,900	26.7	206	40.0	12.32	15.97	26.7
1931	33,700	26.1	216	39.0	12.91	15.60	27.2
1932	29,500	24.4	200	36.0	12.09	14.75	23.6
1933	31,363	24.2	201	35.0	12.96	15.60	25.0
1934	36,101	25.3	216	37.0	14.27	16.71	28.6
1935	36,369	26.5	229	39.0	13.72	15.88	28.6
1936	38,089	28.5	252	42.0	13.36	15.11	29.7
1937	39,643	30.1	270	44.0	13.19	14.68	30.8
1938	32,582	29.8	271	44.0	10.93	12.02	25.1
1939	32,386	31.0	285	46.0	10.44	11.35	24.7
1940	34,501	32.5	302	48.0	10.63	11.42	26.1
1941	39,969	34.9	334	52.0	11.45	11.98	30.0
1942	28,309	33.0	268	49.0	8.58	10.55	21.1
1943	23,823	30.9	208	46.0	7.71	11.44	17.8
1944	24,282	30.5	213	45.0	7.97	11.42	18.3
1945	28,076	31.0	250	46.0	9.05	11.22	21.2
1946	33,411	34.4	341	50.0	9.72	9.80	23.9
1947	32,697	37.8	371	53.0	8.64	8.82	22.8
1948	32,259	41.1	398	55.0	7.85	8.11	22.1
1949	31,701	44.7	424	59.3	7.09	7.47	21.3
1950	34,763	49.2	458	62.2	7.07	7.59	23.0
1951	36,996	51.9	491	64.4	7.13	7.53	24.1
1952	37,794	53.3	514	66.8	7.10	7.36	24.3
1953	37,956	56.3	544	69.9	6.74	6.97	24.0
1954	35,586	58.6	562	72.2	6.07	6.33	22.1
1955	38,426	62.8	606	74.7	6.12	6.34	23.4
1956	39,628	65.2	631	77.9	6.07	6.28	23.7
1957	38,702	67.6	647	79.6	5.73	5.98	22.7
1958	36,981	68.8	665	81.5	5.37	5.56	21.3
1959	37,910	72.1	700	84.5	5.26	5.41	21.5
1960	38,137	74.5	719	87.4	5.12	5.31	21.2
1961	38,091	76.4	738	88.9	4.98	5.16	20.8
1962	40,804	79.7	767	92.0	5.12	5.32	22.0
1963	43,564	83.5	805	93.7	5.22	5.41	23.1
1964	47,700	87.3	847	95.6	5.46	5.63	25.0
1965	49,163	91.8	888	99.0	5.36	5.54	25.4
1966	53,041	95.9	930	101.0	5.53	5.70	27.1
1967	52,924	98.9	962	103.2	5.35	5.50	26.8
1968	54,862	103.1	1,016	105.4	5.32	5.40	27.5
1969	55,791	107.4	1,071	108.3	5.19	5.21	27.7
1970	54,633	111.2	1,120	111.5	4.92	4.88	26.8
1971	54,381	116.3	1,186	114.4	4.68	4.57	26.3
1972	56,278	122.3	1,268	118.4	4.60	4.43	26.9
1973	55,511	129.8	1,309	121.6	4.28	4.24	26.3
1974	46,402	134.9	1,290	125.6	3.44	3.59	21.8
1975	45,853	137.9	1,330	129.8	3.33	3.45	21.3
1976	47,038	143.5	1,412	133.9	3.28	3.33	21.6

See source and footnotes on page 111.

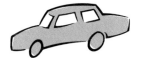

MOTOR-VEHICLE DEATHS AND RATES, UNITED STATES, 1913–2003, Cont.

Year	No. of Deaths	Estimated No. of Vehicles (Millions)	Estimated Vehicle Miles (Billions)	Estimated No. of Drivers (Millions)	Death Rates Per 10,000 Motor Vehicles	Per 100,000,000 Vehicle Miles	Per 100,000 Population
1977	49,510	148.8	1,477	138.1	3.33	3.35	22.5
1978	52,411	153.6	1,548	140.8	3.41	3.39	23.6
1979	53,524	159.6	1,529	143.3	3.35	3.50	23.8
1980	53,172	161.6	1,521	145.3	3.29	3.50	23.4
1981	51,385	164.1	1,556	147.1	3.13	3.30	22.4
1982	45,779	165.2	1,592	150.3	2.77	2.88	19.8
1983	44,452	169.4	1,657	154.2	2.62	2.68	19.0
1984	46,263	171.8	1,718	155.4	2.69	2.69	19.6
1985	45,901	177.1	1,774	156.9	2.59°	2.59	19.3
1986	47,865	181.4	1,835	159.5	2.63	2.60	19.9
1987	48,290	183.9	1,924	161.8	2.63	2.51	19.9
1988	49,078	189.0	2,026	162.9	2.60	2.42	20.1
1989	47,575	191.7	2,107	165.6	2.48	2.26	19.3
1990	46,814	192.9	2,148	167.0	2.43	2.18	18.8
1991	43,536	192.5	2,172	169.0	2.26	2.00	17.3
1992	40,982	194.4	2,240	173.1	2.11	1.83	16.1
1993	41,893	198.0	2,297	173.1	2.12	1.82	16.3
1994	42,524	201.8	2,360	175.4	2.11	1.80	16.3
1995	43,363	205.3	2,423	176.6	2.11	1.79	16.5
1996	43,649	210.4	2,486	179.5	2.07	1.76	16.5
1997	43,458	211.5	2,562	182.7	2.05	1.70	16.2
1998	43,501	215.0	2,632	185.2	2.02	1.65	16.1
1999	42,401	220.5	2,691	187.2	1.92	1.58	15.5
2000	43,354	225.8	2,747	190.6	1.92	1.58	15.8
2001[b]	43,788	235.3	2,797	191.3	1.86	1.57	15.4
2002[b]	44,100	234.6	2,856	194.3	1.88	1.54	15.3
2003[c]	44,800	239.6	2,880	196.7	1.87	1.56	15.4
Changes							
1993 to 2003	+7%	+21%	+25%	+14%	−12%	−14%	−6%
2002 to 2003	+2%	+2%	+1%	+1%	−1%	+1%	+1%

Source: Deaths from National Center for Health Statistics except 1964, 2002, and 2003, which are National Safety Council estimates based on data from state traffic authorities. See Technical Appendix for comparability. Motor-vehicle registrations, mileage, and drivers estimated by Federal Highway Administration except 2003 registrations and drivers which are National Safety Council estimates.
[a] Mileage data inadequate prior to 1923.
[b] Revised.
[c] Preliminary.

MOTOR-VEHICLE DEATHS BY TYPE OF ACCIDENT

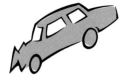

MOTOR-VEHICLE DEATHS BY TYPE OF ACCIDENT, UNITED STATES, 1913–2003

Year	Total Deaths	Deaths from Collision with —							Deaths from Noncollision Accidents	Nontraffic Deaths[a]
		Pedestrians	Other Motor Vehicles	Railroad Trains	Streetcars	Pedal-cycles	Animal-Drawn Vehicle or Animal	Fixed Objects		
1913	4,200	(b)	(b)	(b)	(b)	(b)	(b)	(b)	(b)	(c)
1914	4,700	(b)	(b)	(b)	(b)	(b)	(b)	(b)	(b)	(c)
1915	6,600	(b)	(b)	(b)	(b)	(b)	(b)	(b)	(b)	(c)
1916	8,200	(b)	(b)	(b)	(b)	(b)	(b)	(b)	(b)	(c)
1917	10,200	(b)	(b)	(b)	(b)	(b)	(b)	(b)	(b)	(c)
1918	10,700	(b)	(b)	(b)	(b)	(b)	(b)	(b)	(b)	(c)
1919	11,200	(b)	(b)	(b)	(b)	(b)	(b)	(b)	(b)	(c)
1920	12,500	(b)	(b)	(b)	(b)	(b)	(b)	(b)	(b)	(c)
1921	13,900	(b)	(b)	(b)	(b)	(b)	(b)	(b)	(b)	(c)
1922	15,300	(b)	(b)	(b)	(b)	(b)	(b)	(b)	(b)	(c)
1923	18,400	(b)	(b)	(b)	(b)	(b)	(b)	(b)	(b)	(c)
1924	19,400	(b)	(b)	1,130	410	(b)	(b)	(b)	(b)	(c)
1925	21,900	(b)	(b)	1,410	560	(b)	(b)	(b)	(b)	(c)
1926	23,400	(b)	(b)	1,730	520	(b)	(b)	(b)	(b)	(c)
1927	25,800	10,820	3,430	1,830	520	(b)	(b)	(b)	(b)	(c)
1928	28,000	11,420	4,310	2,140	570	(b)	(b)	540	8,070	(c)
1929	31,200	12,250	5,400	2,050	530	(b)	(b)	620	9,380	(c)
1930	32,900	12,900	5,880	1,830	480	(b)	(b)	720	9,970	(c)
1931	33,700	13,370	6,820	1,710	440	(b)	(b)	870	9,570	(c)
1932	29,500	11,490	6,070	1,520	320	350	400	800	8,500	(c)
1933	31,363	12,840	6,470	1,437	318	400	310	900	8,680	(c)
1934	36,101	14,480	8,110	1,457	332	500	360	1,040	9,820	(c)
1935	36,369	14,350	8,750	1,587	253	450	250	1,010	9,720	(c)
1936	38,089	15,250	9,500	1,697	269	650	250	1,060	9,410	(c)
1937	39,643	15,500	10,320	1,810	264	700	200	1,160	9,690	(c)
1938	32,582	12,850	8,900	1,490	165	720	170	940	7,350	(c)
1939	32,386	12,400	8,700	1,330	150	710	200	1,000	7,900	(c)
1940	34,501	12,700	10,100	1,707	132	750	210	1,100	7,800	(c)
1941	39,969	13,550	12,500	1,840	118	910	250	1,350	9,450	(c)
1942	28,309	10,650	7,300	1,754	124	650	240	850	6,740	(c)
1943	23,823	9,900	5,300	1,448	171	450	160	700	5,690	(c)
1944	24,282	9,900	5,700	1,663	175	400	140	700	5,600	(c)
1945	28,076	11,000	7,150	1,703	163	500	130	800	6,600	(c)
1946	33,411	11,600	9,400	1,703	174	450	130	950	8,900	(c)
1947	32,697	10,450	9,900	1,736	102	550	150	1,000	8,800	(c)
1948	32,259	9,950	10,200	1,474	83	500	100	1,000	8,950	(c)
1949	31,701	8,800	10,500	1,452	56	550	140	1,100	9,100	838
1950	34,763	9,000	11,650	1,541	89	440	120	1,300	10,600	900
1951	36,996	9,150	13,100	1,573	46	390	100	1,400	11,200	966
1952	37,794	8,900	13,500	1,429	32	430	130	1,450	11,900	970
1953	37,956	8,750	13,400	1,506	26	420	120	1,500	12,200	1,026
1954	35,586	8,000	12,800	1,289	28	380	90	1,500	11,500	1,004
1955	38,426	8,200	14,500	1,490	15	410	90	1,600	12,100	989
1956	39,628	7,900	15,200	1,377	11	440	100	1,600	13,000	888
1957	38,702	7,850	15,400	1,376	13	460	80	1,700	11,800	1,016
1958	36,981	7,650	14,200	1,316	9	450	80	1,650	11,600	929
1959	37,910	7,850	14,900	1,202	6	480	70	1,600	11,800	948
1960	38,137	7,850	14,800	1,368	5	460	80	1,700	11,900	995
1961	38,091	7,650	14,700	1,267	5	490	80	1,700	12,200	1,065
1962	40,804	7,900	16,400	1,245	3	500	90	1,750	12,900	1,029
1963	43,564	8,200	17,600	1,385	10	580	80	1,900	13,800	990
1964	47,700	9,000	19,600	1,580	5	710	100	2,100	14,600	1,123
1965	49,163	8,900	20,800	1,556	5	680	120	2,200	14,900	1,113
1966	53,041	9,400	22,200	1,800	2	740	100	2,500	16,300	1,108
1967	52,924	9,400	22,000	1,620	3	750	100	2,350	16,700	1,165
1968	54,862	9,900	22,400	1,570	4	790	100	2,700	17,400	1,061
1969	55,791	10,100	23,700	1,495	2	800	100	3,900d	15,700d	1,155
1970	54,633	9,900	23,200	1,459	3	780	100	3,800	15,400	1,140
1971	54,381	9,900	23,100	1,378	2	800	100	3,800	15,300	1,015
1972	56,278	10,300	23,900	1,260	2	1,000	100	3,900	15,800	1,064
1973	55,511	10,200	23,600	1,194	2	1,000	100	3,800	15,600	1,164
1974	46,402	8,500	19,700	1,209	1	1,000	100	3,100	12,800	1,088
1975	45,853	8,400	19,550	979	1	1,000	100	3,130	12,700	1,033
1976	47,038	8,600	20,100	1,033	2	1,000	100	3,200	13,000	1,026

See source and footnotes on page 113.

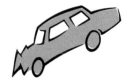

MOTOR-VEHICLE DEATHS BY TYPE OF ACCIDENT, UNITED STATES, 1913–2003, Cont.

Year	Total Deaths	Deaths from Collision with —							Deaths from Noncollision Accidents	Nontraffic Deaths[a]
		Pedestrians	Other Motor Vehicles	Railroad Trains	Streetcars	Pedal-cycles	Animal-Drawn Vehicle or Animal	Fixed Objects		
1977	49,510	9,100	21,200	902	3	1,100	100	3,400	13,700	1,053
1978	52,411	9,600	22,400	986	1	1,200	100	3,600	14,500	1,074
1979	53,524	9,800	23,100	826	1	1,200	100	3,700	14,800	1,271
1980	53,172	9,700	23,000	739	1	1,200	100	3,700	14,700	1,242
1981	51,385	9,400	22,200	668	1	1,200	100	3,600	14,200	1,189
1982	45,779	8,400	19,800	554	1	1,100	100	3,200	12,600	1,066
1983	44,452	8,200	19,200	520	1	1,100	100	3,100	12,200	1,024
1984	46,263	8,500	20,000	630	0	1,100	100	3,200	12,700	1,055
1985	45,901	8,500	19,900	538	2	1,100	100	3,200	12,600	1,079
1986	47,865	8,900	20,800	574	2	1,100	100	3,300	13,100	998
1987	48,290	7,500[e]	20,700	554	1	1,000[e]	100	13,200[e]	5,200[e]	993
1988	49,078	7,700	20,900	638	2	1,000	100	13,400	5,300	1,054
1989	47,575	7,800	20,300	720	2	900	100	12,900	4,900	989
1990	46,814	7,300	19,900	623	2	900	100	13,100	4,900	987
1991	43,536	6,600	18,200	541	1	800	100	12,600	4,700	915
1992	40,982	6,300	17,600	521	2	700	100	11,700	4,100	997
1993	41,893	6,400	18,300	553	3	800	100	11,500	4,200	994
1994	42,524	6,300	18,900	549	1	800	100	11,500	4,400	1,017
1995	43,363	6,400	19,000	514	(c)	800	100	12,100	4,400	1,032
1996	43,649	6,100	19,600	373	(c)	800	100	12,100	4,600	1,127
1997	43,458	5,900	19,900	371	(c)	800	100	12,000	4,400	1,118
1998	43,501	5,900	19,700	309	(c)	700	100	12,200	4,600	1,310
1999	42,401	6,100	18,600	314	1	800	100	11,800	4,700	1,436
2000	43,354	5,900	19,100	321	(c)	800	100	12,300	4,800	1,360
2001[f]	43,788	6,100	18,800	324	3	800	100	12,800	4,900	1,345
2002[f]	44,100	5,700	18,700	300	(c)	700	100	13,400	5,200	1,400
2003[g]	44,800	5,600	19,900	300	(c)	700	100	13,000	5,200	1,400

Changes in Deaths										
1993 to 2003	+7%	−12%	+9%	−46%	—	−12%	0%	+13%	+24%	+41%
2002 to 2003	+2%	−2%	+6%	0%	—	0%	0%	−3%	0%	0%

Source: Total deaths from National Center for Health Statistics except 1964 and 2002–2003, which are National Safety Council estimates based on data from state traffic authorities. Most totals by type are estimated and may not add to the total deaths. See Technical Appendix for comparability.
[a] *See definition, page 175. Nontraffic deaths are included in appropriate accident type totals in table; in 2001, 35% of the nontraffic deaths were pedestrians.*
[b] *Insufficient data for approximations.*
[c] *Data not available.*
[d] *1969 through 1986 totals are not comparable to previous years.*
[e] *Procedures and benchmarks for estimating deaths for certain types of accidents were changed for the 1990 edition. Estimates for 1987 and later years are not comparable to earlier years.*
[f] *Revised.*
[g] *Preliminary.*

MOTOR-VEHICLE DEATHS BY AGE

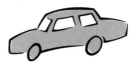

MOTOR-VEHICLE DEATHS BY AGE, UNITED STATES, 1913–2003

Year	All Ages	Under 5 Years	5–14 Years	15–24 Years	25–44 Years	45–64 Years	65–74 Years	75 & Over[a]
1913	4,200	300	1,100	600	1,100	800	300	
1914	4,700	300	1,200	700	1,200	900	400	
1915	6,600	400	1,500	1,000	1,700	1,400	600	
1916	8,200	600	1,800	1,300	2,100	1,700	700	
1917	10,200	700	2,400	1,400	2,700	2,100	900	
1918	10,700	800	2,700	1,400	2,500	2,300	1,000	
1919	11,200	900	3,000	1,400	2,500	2,100	1,300	
1920	12,500	1,000	3,300	1,700	2,800	2,300	1,400	
1921	13,900	1,100	3,400	1,800	3,300	2,700	1,600	
1922	15,300	1,100	3,500	2,100	3,700	3,100	1,800	
1923	18,400	1,200	3,700	2,800	4,600	3,900	2,200	
1924	19,400	1,400	3,800	2,900	4,700	4,100	2,500	
1925	21,900	1,400	3,900	3,600	5,400	4,800	2,800	
1926	23,400	1,400	3,900	3,900	5,900	5,200	3,100	
1927	25,800	1,600	4,000	4,300	6,600	5,800	3,500	
1928	28,000	1,600	3,800	4,900	7,200	6,600	3,900	
1929	31,200	1,600	3,900	5,700	8,000	7,500	4,500	
1930	32,900	1,500	3,600	6,200	8,700	8,000	4,900	
1931	33,700	1,500	3,600	6,300	9,100	8,200	5,000	
1932	29,500	1,200	2,900	5,100	8,100	7,400	4,800	
1933	31,363	1,274	3,121	5,649	8,730	7,947	4,642	
1934	36,101	1,210	3,182	6,561	10,232	9,530	5,386	
1935	36,369	1,253	2,951	6,755	10,474	9,562	5,374	
1936	38,089	1,324	3,026	7,184	10,807	10,089	5,659	
1937	39,643	1,303	2,991	7,800	10,877	10,475	6,197	
1938	32,582	1,122	2,511	6,016	8,772	8,711	5,450	
1939	32,386	1,192	2,339	6,318	8,917	8,292	5,328	
1940	34,501	1,176	2,584	6,846	9,362	8,882	5,651	
1941	39,969	1,378	2,838	8,414	11,069	9,829	6,441	
1942	28,309	1,069	1,991	5,932	7,747	7,254	4,316	
1943	23,823	1,132	1,959	4,522	6,454	5,996	3,760	
1944	24,282	1,203	2,093	4,561	6,514	5,982	3,929	
1945	28,076	1,290	2,386	5,358	7,578	6,794	4,670	
1946	33,411	1,568	2,508	7,445	8,955	7,532	5,403	
1947	32,697	1,502	2,275	7,251	8,775	7,468	5,426	
1948	32,259	1,635	2,337	7,218	8,702	7,190	3,173	2,004
1949	31,701	1,667	2,158	6,772	8,892	7,073	3,116	2,023
1950	34,763	1,767	2,152	7,600	10,214	7,728	3,264	2,038
1951	36,996	1,875	2,300	7,713	11,253	8,276	3,444	2,135
1952	37,794	1,951	2,295	8,115	11,380	8,463	3,472	2,118
1953	37,956	2,019	2,368	8,169	11,302	8,318	3,508	2,271
1954	35,586	1,864	2,332	7,571	10,521	7,848	3,247	2,203
1955	38,426	1,875	2,406	8,656	11,448	8,372	3,455	2,214
1956	39,628	1,770	2,640	9,169	11,551	8,573	3,657	2,268
1957	38,702	1,785	2,604	8,667	11,230	8,545	3,560	2,311
1958	36,981	1,791	2,710	8,388	10,414	7,922	3,535	2,221
1959	37,910	1,842	2,719	8,969	10,358	8,263	3,487	2,272
1960	38,137	1,953	2,814	9,117	10,189	8,294	3,457	2,313
1961	38,091	1,891	2,802	9,088	10,212	8,267	3,467	2,364
1962	40,804	1,903	3,028	10,157	10,701	8,812	3,696	2,507
1963	43,564	1,991	3,063	11,123	11,356	9,506	3,786	2,739
1964	47,700	2,120	3,430	12,400	12,500	10,200	4,150	2,900
1965	49,163	2,059	3,526	13,395	12,595	10,509	4,077	3,002
1966	53,041	2,182	3,869	15,298	13,282	11,051	4,217	3,142
1967	52,924	2,067	3,845	15,646	12,987	10,902	4,285	3,192
1968	54,862	1,987	4,105	16,543	13,602	11,031	4,261	3,333
1969	55,791	2,077	4,045	17,443	13,868	11,012	4,210	3,136
1970	54,633	1,915	4,159	16,720	13,446	11,099	4,084	3,210
1971	54,381	1,885	4,256	17,103	13,307	10,471	4,108	3,251
1972	56,278	1,896	4,258	17,942	13,758	10,836	4,138	3,450
1973	55,511	1,998	4,124	18,032	14,013	10,216	3,892	3,236
1974	46,402	1,546	3,332	15,905	11,834	8,159	3,071	2,555
1975	45,853	1,576	3,286	15,672	11,969	7,663	3,047	2,640
1976	47,038	1,532	3,175	16,650	12,112	7,770	3,082	2,717

See source and footnotes on page 115.

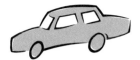
MOTOR-VEHICLE DEATHS BY AGE, UNITED STATES, 1913–2003, Cont.

Year	All Ages	Under 5 Years	5–14 Years	15–24 Years	25–44 Years	45–64 Years	65–74 Years	75 & Over[a]
1977	49,510	1,472	3,142	18,092	13,031	8,000	3,060	2,713
1978	52,411	1,551	3,130	19,164	14,574	8,048	3,217	2,727
1979	53,524	1,461	2,952	19,369	15,658	8,162	3,171	2,751
1980	53,172	1,426	2,747	19,040	16,133	8,022	2,991	2,813
1981	51,385	1,256	2,575	17,363	16,447	7,818	3,090	2,836
1982	45,779	1,300	2,301	15,324	14,469	6,879	2,825	2,681
1983	44,452	1,233	2,241	14,289	14,323	6,690	2,827	2,849
1984	46,263	1,138	2,263	14,738	15,036	6,954	3,020	3,114
1985	45,901	1,195	2,319	14,277	15,034	6,885	3,014	3,177
1986	47,865	1,188	2,350	15,227	15,844	6,799	3,096	3,361
1987	48,290	1,190	2,397	14,447	16,405	7,021	3,277	3,553
1988	49,078	1,220	2,423	14,406	16,580	7,245	3,429	3,775
1989	47,575	1,221	2,266	12,941	16,571	7,287	3,465	3,824
1990	46,814	1,123	2,059	12,607	16,488	7,282	3,350	3,905
1991	43,536	1,076	2,011	11,664	15,082	6,616	3,193	3,894
1992	40,982	1,020	1,904	10,305	14,071	6,597	3,247	3,838
1993	41,893	1,081	1,963	10,500	14,283	6,711	3,116	4,239
1994	42,524	1,139	2,026	10,660	13,966	7,097	3,385	4,251
1995	43,363	1,004	2,055	10,600	14,618	7,428	3,300	4,358
1996	43,649	1,035	1,980	10,576	14,482	7,749	3,419	4,408
1997	43,458	933	1,967	10,208	14,167	8,134	3,370	4,679
1998	43,501	921	1,868	10,026	14,095	8,416	3,410	4,765
1999	42,401	834	1,771	10,128	13,516	8,342	3,276	4,534
2000	43,354	819	1,772	10,560	13,811	8,867	3,038	4,487
2001[b]	43,788	770	1,686	10,725	14,020	9,029	2,990	4,568
2002[b]	44,100	700	1,700	11,100	13,700	9,500	3,000	4,400
2003[c]	44,800	700	1,800	10,900	13,500	10,300	3,100	4,500
Changes in Deaths								
1993 to 2003	+7%	−35%	−8%	+4%	−5%	+53%	−1%	+6%
2002 to 2003	+2%	0%	+6%	−2%	−1%	+8%	+3%	+2%

Source: 1913 to 1932 calculated from National Center for Health Statistics data for registration states; 1933 to 1963, 1965 to 2001 are NCHS totals. All other figures are National Safety Council estimates. See Technical Appendix for comparability.
[a] Includes "age unknown." In 2001 these deaths numbered 33.
[b] Revised.
[c] Preliminary.

MOTOR-VEHICLE DEATH RATES BY AGE

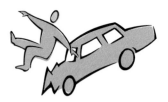

MOTOR-VEHICLE DEATH RATES[a] BY AGE, UNITED STATES, 1913–2003

Year	All Ages	Under 5 Years	5–14 Years	15–24 Years	25–44 Years	45–64 Years	65–74 Years	75 & Over
1913	4.4	2.3	5.5	3.1	3.8	5.3	8.5	
1914	4.8	2.5	5.7	3.5	4.1	6.2	9.3	
1915	6.6	3.5	7.3	5.0	5.6	8.8	13.5	
1916	8.1	4.7	8.6	6.0	7.0	10.7	15.8	
1917	10.0	5.6	10.6	7.4	8.6	12.6	18.6	
1918	10.3	6.9	12.3	7.7	8.3	13.7	21.2	
1919	10.7	7.5	13.9	7.5	8.1	12.4	24.1	
1920	11.7	8.6	14.6	8.7	8.8	13.5	27.0	
1921	12.9	9.0	14.5	9.2	10.2	15.4	31.0	
1922	13.9	9.2	15.0	10.8	11.1	17.2	34.9	
1923	16.5	9.7	15.6	13.4	13.6	21.0	40.5	
1924	17.1	11.1	16.1	14.3	13.7	21.8	43.7	
1925	19.1	11.0	15.6	17.2	15.8	25.0	48.9	
1926	20.1	11.0	15.9	18.6	17.1	26.3	51.4	
1927	21.8	12.8	16.0	20.0	18.8	28.9	56.9	
1928	23.4	12.7	15.5	21.9	20.2	32.4	62.2	
1929	25.7	13.4	15.6	25.6	22.3	35.6	68.6	
1930	26.7	13.0	14.7	27.4	23.9	37.0	72.5	
1931	27.2	13.3	14.5	27.9	24.8	37.4	70.6	
1932	23.6	11.3	12.0	22.6	22.0	32.9	63.6	
1933	25.0	12.0	12.7	24.8	23.4	34.7	63.1	
1934	28.6	11.7	13.0	28.6	27.2	40.7	71.0	
1935	28.6	12.3	12.2	29.2	27.6	39.9	68.9	
1936	29.7	13.2	12.6	30.8	28.2	41.3	70.5	
1937	30.8	13.0	12.7	33.2	28.2	42.0	75.1	
1938	25.1	11.0	10.8	25.4	22.5	34.3	64.1	
1939	24.7	11.2	10.4	26.5	22.6	32.2	60.2	
1940	26.1	11.1	11.5	28.7	23.5	33.9	62.1	
1941	30.0	12.7	12.6	35.7	27.5	37.0	68.6	
1942	21.1	9.5	8.8	25.8	19.2	26.9	44.5	
1943	17.8	9.4	8.6	20.6	16.1	21.9	37.6	
1944	18.3	9.6	9.1	22.5	16.6	21.6	38.2	
1945	21.2	10.0	10.3	27.8	19.7	24.2	44.1	
1946	23.9	11.9	10.8	34.4	21.1	26.4	49.6	
1947	22.8	10.5	9.7	32.8	20.3	25.7	48.2	
1948	22.1	11.0	9.8	32.5	19.8	24.3	39.6	55.4
1949	21.3	10.7	9.0	30.7	19.9	23.4	37.8	53.9
1950	23.0	10.8	8.8	34.5	22.5	25.1	38.8	52.4
1951	24.1	10.9	9.2	36.0	24.7	26.5	39.5	53.0
1952	24.3	11.3	8.7	38.6	24.7	26.7	38.5	50.8
1953	24.0	11.5	8.5	39.1	24.5	25.8	37.7	52.6
1954	22.1	10.4	8.1	36.2	22.6	24.0	33.9	49.0
1955	23.4	10.2	8.0	40.9	24.5	25.2	35.1	47.1
1956	23.7	9.4	8.4	42.9	24.6	25.3	36.2	46.4
1957	22.7	9.2	8.0	39.7	23.9	24.8	34.4	45.5
1958	21.3	9.1	8.1	37.0	22.3	22.6	33.5	42.3
1959	21.5	9.1	7.9	38.2	22.2	23.2	32.3	41.8
1960	21.2	9.6	7.9	37.7	21.7	22.9	31.3	41.1
1961	20.8	9.2	7.6	36.5	21.8	22.5	30.7	40.5
1962	22.0	9.3	8.1	38.4	22.9	23.7	32.2	41.7
1963	23.1	9.8	8.0	40.0	24.3	25.2	32.6	44.3
1964	25.0	10.5	8.8	42.6	26.8	26.6	35.5	45.2
1965	25.4	10.4	8.9	44.2	27.0	27.0	34.6	45.4
1966	27.1	11.4	9.7	48.7	28.5	27.9	35.4	46.2
1967	26.8	11.2	9.5	48.4	27.8	27.1	35.6	45.4
1968	27.5	11.1	10.1	49.8	28.8	27.0	35.1	46.0
1969	27.7	12.0	9.9	50.7	29.1	26.6	34.3	42.0
1970	26.8	11.2	10.2	46.7	27.9	26.4	32.7	42.2
1971	26.3	10.9	10.5	45.7	27.4	24.7	32.4	41.3
1972	26.9	11.1	10.7	47.1	27.4	25.3	32.0	42.6
1973	26.3	11.9	10.5	46.3	27.2	23.6	29.4	39.1
1974	21.8	9.4	8.6	40.0	22.4	18.8	22.6	30.1
1975	21.3	9.8	8.6	38.7	22.1	17.5	21.9	30.1
1976	21.6	9.8	8.4	40.3	21.8	17.6	21.6	30.1

See source and footnotes on page 117.

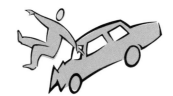

MOTOR-VEHICLE DEATH RATES
BY AGE (CONT.)

MOTOR-VEHICLE DEATH RATES[a] BY AGE, UNITED STATES, 1913–2003, Cont.

Year	All Ages	Under 5 Years	5–14 Years	15–24 Years	25–44 Years	45–64 Years	65–74 Years	75 & Over
1977	22.5	9.5	8.5	43.3	22.7	18.1	20.9	29.3
1978	23.6	9.9	8.6	45.4	24.6	18.2	21.5	28.7
1979	23.8	9.1	8.3	45.6	25.6	18.4	20.7	28.1
1980	23.4	8.7	7.9	44.8	25.5	18.0	19.1	28.0
1981	22.4	7.4	7.5	41.1	25.2	17.6	19.4	27.5
1982	19.8	7.5	6.7	36.8	21.5	15.5	17.5	25.2
1983	19.0	7.0	6.6	34.8	20.6	15.0	17.2	26.0
1984	19.6	6.4	6.7	36.4	21.0	15.6	18.2	27.7
1985	19.3	6.7	6.9	35.7	20.5	15.4	17.9	27.5
1986	19.9	6.6	7.0	38.5	21.0	15.2	18.1	28.3
1987	19.9	6.6	7.1	37.1	21.3	15.7	18.8	29.1
1988	20.1	6.7	7.1	37.8	21.2	15.9	19.5	30.2
1989	19.3	6.6	6.5	34.6	20.8	15.9	19.4	29.8
1990	18.8	6.0	5.8	34.2	20.4	15.7	18.5	29.7
1991	17.3	5.6	5.6	32.1	18.3	14.2	17.5	28.9
1992	16.1	5.2	5.2	28.5	17.1	13.6	17.6	27.8
1993	16.3	5.5	5.3	29.1	17.3	13.5	16.7	30.0
1994	16.3	5.8	5.4	29.5	16.8	13.9	18.1	29.4
1995	16.5	5.1	5.4	29.3	17.5	14.2	17.6	29.4
1996	16.5	5.4	5.2	29.2	17.3	14.4	18.3	29.0
1997	16.2	4.9	5.1	27.9	17.0	14.7	18.2	29.9
1998	16.1	4.9	4.8	26.9	16.9	14.7	18.5	29.8
1999	15.5	4.4	4.5	26.8	16.3	14.1	18.0	27.8
2000	15.7	4.3	4.5	27.5	16.8	14.5	16.7	27.0
2001[b]	15.4	4.0	4.1	26.8	16.5	14.0	16.3	26.8
2002[b]	15.3	3.6	4.1	27.3	16.4	14.1	16.4	25.4
2003[c]	15.4	3.5	4.4	26.5	16.1	15.0	16.9	25.6
Changes in Rates								
1993 to 2003	−6%	−36%	−17%	−9%	−7%	+11%	+1%	−15%
2002 to 2003	+1%	−3%	+7%	−3%	−2%	+6%	+3%	+1%

Source: 1913 to 1932 calculated from National Center for Health Statistics data for registration states; 1933 to 1963, 1965 to 2001 are NCHS totals. All other figures are National Safety Council estimates. See Technical Appendix for comparability.
[a] Death rates are deaths per 100,000 population in each age group.
[b] Revised.
[c] Preliminary.

INJURY FACTS®

NATIONAL SAFETY COUNCIL

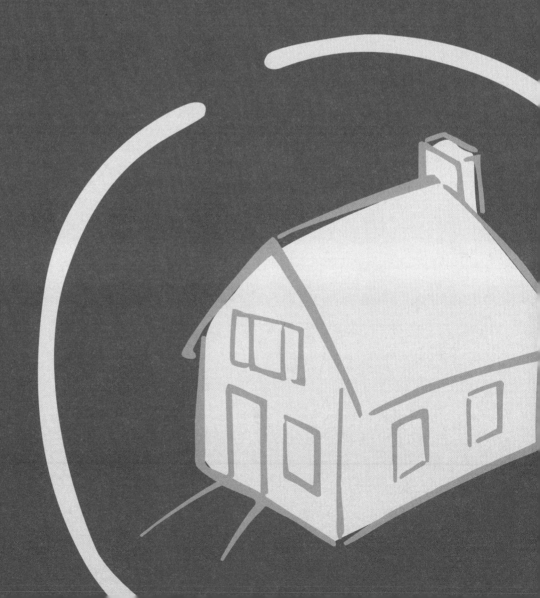

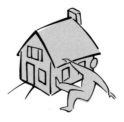

The Home and Community venue is the combination of the Home class and the Public class. Home and Community together with the Occupational and Transportation venues make up the totality of unintentional injuries. Home and Community includes all unintentional injuries that are not work related and do not involve motor vehicles on streets and highways.

In 2003, an estimated 54,400 unintentional-injury deaths occurred in the Home and Community venue, or 54% of all unintentional-injury deaths that year. The number of deaths decreased by 4% from the revised 2002 total of 56,900. Another 15,000,000 people suffered nonfatal disabling injuries. The death rate per 100,000 population was 18.7, a decrease of 6% from the revised 2002 rate of 19.8.

About 1 out of 19 people experience an unintentional injury in the Home and Community venue each year and about 1 out of 5,300 people die from such an injury. About 35% of the deaths and disabling injuries involve workers while they are away from work (off the job).

The graph on the next page shows the five leading causes of unintentional-injury deaths in the Home and Community venue and the broad age groups (children, youths and adults, and the elderly) affected by them. This is one way to prioritize issues in this venue. Also shown on the next page is a graph of the trend in deaths and death rates from 1993 to the present. Similar graphs for the Public and Home classes are on pages 122 and 126.

The Council adopted the Bureau of Labor Statistics' Census of Fatal Occupational Injuries count for work-related unintentional injuries retroactive to 1992 data. Because of the lower Work class total resulting from this change, several thousand unintentional-injury deaths that had been classified by the Council as work related had to be reassigned to the Home and Public classes. Long-term historical comparisons for these three classes should be made with caution. Also, beginning with 1999 data, deaths are now classified according to the 10th revision of the *International Classification of Diseases*. Caution should be used in comparing data classified under the two systems. See the Technical Appendix for more information about both changes.

Deaths **54,400**
Disabling Injuries **15,000,000**
Death Rate per 100,000 Population **18.7**
Costs . . . . **$230.5 billion**

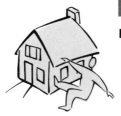

LEADING CAUSES OF UNINTENTIONAL-INJURY DEATHS IN HOME AND COMMUNITY, UNITED STATES, 2003

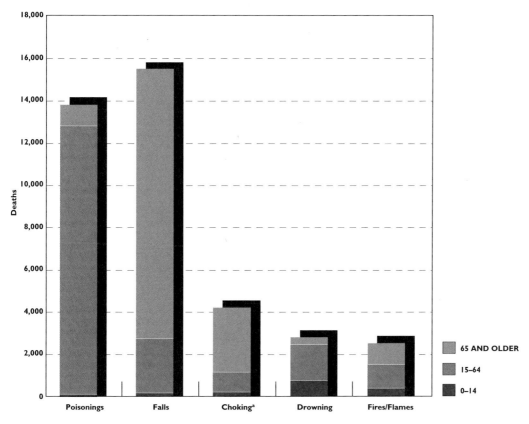

ᵃInhalation and ingestion of food or other object that obstructs breathing.

HOME AND COMMUNITY DEATHS AND DEATH RATES, UNITED STATES, 1993–2003

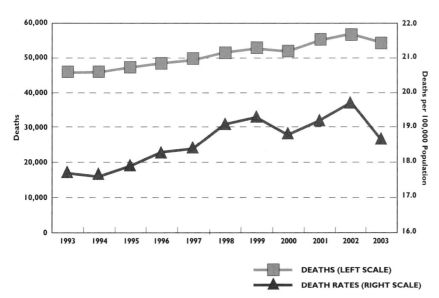

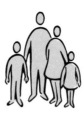

Between 1912 and 2003, public unintentional-injury deaths per 100,000 population were reduced 74% from 30 to 7.3 (after adjusting for the 1948 change in classification). In 1912, an estimated 28,000 to 30,000 persons died from public nonmotor-vehicle injuries. In 2003, with a population tripled, and travel and recreational activity greatly increased, only 21,300 persons died of public unintentional injuries and 7,100,000 suffered disabling injuries. The public class excludes deaths and injuries involving motor vehicles and persons at work or at home.

The number of public unintentional-injury deaths decreased by 300, or 1%, from the revised 2002 figure of 21,600. The death rate per 100,000 population decreased from 7.5 to 7.3, or 3%.

With an estimated 7,100,000 disabling unintentional injuries occurring in public places and a population of more than 290 million people, on average about 1 person in 41 experienced such an injury.

The Council adopted the Bureau of Labor Statistics' Census of Fatal Occupational Injuries count for work-related unintentional injuries retroactive to 1992 data. Because of the lower Work class total resulting from this change, several thousand unintentional-injury deaths that had been classified by the Council as work related had to be reassigned to the Home and Public classes. For this reason, long-term historical comparisons for these three classes should be made with caution. See the Technical Appendix for an explanation of the methodological changes.

Beginning with 1999 data, which became available in September 2001, deaths are now classified according to the 10th revision of the *International Classification of Diseases*. Overall, about 3% more deaths are classified as due to "unintentional injuries" under the new classification system than under the 9th revision. The difference varies across causes of death. See the Technical Appendix for more information on comparability. Caution should be used in comparing data classified under the two systems.

Deaths **21,300**
Disabling Injuries **7,100,000**
Death Rate per 100,000 Population **7.3**
Costs . . . . **$95.4 billion**

PUBLIC DEATHS AND DEATH RATES, UNITED STATES, 1993–2003

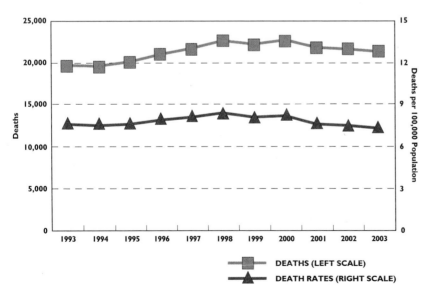

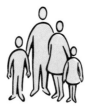

PUBLIC, 2003 (CONT.)

PRINCIPAL TYPES OF PUBLIC UNINTENTIONAL-INJURY DEATHS, UNITED STATES, 1983–2003

Year	Total Public[a]	Falls	Drowning	Poisoning	Suffocation by Ingestion	Fires/ Burns	Firearms	Mechanical Suffocation	Air Transport	Water Transport	Rail Transport[b]
1983	19,400	4,100	4,000	(c)	(c)	500	700	(c)	1,000	1,100	400
1984	18,300	4,100	3,300	(c)	(c)	500	700	(c)	900	900	400
1985	18,800	4,100	3,300	(c)	(c)	500	600	(c)	1,000	900	400
1986	18,700	3,900	3,600	(c)	(c)	500	600	(c)	800	900	400
1987	18,400	4,000	3,200	(c)	(c)	500	600	(c)	900	800	400
1988	18,400	4,100	3,100	(c)	(c)	500	600	(c)	700	800	400
1989	18,200	4,200	3,000	(c)	(c)	500	600	(c)	800	700	400
1990	17,400	4,300	2,800	(c)	(c)	400	500	(c)	700	800	400
1991	17,600	4,500	2,800	(c)	(c)	400	600	(c)	700	700	500
1992	19,000	4,400	2,500	(c)	(c)	200	400	(c)	700	700	600
1993	19,700	4,600	2,800	(c)	(c)	200	400	(c)	600	700	600
1994	19,600	4,700	2,400	(c)	(c)	200	400	(c)	600	600	600
1995	20,100	5,000	2,800	(c)	(c)	200	300	(c)	600	700	500
1996	21,000	5,300	2,500	(c)	(c)	200	300	(c)	700	600	500
1997	21,700	5,600	2,600	(c)	(c)	200	300	(c)	500	600	400
1998	22,600	6,000	2,900	(c)	(c)	200	300	(c)	500	600	500
1999[d]	22,200	4,800	2,600	2,800	2,000	200	300	500	500	600	400
2000	22,700	5,500	2,400	2,900	2,200	(c)	(c)	300	500	500	400
2001[e]	21,800	5,600	2,400	2,700	2,100	(c)	(c)	300	700	500	400
2002[e]	21,600	6,000	2,100	3,000	2,100	(c)	(c)	200	600	600	600
2003[f]	21,300	6,500	2,100	2,600	2,000	(c)	(c)	200	600	700	500

Source: National Safety Council estimates based on data from the National Center for Health Statistics and state vital statistics departments. The Council adopted the Bureau of Labor Statistics' Census of Fatal Occupational Injuries count for work-related unintentional injuries retroactive to 1992 data. Because of the lower Work class total resulting from this change, several thousand unintentional-injury deaths that had been classified by the Council as work-related, had to be reassigned to the Home and Public classes. For this reason long-term historical comparisons for these three classes should be made with caution. See the Technical Appendix for an explanation of the methodological changes.
[a] *Includes some deaths not shown separately.*
[b] *Includes subways and elevateds.*
[c] *Estimates not available.*
[d] *In 1999, a revision was made in the International Classification of Diseases. See the Technical Appendix for comparability with earlier years.*
[e] *Revised.*
[f] *Preliminary.*

PRINCIPAL TYPES OF PUBLIC UNINTENTIONAL-INJURY DEATHS, UNITED STATES, 2003

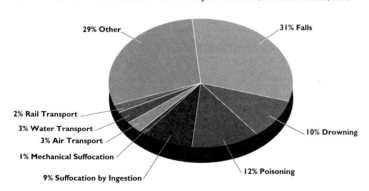

29% Other
31% Falls
10% Drowning
12% Poisoning
9% Suffocation by Ingestion
1% Mechanical Suffocation
3% Air Transport
3% Water Transport
2% Rail Transport

DEATHS DUE TO UNINTENTIONAL PUBLIC INJURIES, 2003

TYPE OF EVENT AND AGE OF VICTIM

All Public

Includes deaths in public places or places used in a public way and not involving motor vehicles. Most sports, recreation, and transportation deaths are included. Excludes deaths in the course of employment.

	Total	Change from 2002	Death Rate[a]
Deaths	21,300	−1%	7.3

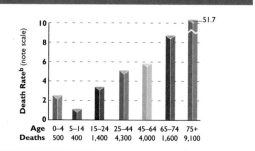

Falls

Includes deaths from falls from one level to another or on the same level in public places. Excludes deaths from falls in moving vehicles.

	Total	Change from 2002	Death Rate[a]
Deaths	6,500	+8%	2.2

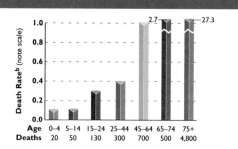

Poisoning

Includes deaths from drugs, medicines, other solid and liquid substances, and gases and vapors. Excludes poisonings from spoiled foods, salmonella, etc., which are classified as disease deaths.

	Total	Change from 2002	Death Rate[a]
Deaths	2,600	−13%	0.9

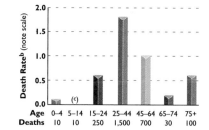

Drowning

Includes drownings of person swimming or playing in water, or falling into water, except on home premises or at work. Excludes drownings involving boats, which are in water transportation.

	Total	Change from 2002	Death Rate[a]
Deaths	2,100	0%	0.7

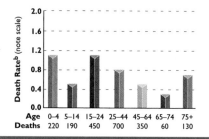

Choking

Includes deaths from unintentional ingestion or inhalation of food or other objects resulting in the obstruction of respiratory passages.

	Total	Change from 2002	Death Rate[a]
Deaths	2,000	−5%	0.7

See footnotes on page 125.

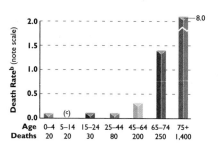

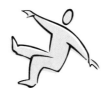

TYPE OF EVENT AND AGE OF VICTIM

Water Transport

Includes deaths in water transport accidents from falls, burns, etc., as well as drownings. Excludes crews and persons traveling in the course of employment.

	Total	Change from 2002	Death Rate[a]
Deaths	700	+17%	0.2

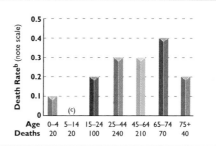

Age	0–4	5–14	15–24	25–44	45–64	65–74	75+
Deaths	20	20	100	240	210	70	40

Air Transport

Includes deaths in private flying, passengers in commercial aviation, and deaths of military personnel in the U.S. Excludes crews and persons traveling in the course of employment.

	Total	Change from 2002	Death Rate[a]
Deaths	600	0%	0.2

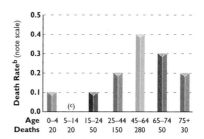

Age	0–4	5–14	15–24	25–44	45–64	65–74	75+
Deaths	20	20	50	150	280	50	30

Railroad

Includes deaths arising from railroad vehicles in motion (except involving motor vehicles), subway and elevated trains, and persons boarding or alighting from standing train. Excludes crews and persons traveling in the course of employment.

	Total	Change from 2002	Death Rate[a]
Deaths	500	–17%	0.2

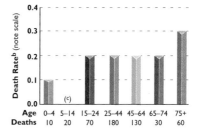

Age	0–4	5–14	15–24	25–44	45–64	65–74	75+
Deaths	10	20	70	180	130	30	60

Mechanical Suffocation

Includes deaths from hanging and strangulation, and suffocation in enclosed or confined spaces, cave-ins, or by bed clothes, plastic bags, or similar materials.

	Total	Change from 2002	Death Rate[a]
Deaths	200	0%	0.1

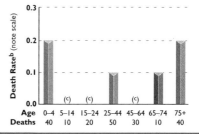

Age	0–4	5–14	15–24	25–44	45–64	65–74	75+
Deaths	40	10	20	50	30	10	40

All Other Public

Most important types included are: excessive natural heat or cold, firearms, fires and flames, and machinery.

	Total	Change from 2002	Death Rate[a]
Deaths	6,100	–5%	2.1

[a]Deaths per 100,000 population.
[b]Deaths per 100,000 population in each age group.
[c]Death rate less than 0.05.

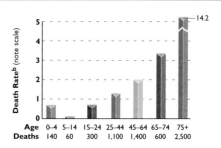

Age	0–4	5–14	15–24	25–44	45–64	65–74	75+
Deaths	140	60	300	1,100	1,400	600	2,500

Between 1912 and 2003, unintentional–home-injury deaths per 100,000 population were reduced 54% from 28 to 11.4 (after adjusting for the 1948 classification change). In 1912, when there were 21 million households, an estimated 26,000 to 28,000 persons were killed by unintentional home injuries. In 2003, with more than 107 million households and the population tripled, home deaths numbered 33,100.

The injury total of 7,900,000 means that 1 person in 37 in the United States was disabled one full day or more by unintentional injuries received in the home in 2003. Disabling injuries are more numerous in the home than in the workplace and in motor-vehicle crashes combined.

The National Health Interview Survey indicates that about 9,913,000 episodes of medically-attended home injuries occurred in 2002 (the latest year available). This means that about 1 person in 21 incurred a home injury requiring medical attention. About 42% of all medically attended injuries occurred at home. See page 23 for definitions and numerical differences between National Health Interview Survey and National Safety Council figures.

The Council adopted the Bureau of Labor Statistics' Census of Fatal Occupational Injuries count for work-related unintentional injuries retroactive to 1992 data. Because of the lower Work class total resulting from this change, several thousand unintentional-injury deaths that had been classified by the Council as work related had to be reassigned to the Home and Public classes. For this reason long-term historical comparisons for these three classes should be made with caution. See the Technical Appendix for an explanation of the methodological changes.

Beginning with 1999 data, which became available in September 2001, deaths are now classified according to the 10th revision of the *International Classification of Diseases*. Overall, about 3% more deaths are classified as due to "unintentional injuries" under the new classification system than under the 9th revision. The difference varies across causes of death. See the Technical Appendix for more information on comparability. Caution should be used in comparing data classified under the two systems.

Deaths **33,100**
Disabling Injuries **7,900,000**
Death Rate per 100,000 Population **11.4**
Costs . . . . **$135.1 billion**

HOME DEATHS AND DEATH RATES, UNITED STATES, 1993–2003

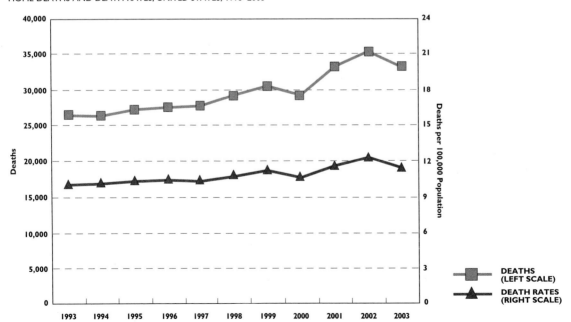

PRINCIPAL TYPES OF HOME UNINTENTIONAL-INJURY DEATHS, UNITED STATES, 1983–2003

Year	Total Home	Falls	Fires/Burns[a]	Suffocation, Ing. Obj.	Suffocation, Mechanical	Drowning	Poisoning	Natural Heat/Cold	Firearms	Other
1983	21,200	6,500	4,100	2,200	600	(b)	3,500	(b)	900	3,400
1984	21,200	6,400	4,100	2,300	600	(b)	3,700	(b)	900	3,200
1985	21,600	6,500	4,000	2,400	600	(b)	3,900	(b)	900	3,300
1986	21,700	6,100	4,000	2,500	600	(b)	4,300	(b)	800	3,400
1987	21,400	6,300	3,900	2,500	600	(b)	4,100	(b)	800	3,200
1988	22,700	6,600	4,100	2,600	600	(b)	4,800	(b)	800	3,200
1989	22,500	6,600	3,900	2,500	600	(b)	5,000	(b)	800	3,100
1990	21,500	6,700	3,400	2,300	600	(b)	4,500	(b)	800	3,200
1991	22,100	6,900	3,400	2,200	700	(b)	5,000	(b)	800	3,100
1992	24,000	7,700	3,700	1,500	700	900	5,200	(b)	1,000	3,300
1993	26,100	7,900	3,700	1,700	700	900	6,500	(b)	1,100	3,600
1994	26,300	8,100	3,700	1,600	800	900	6,800	(b)	900	3,500
1995	27,200	8,400	3,500	1,500	800	900	7,000	(b)	900	4,200
1996	27,500	9,000	3,500	1,500	800	900	7,300	(b)	800	3,700
1997	27,700	9,100	3,200	1,500	800	900	7,800	(b)	700	3,500
1998	29,000	9,500	2,900	1,800	800	1,000	8,400	(b)	600	4,000
1999c	30,500	7,600	3,000	1,900	1,100	900	9,300	700	600	5,400
2000	29,200	7,100	2,700	2,100	1,000	1,000	9,800	400	500	4,600
2001d	33,200	8,600	3,000	2,000	1,100	900	11,300	400	600	5,300
2002d	35,300	8,600	2,500	2,200	1,300	900	13,000	300	500	6,000
2003e	33,100	9,000	2,300	2,200	1,000	700	11,200	300	400	6,000

Source: National Safety Council estimates based on data from National Center for Health Statistics and state vital statistics departments. The Council adopted the Bureau of Labor Statistics' Census of Fatal Occupational Injuries count for work-related unintentional injuries retroactive to 1992 data. Because of the lower Work class total resulting from this change, several thousand unintentional-injury deaths that had been classified by the Council as work-related, had to be reassigned to the Home and Public classes. For this reason long-term historical comparisons for these three classes should be made with caution. See the Technical Appendix for an explanation of the methodological changes.
a Includes deaths resulting from conflagration, regardless of nature of injury.
b Included in Other.
c In 1999, a revision was made in the International Classification of Diseases. See the Technical Appendix for comparability with earlier years.
d Revised.
e Preliminary.

PRINCIPAL TYPES OF HOME UNINTENTIONAL-INJURY DEATHS, UNITED STATES, 2003

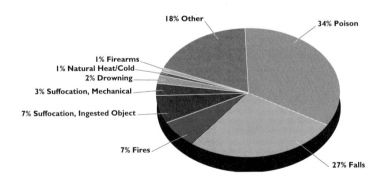

18% Other
34% Poison
1% Firearms
1% Natural Heat/Cold
2% Drowning
3% Suffocation, Mechanical
7% Suffocation, Ingested Object
7% Fires
27% Falls

DEATHS DUE TO UNINTENTIONAL HOME INJURIES, 2003

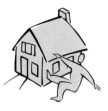

TYPE OF EVENT AND AGE OF VICTIM

All Home

Includes deaths in the home and on home premises to occupants, guests, and trespassers. Also includes hired household workers but excludes other persons working on home premises.

	Total	Change from 2002	Death Rate[a]
Deaths	33,100	–6%	11.4

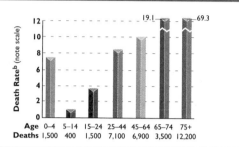

Poisoning

Includes deaths from drugs, medicines, other solid and liquid substances, and gases and vapors. Excludes poisonings from spoiled foods, salmonella, etc., which are classified as disease deaths.

	Total	Change from 2002	Death Rate[a]
Deaths	11,200	–14%	3.9

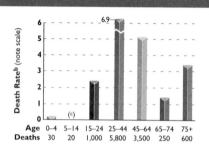

Falls

Includes deaths from falls from one level to another or on the same level in the home or on home premises.

	Total	Change from 2002	Death Rate[a]
Deaths	9,000	+5%	3.1

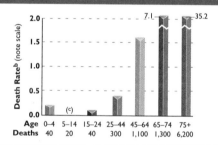

Fires, Flames, and Smoke

Includes deaths from fires, smoke, and injuries in conflagrations in the home — such as asphyxiation, falls, and struck by falling objects. Excludes burns from hot objects or liquids.

	Total	Change from 2002	Death Rate[a]
Deaths	2,300	–8%	0.8

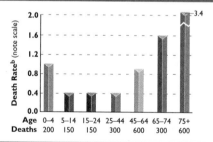

Choking

Includes deaths from unintentional ingestion or inhalation of objects or food resulting in the obstruction of respiratory passages.

	Total	Change from 2002	Death Rate[a]
Deaths	2,200	0%	0.8

See footnotes on page 137.

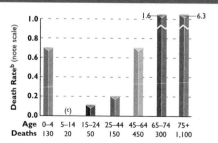

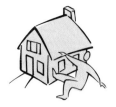

TYPE OF EVENT AND AGE OF VICTIM

Mechanical Suffocation

Includes deaths from smothering by bed clothes, thin plastic materials, etc.; suffocation by cave-ins or confinement in closed spaces; and mechanical strangulation and hanging.

	Total	Change from 2002	Death Rate[a]
Deaths	1,000	−23%	0.3

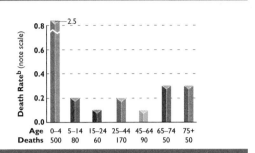

Age	0–4	5–14	15–24	25–44	45–64	65–74	75+
Deaths	500	80	60	170	90	50	50

Drowning

Includes drownings of persons in or on home premises — such as in swimming pools and bathtubs. Excludes drowning in floods and other cataclysms.

	Total	Change from 2002	Death Rate[a]
Deaths	700	−22%	0.2

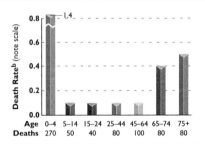

Age	0–4	5–14	15–24	25–44	45–64	65–74	75+
Deaths	270	50	40	80	100	80	80

Firearms

Includes firearms injuries in or on home premises — such as while cleaning or playing with guns. Excludes deaths from explosive materials.

	Total	Change from 2002	Death Rate[a]
Deaths	400	−20%	0.1

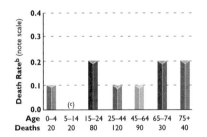

Age	0–4	5–14	15–24	25–44	45–64	65–74	75+
Deaths	20	20	80	120	90	30	40

Natural Heat or Cold

Includes deaths resulting from exposure to excessive natural heat and cold (e.g., extreme weather conditions).

	Total	Change from 2002	Death Rate[a]
Deaths	300	0%	0.1

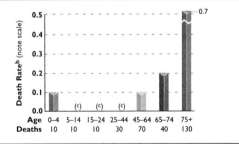

Age	0–4	5–14	15–24	25–44	45–64	65–74	75+
Deaths	10	10	10	30	70	40	130

All Other Home

Most important types included are: struck by or against objects, machinery, and electric current.

	Total	Change from 2002	Death Rate[a]
Deaths	6,000	0%	2.1

[a]Deaths per 100,000 population.
[b]Deaths per 100,000 population in each age group.
[c]Death rate less than 0.05.

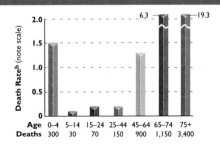

Age	0–4	5–14	15–24	25–44	45–64	65–74	75+
Deaths	300	30	70	150	900	1,150	3,400

SPORTS AND RECREATION INJURIES

Basketball injuries accounted for more than 615,000 emergency department visits in 2002.

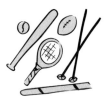

The table below shows estimates of injuries treated in hospital emergency departments and participants associated with various sports and recreational activities. Differences between the two sources in methods, coverage, classification systems, and definitions can affect comparisons among sports. Because this list of sports is not complete, because the frequency and duration of participation is not known, and because the number of participants varies greatly, no inference should be made concerning the relative hazard of these sports or rank with respect to risk of injury. In particular, it is *not* appropriate to calculate injury rates from these data.

SPORTS PARTICIPATION AND INJURIES, UNITED STATES, 2002

Sport or Activity	Participants	Injuries	Percent of Injuries by Age				
			0–4	5–14	15–24	25–64	65 & Over
Archery	4,200,000	4,306	2.3	17.7	17.1	61.4	1.6
Baseball	15,600,000	178,668	3.7	50.2	26.1	19.6	0.3
Basketball	28,900,000	615,546	0.3	33.7	45.3	20.5	0.1
Bicycle riding[a]	41,400,000	521,328	6.1	52.3	14.7	24.6	2.3
Billiards, pool	35,300,000	6,235	7.8	20.3	23.9	43.6	4.4
Bowling	43,900,000	21,133	7.9	16.5	16.9	50.9	7.8
Boxing	1,700,000[b]	11,811	1.0	13.2	55.7	29.9	0.1
Exercise	[c]	191,502[d]	3.5	17.9	21.0	49.3	8.1
Fishing	44,200,000	68,743	3.6	21.9	14.3	51.3	8.8
Football	17,700,000[e]	387,948	0.2	48.4	41.4	9.9	0.1
Golf	28,300,000	39,470[f]	6.5	23.0	8.2	45.3	17.0
Gymnastics	[c]	29,678[g]	3.9	71.4	20.0	4.7	0.0
Hockey, street, roller & field	[c]	11,073[h]	0.2	44.8	39.4	15.6	0.0
Horseback riding	9,500,000[i]	70,704	1.7	17.3	20.7	58.4	1.9
Horseshoe pitching	9,100,000[i]	2,125	19.6	16.8	10.4	45.6	7.5
Ice hockey	2,100,000	16,435[j]	0.2	29.4	47.5	22.7	0.3
Ice skating	5,300,000[b]	26,118	2.6	52.6	15.4	27.2	2.2
Martial arts	4,200,000	28,607	1.3	25.5	30.6	42.0	0.6
Mountain climbing	3,400,000[i]	4,056	0.1	10.4	39.2	50.2	0.0
Racquetball, squash & paddleball	3,400,000[b]	8,948	0.2	7.6	27.5	63.2	1.6
Roller skating	26,900,000[b]	106,531[k,l]	0.9	60.7	14.6	23.4	0.4
Rugby	[c]	12,253	0.0	2.6	72.8	24.6	0.0
Scuba diving	[c]	2,335	0.0	3.8	7.9	84.1	4.2
Skateboarding	9,700,000	113,192	1.9	53.1	36.1	8.7	0.2
Snowboarding	5,600,000	63,014	0.0	36.3	42.9	20.7	0.1
Snowmobiling	4,600,000[b]	12,862	1.1	9.7	24.1	64.6	0.5
Soccer	14,500,000	173,519	0.5	43.9	37.5	18.0	0.0
Softball	13,600,000	125,875	0.4	21.6	29.7	47.4	0.9
Swimming	54,700,000	168,529[m]	8.8	43.7	18.2	26.5	2.8
Tennis	11,000,000	19,633	0.8	15.0	17.7	51.4	15.1
Track & field	[c]	19,608	0.0	44.8	50.8	4.1	0.3
Volleyball	11,500,000	59,225	0.2	28.0	39.0	32.3	0.5
Water skiing	6,900,000	9,515	0.1	9.0	36.4	54.6	0.0
Weight lifting	21,200,000[b]	71,699	3.9	10.6	36.7	46.9	1.9
Wrestling	3,500,000[b]	36,702	0.1	37.0	55.8	6.9	0.2

Source: Participants — National Sporting Goods Association; figures include those seven years of age or older who participated more than once per year except for bicycle riding and swimming, which include those who participated six or more time per year. Injuries — Consumer Product Safety Commission; figures include only injuries treated in hospital emergency departments.
[a] Excludes mountain biking.
[b] Participation for 2001.
[c] Data not available.
[d] Includes exercise equipment (38,098 injuries) and exercise activity (153,404 injuries).
[e] Includes 10,300,000 in touch football and 7,400,000 tackle football.
[f] Excludes golf carts (10,623 injuries).
[g] Excludes trampolines (89,393 injuries).
[h] There were 4,621 injuries in field hockey, 3,289 in roller hockey, and 3,163 in street hockey.
[i] Participation for 2000.
[j] Excludes 35,447 injuries in hockey, unspecified.
[k] Excludes 21,049 injuries in skating, unspecified.
[l] Includes 2x2 (45,959 injuries) and in-line (60,572 injuries).
[m] Includes injuries associated with swimming, swimming pools, pool slides, diving or diving boards, and swimming pool equipment.

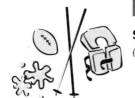

Paintball

A recent study quantified and characterized injuries associated with paintball games and treated in hospital emergency departments. Data on injuries were collected through the National Electronic Injury Surveillance System from 1997 to 2001. Over the five-year period, an estimated 11,998 persons ages seven and older were treated in emergency departments. Almost all (94.0%) were males and 95.5% were treated and released. As with other sports, there are probably many more cases treated in outpatient clinics or physician's offices, or not medically attended.

Overall, about 59.8% of the injuries were from being shot by a paintball, but the proportion was greater among players 7–17 years old (76.9%) compared to players 18 and older (45.5%). Overexertion was the second most common cause of injury accounting for 17.9% of all cases. Overexertion was more common among older players (39.1%) than younger players (12.6%). Falls were the third most common type of injury — 9.3% of all cases.

The locale where the injury occurred was home or home premises in 28.4% of the cases, a sports arena in 26.3%, a public street in 7.6%, and unknown in 37.7%.

Source: Conn, J.M., Annest, J.L., Gilchrist, J., & Ryan, G.W. (2004). Injuries from paintball game related activities in the United States, 1997–2001. Injury Prevention, 10, 139–143.

ESTIMATED PAINTBALL GAME–RELATED INJURIES TREATED IN HOSPITAL EMERGENCY DEPARTMENTS, UNITED STATES, 1997–2001

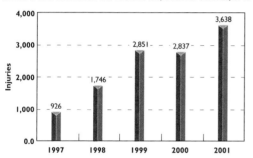

PAINTBALL GAME–RELATED INJURIES BY AGE GROUP, UNITED STATES, 1997–2001

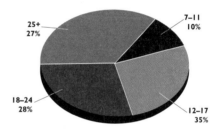

Older Americans' Recreational Injuries

Americans ages 65 and older are a growing segment of the population, and they are urged to participate in recreational activities to maintain health. A consequence of these two factors could be a growth in recreational injuries among this age group. A new study developed a profile of the recreational injuries currently experienced by older adults. Data for 2001 from the National Electronic Injury Surveillance System — All Injury Program was used to characterize the injuries.

There were an estimated 62,164 injuries sustained while participating in recreational activities and treated in

hospital emergency departments. Two thirds of the cases (66.3%) involved persons 65–74 years old, 29.3% were 75–84 years old, and 4.4% were 85 or older. About one fourth (26.5%) of the injuries were fractures, 21.8% were sprains/strains, 16.2% were contusions/abrasions, 12.6% lacerations, 4.5% internal injuries, and 18.5% other kinds of injuries.

The authors point out that even seemingly minor injuries in this age group may have long-term consequences affecting the person's ability to perform activities of daily living and thus to function independently.

ACTIVITIES ASSOCIATED WITH RECREATIONAL INJURIES TO PERSONS 65 AND OLDER, UNITED STATES, 2001

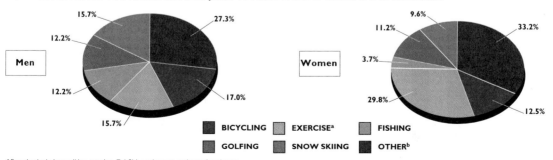

[a] Exercise includes walking, running, Tai Chi, equipment, and exercise classes.
[b] Includes more than 30 different activities.

Source: Gerson, L.W., & Stevens, J.A. (2004). Recreational injuries among older Americans, 2001. Injury Prevention, 10, 134–138.

WEATHER

Floods caused 23% of weather-related deaths in 2003.

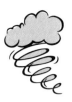

A variety of weather events resulted in 348 deaths in the 50 United States and District of Columbia in 2003, according to data compiled by the National Climatic Data Center (NCDC), which is part of the National Oceanic and Atmospheric Administration. Twenty three percent of those deaths were due to floods. Temperature extremes and tornadoes each accounted for 16%. Data

compiled by the NCDC may differ from data based on death certificates that appears elsewhere in *Injury Facts*.

May had the most weather-related deaths because of the high number of deaths associated with tornadoes. July ranked second because of deaths related to temperature extremes and lightning that month. August was third highest due mainly to floods and lightning.

WEATHER-RELATED FATALITIES BY MONTH, UNITED STATES, 2003

Event	Total	Jan	Feb	Mar	Apr	May	Jun	Jul	Aug	Sep	Oct	Nov	Dec
Total	**348**	**22**	**29**	**17**	**16**	**64**	**28**	**58**	**41**	**20**	**9**	**28**	**16**
Flood	81	0	7	0	5	14	14	11	15	1	2	10	2
Temperature extreme	56	14	4	3	0	0	7	21	7	0	0	0	0
Tornado	55	0	2	8	0	42	2	0	0	0	1	0	0
Lightning	43	0	1	0	3	1	4	14	13	5	2	0	0
Thunderstorm and high wind	41	2	1	3	1	2	1	11	3	1	2	12	2
Snow and ice	36	2	12	3	5	0	0	0	0	0	2	0	12
Hurricane and tropical storm	12	0	0	0	0	0	0	1	0	11	0	0	0
Ocean/lake surf	12	0	1	0	2	4	0	0	0	2	0	3	0
Fog	5	2	0	0	0	0	0	0	0	0	0	3	0
Precipitation (without flood)	5	0	1	0	0	1	0	0	3	0	0	0	0
Dust storm	2	2	0	0	0	0	0	0	0	0	0	0	0
Hail	0	0	0	0	0	0	0	0	0	0	0	0	0
Wild/forest fire	0	0	0	0	0	0	0	0	0	0	0	0	0
Drought	0	0	0	0	0	0	0	0	0	0	0	0	0

Source: National Safety Council tabulations of National Climatic Data Center data.

WEATHER-RELATED FATALITIES BY MONTH, UNITED STATES, 2003

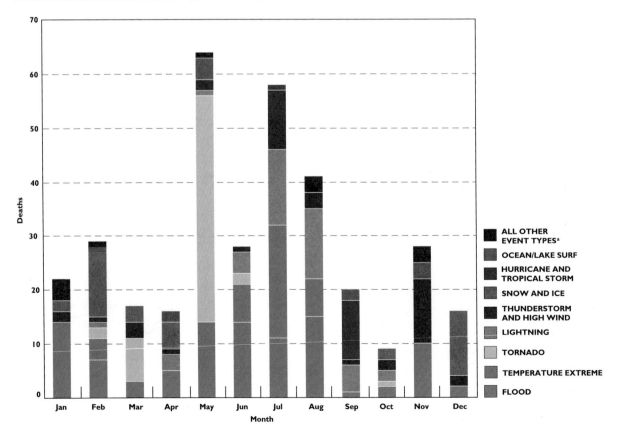

[a] Includes fog, precipitation (without flood), and dust storm.

Firearm-related deaths from unintentional, intentional, and undetermined causes totaled 29,573 in 2001, an increase of 3.2% from 2000. Suicides accounted for 57% of firearms deaths, about 38% were homicides, and almost 3% were unintentional deaths. Males dominate all categories of firearms deaths and accounted for more than 86% of the total.

The numbers of homicide, suicide, and unintentional deaths by firearms increased in 2001 following 7 years of decreases. Compared to 2000, homicides were up

5.1%, suicides were up 1.7%, and unintentional deaths increased 3.4%.

Hospital emergency department surveillance data indicate an estimated 17,696 nonfatal unintentional firearm-related injuries in 2001. For assault there were an estimated 41,044 nonfatal injuries and 3,267 intentionally self-inflicted nonfatal injuries.

Source: National Safety Council analysis of National Center for Health Statistics mortality data and National Center for Injury Prevention and Control injury surveillance data using WISQARS™ (http://www.cdc.gov/ncipc/wisqars/).

DEATHS INVOLVING FIREARMS, BY AGE AND SEX, UNITED STATES, 2001

Type & Sex	All Ages	Under 5 Years	5–14 Years	15–19 Years	20–24 Years	25–44 Years	45–64 Years	65–74 Years	75 & Over
Total Firearms Deaths	29,573	81	333	2,523	4,164	11,425	6,664	1,998	2,385
Male	25,480	46	249	2,270	3,796	9,659	5,532	1,754	2,174
Female	4,093	35	84	253	368	1,766	1,132	244	211
Unintentional	802	15	57	110	96	268	172	33	51
Male	690	12	49	102	91	224	142	26	44
Female	112	3	8	8	5	44	30	7	7
Suicide	16,869	—	90	838	1,292	5,594	5,106	1,758	2,191
Male	14,758	—	69	743	1,192	4,797	4,322	1,592	2,043
Female	2,111	—	21	95	100	797	784	166	148
Homicide	11,348	66	180	1,525	2,675	5,286	1,298	192	126
Male	9,532	34	125	1,377	2,419	4,392	990	123	72
Female	1,816	32	55	148	256	894	308	69	54
Legal Intervention	323	0	0	26	61	179	47	5	5
Male	310	0	0	25	58	171	46	5	5
Female	13	0	0	1	3	8	1	0	0
Undetermined[a]	231	0	6	24	40	98	41	10	12
Male	190	0	6	23	36	75	32	8	10
Female	41	0	0	1	4	23	9	2	2

[a]*Undetermined means the intentionality of the deaths (unintentional, homicide, suicide) was not determined.*

FIREARMS DEATHS BY INTENTIONALITY AND YEAR, UNITED STATES, 1992–2001

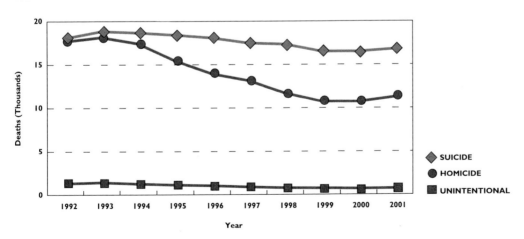

TRANSPORTATION MODE COMPARISONS

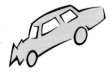

Passenger transportation incidents account for over one-fifth of all unintentional-injury deaths. But the risk of death to the passenger, expressed on a per mile basis, varies greatly by transportation mode. Highway travel by personal vehicle presents the greatest risk; air, rail, and bus travel have much lower death rates. The tables below show the latest information on passenger transportation deaths and death rates.

The statistics for automobiles, vans, sport utility vehicles (SUVs), pickups, and other light trucks shown in the tables below represent all passenger vehicle usage, both intercity and local. The bus data also include intercity and local (transit) bus travel. Railroad includes both intercity (Amtrak) and local commuting travel. Scheduled airlines includes both large airlines and commuter airlines but excludes on-demand air taxis and charter operations. In comparing the four modes, drivers of automobiles (except taxis), vans, SUVs, and pickup trucks are considered passengers. Bus drivers and airline or railroad crews are not considered passengers.

Other comparisons are possible based on passenger-trips, vehicle-miles, or vehicle-trips, but passenger-miles is the most commonly used basis for comparing the safety of various modes of travel.

TRANSPORTATION ACCIDENT DEATH RATES, 2000–2002

Mode of Transportation	2002			2000–2002 Average Death Rate
	Passenger Deaths	Passenger Miles (billions)	Deaths per 100.000.000 Passenger Miles	
Passenger automobiles[a]	20,408	2,637.2	0.77	0.79
Vans, SUVs, pickup trucks[b]	12,186	1,584.0	0.77	0.76
Buses[c]	36	62.2	0.06	0.03
Transit buses	6	22.0	0.03	0.01
Intercity buses	18	40.2	0.05	0.02
Railroad passenger trains[d]	7	15.7	0.04	0.03
Scheduled airlines[e]	0	518.3	0.00	0.02

Source: Highway passenger deaths — Fatality Analysis Reporting System data. Railroad passenger deaths — Federal Railroad Administration. Airline passenger deaths — National Transportation Safety Board. Passenger miles for transit buses — American Public Transit Association. All other figures — National Safety Council estimates.
[a]Includes taxi passengers. Drivers of passenger automobiles are considered passengers.
[b]Includes 2-axle, 4-tire vehicles under 10,000 lbs GVWR other than automobiles.
[c]Figures exclude school buses but include "other" and "unknown" bus types.
[d]Includes Amtrak and commuter rail service.
[e]Includes large airlines and scheduled commuter airlines; excludes charter, cargo, and on-demand service and suicide/sabotage.

PASSENGER DEATHS AND DEATH RATES, UNITED STATES, 1993–2002

Year	Passenger Automobiles		Vans, SUVs, Pickup Trucks		Buses		Railroad Passenger Trains		Scheduled Airlines	
	Deaths	Rate[a]	Deaths	Rate[a]	Deaths	Rate[a]	Deaths	Rate[a]	Deaths	Rate[a]
1993	21,414	0.86	—	—	9	0.02	58	0.45	19	0.01
1994	21,813	0.91	—	—	13	0.03	5	0.04	245	0.06
1995	22,288	0.97	—	—	16	0.03	0	0.00	159	0.04
1996	22,359	0.96	—	—	10	0.02	12	0.09	329	0.08
1997	21,920	0.92	—	—	4	0.01	6	0.05	42	0.01
1998	21,099	0.86	—	—	26	0.05	4	0.03	0	0.00
1999	20,763	0.83	10,666	0.72	39	0.07	14	0.10	17	0.003
2000	20,444	0.80	11,435	0.76	3	0.01	4	0.03	87	0.02
2001	20,221	0.79	11,690	0.76	11	0.02	3	0.02	279	0.06
2002	20,408	0.77	12,186	0.77	36	0.06	7	0.04	0	0.00
10-year average	21,273	0.86	—	—	17	0.03	11	0.08	118	0.03

Source: See table above. Note: Dashes (—) indicate data not available.
[a]Deaths per 100,000,000 passenger miles.

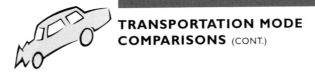
PASSENGER DEATH RATES, UNITED STATES, 2000–2002

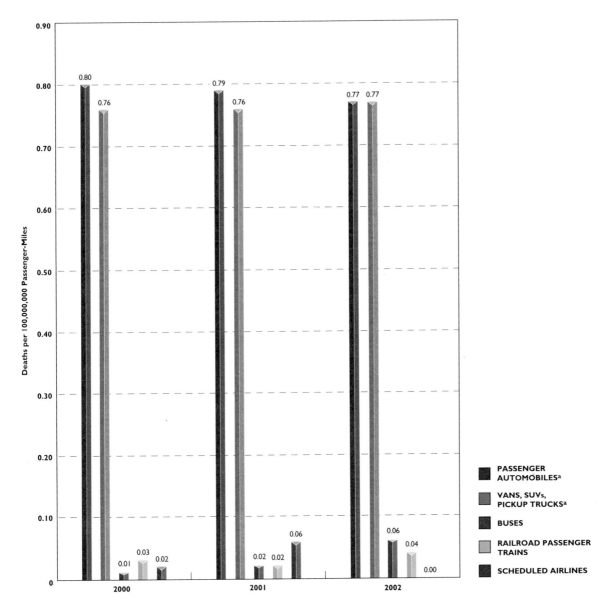

PASSENGER
AUTOMOBILES[a]

VANS, SUVs,
PICKUP TRUCKS[a]

BUSES

RAILROAD PASSENGER
TRAINS

SCHEDULED AIRLINES

[a]Drivers of these vehicles are considered passengers.

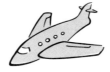
International Civil Aviation Organization (ICAO) data show that in 2003, there were 334 passenger fatalities. This figure is the lowest since 1984 and represents a 58% decrease compared to 2002, when 791 passenger deaths were recorded. ICAO, a specialized United Nations agency with 188 member states, reported a total of six aircraft accidents with passenger fatalities — the lowest since 1945. The death rate per 100 million passenger-kilometers showed a great improvement, declining from 0.025 in 2002 to 0.01 in 2003.

WORLDWIDE SCHEDULED AIR SERVICE ACCIDENTS, DEATHS, AND DEATH RATES, 1988–2003

Year	Fatal Accidents[a]	Passenger Deaths	Death Rate[b]	Year	Fatal Accidents[a]	Passenger Deaths	Death Rate[b]
1988	29	742	0.04	1996	24	1,146	0.05
1989	29	879	0.05	1997	25	921	0.04
1990	27	544	0.03	1998	20	904	0.03
1991	29	638	0.03	1999	21	499	0.02
1992	28	1,070	0.06	2000	18	757	0.03
1993	33	864	0.04	2001	13	577	0.02
1994	27	1,170	0.05	2002	13	791	0.025
1995	25	711	0.03	2003[c]	6	334	0.01

Source: International Civil Aviation Organization. Figures include the USSR up to 1992 and the Commonwealth of Independent States thereafter.
[a]Involving a passenger fatality and an aircraft with maximum take-off mass >2,250 kg.
[b]Passenger deaths per 100 million passenger kilometers.
[c]Preliminary.

U.S. CIVIL AVIATION ACCIDENTS, DEATHS, AND DEATH RATES, 1999–2003

| | Accidents | | | Accident Rates | | | |
| | | | | Per 100,000 Flight-Hours | | Per Million Aircraft-Miles | |
Year	Total	Fatal	Deaths[a]	Total	Fatal	Total	Fatal
Large Airlines[b]							
1999	46	2	12	0.276	0.012	0.0069	0.0003
2000	50	3	92	0.286	0.017	0.0070	0.0004
2001[c]	42	6	531	0.221	0.012	0.0054	0.0003
2002	34	0	0	0.207	0	0.0050	0
2003	52	2	22	0.313	0.012	0.0076	0.0003
Commuter Airlines[b]							
1999	13	5	12	3.793	1.459	0.2481	0.0954
2000	12	1	5	3.247	0.271	0.2670	0.0222
2001	7	2	13	2.330	0.666	0.1624	0.0464
2002	8	0	0	3.181	0	0.2192	0
2003	2	1	2	0.720	0.360	0.0486	0.0243
On-Demand Air Taxis[b]							
1999	73	12	38	2.28	0.37	—	—
2000	80	22	71	2.04	0.56	—	—
2001	72	18	60	2.40	0.60	—	—
2002	59	18	35	2.03	0.62	—	—
2003	77	19	45	2.61	0.64	—	—
General Aviation[b]							
1999[c]	1,905	340	619	6.50	1.16	—	—
2000[c]	1,837	345	596	6.57	1.21	—	—
2001[c]	1,726	325	562	6.78	1.27	—	—
2002[c]	1,713	345	581	6.69	1.33	—	—
2003	1,732	351	626	6.71	1.36	—	—

Source: National Transportation Safety Board: 2003 preliminary, 1999–2002 revised; exposure data for rates from Federal Aviation Administration.
Note: Dash (—) indicates data not available.
[a]Includes passengers, crew members, and others such as persons on the ground.
[b]Civil aviation accident statistics collected by the National Transportation Safety Board are classified according to the Federal air regulations under which the flights were made. The classifications are (1) large airlines operating scheduled service under Title 14, Code of Federal Regulations, part 121 (14 CFR 121); (2) commuter carriers operating scheduled service under 14 CFR 135; (3) unscheduled, "on-demand" air taxis under 14 CFR 135; and (4) "general aviation," which includes accidents involving aircraft flown under rules other than 14 CFR 121 and 14 CFR 135. Not shown in the table is nonscheduled air carrier operations under 14 CFR 121 which experienced two accidents and no fatalities in 2003. Since 1997, Large Airlines includes aircraft with 10 or more seats, formerly operated as commuter carriers under 14 CFR 135.
[c]Suicide/sabotage and stolen/unauthorized cases are included in "accident" and fatality totals but excluded from rates — Large Airlines, 2001 (4 crashes/265 deaths); General Aviation, 1999 (3/1), 2000 (7/7), 2001 (3/1), 2002 (5/5).

RAILROAD

Between 1994 and 2003, the total number of rail-related deaths and nonfatal conditions[a] declined by 30% and 47%, respectively. During this period, highway-rail crossing accidents/incidents accounted for 56% of all rail-related deaths and 88% of nonfatal conditions. Trespassers represented 90% of deaths and 4% of nonfatal conditions not associated with highway-rail crossing incidents.

In 2003, highway-rail incidents and trespassing resulted in 96% of all rail-related deaths. About 58% of deaths not associated with highway-rail incidents or trespassing were to employees on duty. Passengers on trains[b] and persons lawfully on railroad property accounted for the remainder.

[a]Includes injuries and illnesses. In 2003, injuries to on-duty railroad employees accounted for 68% of all nonfatal conditions.
[b]Passengers on trains are persons on, boarding, or alighting train, other than employees.

DEATHS AND NONFATAL CASES IN RAILROAD ACCIDENTS AND INCIDENTS, UNITED STATES, 1994–2003

Year	Total	Highway-Rail Crossing Incident?		Occuring in Other Than Highway-Rail Crossing Incident		Employees On Duty At Highway-Rail Crossing?		Passengers on Trains[a] At Highway-Rail Crossing?	
		Yes	No	Trespassers	Others	Yes	No	Yes	No
Deaths									
1994	1,226	615	611	529	82	1	30	0	5
1995	1,146	579	567	494	73	2	32	0	0
1996	1,039	488	551	471	80	1	32	0	12
1997	1,063	461	602	533	69	0	37	0	6
1998	1,008	431	577	536	41	4	23	2	2
1999	932	402	530	479	51	2	29	11	3
2000	937	425	512	463	49	2	22	0	4
2001	971	421	550	511	39	1	21	0	3
2002	951	357	594	540	53	1	19	0	7
2003	858	324	534	503	31	1	18	0	2
Nonfatal conditions									
1994	16,812	1,961	14,851	452	14,399	125	12,955	84	413
1995	14,440	1,894	12,546	461	12,085	123	10,654	30	543
1996	12,558	1,610	10,948	474	10,474	79	9,120	24	489
1997	11,767	1,540	10,227	516	9,711	111	8,184	43	558
1998	11,459	1,303	10,156	513	9,643	122	8,276	19	516
1999	11,700	1,396	10,304	445	9,859	140	8,482	43	438
2000	11,643	1,219	10,424	414	10,010	100	8,323	10	648
2001	10,985	1,157	9,828	404	9,424	97	7,718	20	726
2002	11,103	999	10,104	395	9,709	110	6,534	26	851
2003	8,839	995	7,844	394	7,450	73	5,933	59	569

Source: Federal Railroad Administration.
[a]Passengers on trains are persons on, boarding, or alighting, other than railroad employees.

HIGHWAY-RAIL GRADE-CROSSING CASUALTIES, UNITED STATES, 1994–2003

Year	Deaths				Nonfatal Conditions			
	Total	Motor-Vehicles	Pedestrians	Others	Total	Motor-Vehicles	Pedestrians	Others
1994	615	542	50	23	1,961	1,885	30	46
1995	579	508	47	24	1,894	1,825	28	41
1996	488	415	60	13	1,610	1,545	31	34
1997	461	419	38	4	1,540	1,494	33	13
1998	431	369	50	12	1,303	1,257	33	13
1999	402	345	45	12	1,396	1,338	35	23
2000	425	361	51	13	1,219	1,169	34	16
2001	421	345	67	9	1,157	1,110	31	16
2002	357	310	35	12	999	939	29	31
2003	324	263	49	12	996	949	27	20

Source: Federal Railroad Administration. Includes both public and private grade crossings.

UNINTENTIONAL POISONINGS

Poisoning deaths up 10% from 2000 to 2001.

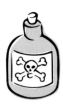

Deaths from unintentional poisoning numbered 14,078 in 2001, the latest year for which data are available. The overall death rate per 100,000 population was 4.9 — 7.1 for males and 2.9 for females. Total poisoning deaths increased approximately 10% from 12,757 in 2000 and have more than doubled since 1991. See pages 42–45 for long-term trends.

Almost half of the poisoning deaths (46%) were classified in the "narcotics and psychodysleptics (hallucinogens), not elsewhere classified," category, which includes many illegal drugs such as cocaine, heroin, cannabinol, and LSD.

Carbon monoxide poisoning is included in the category of "other gases and vapors." Deaths due to alcohol poisoning numbered 303 in 2001, but alcohol may also be present in combination with other drugs.

In 2002, nearly 2.4 million human poisoning exposure cases, both fatal and nonfatal, were reported to 64 poison control centers, which served 99.8% of the U.S. population. That is equivalent to about 8.2 reported exposures per 1,000 population, according to the American Association of Poison Control Centers.

UNINTENTIONAL POISONING DEATHS BY TYPE, AGE, AND SEX, UNITED STATES, 2001

Type of Poison	All Ages	0–4 Years	5–14 Years	15–19 Years	20–24 Years	25–44 Years	45–64 Years	65 Years & Over
Both Sexes								
Total Poisoning Deaths	**14,078**	**46**	**50**	**406**	**956**	**7,543**	**4,345**	**732**
Deaths per 100,000 population	*4.9*	*0.2*	*0.1*	*2.0*	*4.9*	*8.9*	*6.7*	*2.1*
Nonopioid analgesics, antipyretics, and antirheumatics (X40)[a]	208	3	1	1	4	88	68	43
Antiepileptic, sedative-hypnotic, antiparkinsonism, and psychotropic drugs, n.e.c. (X41)	763	3	5	30	49	390	252	34
Narcotics and psychodysleptics (hallucinogens), n.e.c. (X42)	6,509	8	7	180	460	3,711	2,047	96
Other drugs acting on the autonomic nervous system (X43)	19	0	0	1	0	9	7	2
Other and unspecified drugs, medicaments, and biological substances (X44)	5,525	13	10	140	372	2,963	1,658	369
Alcohol (X45)	303	0	0	8	10	154	122	9
Organic solvents and halogenated hydrocarbons and their vapors (X46)	63	1	4	7	5	30	11	5
Other gases and vapors (X47)	593	15	22	35	49	175	148	149
Pesticides (X48)	7	2	0	0	0	3	0	2
Other and unspecified chemical and noxious substances (X49)	88	1	1	4	7	20	32	23
Males								
Total Poisoning Deaths	**9,885**	**29**	**23**	**311**	**769**	**5,384**	**3,003**	**366**
Deaths per 100,000 population	*7.1*	*0.3*	*0.1*	*3.0*	*7.6*	*12.7*	*9.6*	*2.5*
Nonopioid analgesics, antipyretics, and antirheumatics (X40)	86	2	0	1	2	36	30	15
Antiepileptic, sedative-hypnotic, antiparkinsonism, and psychotropic drugs, n.e.c. (X41)	475	3	2	17	37	256	144	16
Narcotics and psychodysleptics (hallucinogens), n.e.c. (X42)	5,001	6	5	146	380	2,827	1,572	65
Other drugs acting on the autonomic nervous system (X43)	13	0	0	0	0	7	6	0
Other and unspecified drugs, medicaments, and biological substances (X44)	3,545	8	4	106	291	1,971	1,016	149
Alcohol (X45)	231	0	0	7	7	118	93	6
Organic solvents and halogenated hydrocarbons and their vapors (X46)	54	1	3	7	4	25	9	5
Other gases and vapors (X47)	425	7	9	24	43	131	117	94
Pesticides (X48)	5	1	0	0	0	3	0	1
Other and unspecified chemical and noxious substances (X49)	50	1	0	3	5	10	16	15
Females								
Total Poisoning Deaths	**4,193**	**17**	**27**	**95**	**187**	**2,159**	**1,342**	**366**
Deaths per 100,000 population	*2.9*	*0.2*	*0.1*	*1.0*	*1.9*	*5.1*	*4.1*	*1.8*
Nonopioid analgesics, antipyretics, and antirheumatics (X40)	122	1	1	0	2	52	38	28
Antiepileptic, sedative-hypnotic, antiparkinsonism, and psychotropic drugs, n.e.c. (X41)	288	0	3	13	12	134	108	18
Narcotics and psychodysleptics (hallucinogens), n.e.c. (X42)	1,508	2	2	34	80	884	475	31
Other drugs acting on the autonomic nervous system (X43)	6	0	0	1	0	2	1	2
Other and unspecified drugs, medicaments, and biological substances (X44)	1,980	5	6	34	81	992	642	220
Alcohol (X45)	72	0	0	1	3	36	29	3
Organic solvents and halogenated hydrocarbons and their vapors (X46)	9	0	1	0	1	5	2	0
Other gases and vapors (X47)	168	8	13	11	6	44	31	55
Pesticides (X48)	2	1	0	0	0	0	0	1
Other and unspecified chemical and noxious substances (X49)	38	0	1	1	2	10	16	8

Source: National Safety Council tabulations of National Center for Health Statistics mortality data.
Note: n.e.c. means not elsewhere classified.
[a]Numbers following titles refer to external cause of injury and poisoning classifications in ICD-10.

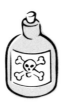

UNINTENTIONAL POISONING DEATHS, UNITED STATES, 1992–2001

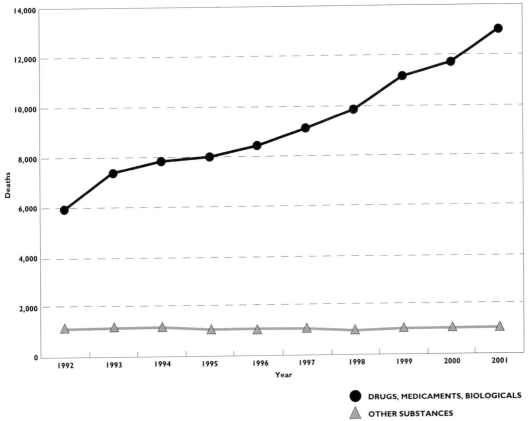

● **DRUGS, MEDICAMENTS, BIOLOGICALS**

△ **OTHER SUBSTANCES**

Note: Classification system changed in 1999 (see the Technical Appendix).

INJURIES ASSOCIATED WITH CONSUMER PRODUCTS

Stairs and steps were associated with more than 1,000,000 emergency department visits in 2002.

The following list of items found in and around the home was selected from the U.S. Consumer Product Safety Commission's National Electronic Injury Surveillance System (NEISS) for 2002. The NEISS estimates are calculated from a statistically representative sample of hospitals in the United States. Injury totals represent estimates of the number of hospital emergency department—treated cases nationwide associated with various products. However, product involvement may or may not be the cause of the injury.

ESTIMATED HOSPITAL EMERGENCY DEPARTMENT VISITS RELATED TO SELECTED CONSUMER PRODUCTS, UNITED STATES, 2002
(excluding most sports or sports equipment; see also page 126)

Description	Injuries[a]
Home Workshop Equipment	
Saws (hand or power)	92,384
Hammers	36,894
Tools, not specified	23,985
Household Packaging & Containers	
Household containers & packaging	216,498
Bottles and jars	76,487
Bags	36,454
Housewares	
Knives	441,250
Tableware and flatware (excl. knives)	106,852
Drinking glasses	86,909
Waste containers, trash baskets, etc.	33,977
Cookware, bowls, and canisters	31,057
Scissors	30,878
Manual cleaning equipment (excl. buckets)	23,211
Home Furnishing, Fixtures, and Accessories	
Beds	495,050
Tables, n.e.c.[b]	307,843
Chairs	298,234
Household cabinets, racks, & shelves	261,622
Bathtubs and showers	216,221
Ladders	163,417
Sofas, couches, davenports, divans, etc.	135,190
Rugs and carpets	115,007
Other furniture[c]	102,601
Toilets	63,969
Misc. decorating items	51,647
Stools	47,466
Benches	26,919
Sinks	23,283
Home Structures and Construction Materials	
Stairs or steps	1,077,853
Floors or flooring materials	953,492
Other doors[d]	328,880
Ceilings and walls	313,925
Nails, screws, tacks, or bolts	164,835
Porches, balconies, open-side floors	135,336
Windows	134,904
Fences or fence posts	113,674
House repair and construction materials	113,669
Door sills or frames	46,612
Poles	44,272
Handrails, railings, or banisters	41,775
Counters or countertops	39,750

Description	Injuries[a]
Home Structures and Construction Materials (CONT.)	
Glass doors	34,469
General Household Appliances	
Refrigerators	30,128
Ranges	25,060
Heating, Cooling, and Ventilating Equipment	
Pipes (excluding smoking pipes)	35,342
Home Communication and Entertainment Equipment	
Televisions	42,811
Personal-Use Items	
Footwear	114,454
Wheelchairs	95,228
Jewelry	73,943
Crutches, canes, walkers	73,615
First aid equipment	53,656
Desk supplies	42,444
Daywear	39,453
Razors and shavers	33,532
Coins	30,377
Other clothing[e]	28,548
Yard and Garden Equipment	
Lawn mowers	72,480
Pruning, trimming, & edging equipment	40,818
Chainsaws	25,557
Other unpowered garden tools[f]	24,440
Recreation Equipment	
All-terrain vehicles	113,900
Trampolines	89,393
Swimming pools	82,304
Monkey bars or other playground climbing	81,745
Toys, n.e.c.	79,684
Swings or swing sets	67,337
Minibikes or trailbikes	66,172
Scooters (unpowered)	59,905
Slides or sliding boards	44,877
Dancing	41,590
Aquariums and other pet supplies	35,643
Other playground equipment[g]	28,197
Sleds	24,998
Miscellaneous Products	
Carts	45,021
Hot water	42,077

Source: U.S. Consumer Product Safety Commission, National Electronic Injury Surveillance System, Product Summary Report, All Products, CY2002. Products are listed above if the estimate was greater than 23,000 cases.
Note: n.e.c. = not elsewhere classified.
[a] Estimated number of product-related injuries in the United States and territories that were treated in hospital emergency departments.

[b] Excludes baby changing and television tables or stands.
[c] Excludes cabinets, racks, shelves, desks, bureaus, chests, buffets, etc.
[d] Excludes glass doors and garage doors.
[e] Excludes costumes, masks, daywear, footwear, nightwear, and outerwear.
[f] Includes cultivators, hoes, pitchforks, rakes, shovels, spades, and trowels.
[g] Excludes monkey bars, seesaws, slides, and swings.

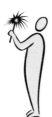

In 2002, there were an estimated 8,800 persons injured by fireworks treated in hospital emergency rooms, the second yearly decrease following an increase in 2000 that was associated with New Year's celebrations of the last year of the millennium. Fireworks-related injuries varied considerably during the ten-year period from 1993–2002, initially climbing from 12,100 in 1993 to a high of 12,500 in 1994 before dropping to a low of 7,300 in 1996. This low was followed by an increase in 1997 to 8,300 and a level period at 8,500 injuries per year for 1998 and 1999 prior to the increase in 2000 to 11,000 injuries and subsequent decline to 9,500 in 2001 and 8,800 in 2002.

The 10–14-year-old age group had the highest injury rate for 2002 of 9.0 injuries per 100,000 population, while those aged 5–9 had the next second highest rate of 6.9 and the 15–19 age group had the third highest rate of 6.2 (see graph below). Over a third of the injuries were associated with sparklers, 17% with fireworks rockets, 14% with small firecrackers, and 7% with illegal firecrackers. Other types of fireworks associated with injuries included roman candles and fountains (7% each), reloadables and novelties (4.5%

each), and homemade or altered fireworks and those used in public displays (2% each). Nearly a third of the injuries in 2002 occurred to the hand or finger, over 21% occurred to the eye, and slightly less than 20% occurred to the leg. Other body parts injured included other head or face locations (17.5%), trunk (7.0%), and arm (3.5%). Over 63% of the injuries were burn injuries, while a further 21% were contusions or lacerations, nearly 2% were fractures or sprains, and 14% were other types of injuries.

According to the latest data from the National Fire Protection Association (NFPA), there were 24,200 fires associated with fireworks in 1999 that resulted in 12 civilian deaths, 55 civilian injuries, and about $17.2 million in property damage. The number of total fires was 24% less than the 20-year average from 1980–1999, while civilian injuries and direct property damage were down 39% and 36%, respectively. The number of civilian deaths in 1999 was more than double the 20-year average.

Source: Hall, J. R., Jr. (2004, April). Fireworks-related injuries, deaths, and fires. Quincy, MA: National Fire Protection Association.

FIREWORKS INJURY RATES[a] BY AGE OF VICTIM, 2002

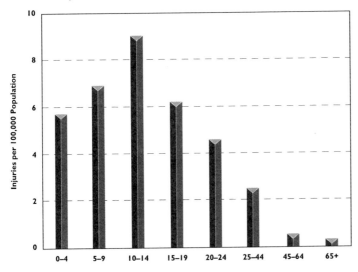

[a]Based on injuries treated in hospital emergency departments during the month around July 4.

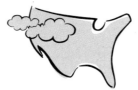

Ozone (O$_3$) is one of the six principal pollutants (also known as criteria pollutants[a]) whose atmospheric levels are regulated by the U.S. Environmental Protection Agency (EPA) through the National Ambient Air Quality Standards (NAAQS) to protect public health. Ozone occurs naturally in the stratosphere where it serves as a shield against solar radiation. It is also formed at ground level as a result of a chemical reaction between oxides of nitrogen and volatile organic compounds.

High concentrations of ground-level ozone are known to be harmful to health, particularly in the summer months. Among known health effects of ozone are irritation of air passages, reduced lung function, and inflammation and damage to the cells lining the lungs. It also may aggravate symptoms of asthma and chronic lung diseases (e.g., emphysema, bronchitis). It may reduce the immune system's ability to fight off bacterial infections in the respiratory system and may cause permanent lung damage.

The Air Quality Index (AQI), a nationally uniform index used for monitoring daily air quality, provides information on air concentrations for ground-level ozone and other principal pollutants.

According to the AQI scale, air pollution is classified into six categories that represent different degrees of health risk due to a specific pollutant. The index is "normalized" across each pollutant so that an AQI value of 100 is set at the level of the short-term, health-based standard for that pollutant. The chart below illustrates the six AQI categories based on daily measurements of ozone concentration in parts per million (ppm) averaged over eight hours.

OZONE AIR QUALITY INDEX DEFINITIONS

Category	AQI	O$_3$,8-hour (ppm)	Health risks
Good	0-50	0.000-0.064	Air quality is satisfactory. Air pollution poses little or no risk.
Moderate	51–100	0.065–0.084	Air quality is acceptable. Some pollutants may cause moderate health problems for a very small number of individuals (e.g., people with high ozone sensitivity).
Unhealthy for Sensitive Groups	101–150	0.085–0.104	People with respiratory problems, children, and other individuals particularly vulnerable to the harmful effects of air pollutants are more likely to be affected at lower levels than is the general public.
Unhealthy	151–200	0.105–0.124	The general public may begin to experience health effects. Health effects among members of sensitive groups may be more serious.
Very Unhealthy	201–300	0.125–0.374	Everyone may experience more serious health effects.
Hazardous	over 300	(b)	Air quality triggers health warnings of emergency conditions.

[a]Other criteria pollutants include nitrogen dioxide (NO$_2$), sulfur dioxide (SO$_2$), particulate matter (PM), carbon monoxide (CO), and lead (Pb).
[b]Health effect information not available. Use 1-hour concentration above 0.405 ppm.

PEOPLE LIVING IN COUNTIES WITH POOR OZONE AIR QUALITY, UNITED STATES, 1998–2003

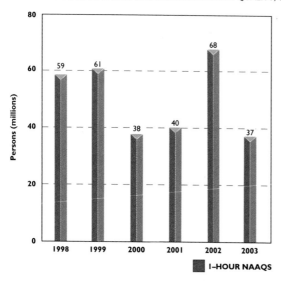

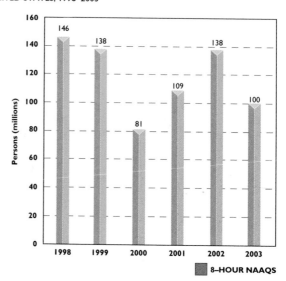

Source: EPA. (2004). The Ozone Report. Measuring Progress through 2003. EPA 454/K-04-001. Research Triangle Park, NC. At http://www.epa.gov/airtrends/ozone.html accessed May 12, 2004.

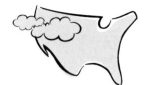

The EPA reports that there has been a marked reduction in concentrations of ground-level ozone since the 1980s. One-hour and eight-hour levels have declined by 29% and 21%, respectively. In 2003, however, over 100 million people residing in 209 counties across the country were exposed to poor quality air as a result of ozone pollution based on the 8-hour ozone standard. Harmful ozone levels are more likely to occur in the Northeast, Mid-Atlantic, Midwest, and California, with a smaller number of areas in the South and south-central United States.

NUMBER OF DAYS WITH AQI VALUES OVER 100 DUE TO OZONE, 2003

Metropolitan Statistical Area[a]	# of days
Bakersfield, CA	116
Riverside-San Bernardino, CA	103
Fresno, CA	97
Los Angeles-Long Beach, CA	86
Sacramento, CA	43
Houston, TX	38
Ventura, CA	31
Fort Worth-Arlington, TX	28
Dallas, TX	20
Denver, CO	17
Baton Rouge, LA	16
Knoxville, TN	14
Philadelphia, PA-NJ	14
Kansas City, MO-KS	14
Atlanta, GA	13
Indianapolis, IN	13
Monmouth-Ocean, NJ	12
Phoenix-Mesa, AZ	12
St. Louis, MO-IL	11
New Haven-Meriden, CT	11
Cincinnati, OH-KY-IN	11
Las Vegas, NV-AZ	11
Baltimore, MD	10
Providence-Fall River-Warwick, RI-MA	10
Orange County, CA	10
Charlotte-Gastonia-Rock Hill, NC-SC	9
Memphis, TN-AR-MS	9
Tulsa, OK	9
Cleveland-Lorain-Elyria, OH	9
Milwaukee-Waukesha, WI	8
New Orleans, LA	8
Raleigh-Durham-Chapel Hill, NC	8
Washington, DC-MD-VA-WV	8
Grand Rapids-Muskegon-Holland, MI	8

Metropolitan Statistical Area[a]	# of days
Pittsburgh, PA	8
Buffalo-Niagara Falls, NY	7
Detroit, MI	7
Hartford, CT	7
Louisville, KY-IN	7
Middlesex-Somerset-Hunterdon, NJ	7
New York, NY	7
Wilmington-Newark, DE-MD	7
Dayton-Springfield, OH	7
Columbus, OH	7
San Antonio, TX	7
Greensboro-Winston Salem-High Point, NC	6
Nashville, TN	6
Nassau-Suffolk, NY	6
San Diego, CA	6
San Jose, CA	6
Toledo, OH	6
Ann Arbor, MI	6
Tampa-St. Petersburg-Clearwater, FL	6
Salt Lake City-Ogden, UT	6
Albany-Schenectady-Troy, NY	5
Youngstown-Warren, OH	5
Boston, MA-NH	5
Gary, IN	5
Richmond-Petersburg, VA	5
Syracuse, NY	5
Akron, OH	4
Allentown-Bethlehem-Easton, PA	4
Chicago, IL	4
Fort Wayne, IN	4
Greenville-Spartanburg-Anderson, SC	4
Newark, NJ	4
Norfolk-Virginia Beach-Newport News, VA-NC	4

Metropolitan Statistical Area[a]	# of days
Austin-San Marcos, TX	4
Birmingham, AL	4
Oakland, CA	4
Harrisburg-Lebanon-Carlisle, PA	3
Rochester, NY	3
Scranton-Wilkes Barre-Hazleton, PA	3
Springfield, MA	3
Albuquerque, NM	3
Sarasota-Bradenton, FL	3
Mobile, AL	3
Jersey City, NJ	2
Oklahoma City, OK	2
Stockton-Lodi, CA	2
Columbia, SC	2
Seattle-Bellevue-Everett, WA	2
Little Rock-North Little Rock, AR	1
McAllen-Edinburg-Mission, TX	1
Miami, FL	1
Minneapolis-St. Paul, MN-WI	1
Tucson, AZ	1
Wichita, KS	1
Worcester, MA	1
El Paso, TX	1
Orlando, FL	1
Tacoma, WA	1
Charleston-North Charleston, SC	0
Fort Lauderdale, FL	0
Jacksonville, FL	0
Omaha, NE-IA	0
Portland-Vancouver, OR-WA	0
San Francisco, CA	0
Vallejo-Fairfield-Napa, CA	0
West Palm Beach-Boca Raton, FL	0

Source: U.S. Environmental Protection Agency. (2004). Fact Book & Related Information. At http://www.epa.gov/airtrends/factbook.html accessed May 12, 2004.
[a] *Metropolitan Statistical Areas have at least one urbanized area of 50,000 or more population, plus adjacent territory that has a high degree of social and economic integration with the core as measured by commuting ties.*

Asthma is the most common chronic disease of childhood. Asthma attacks are typically presented as repeated episodes of wheezing, coughing, breathlessness, and chest tightness. Among known triggers of asthma are infections, strenuous exercise, adverse weather conditions, environmental pollutants (e.g., sulfur dioxide), dust mites, cockroaches, animal dander, environmental tobacco smoke, and mold.

In the United States, the prevalence of asthma is estimated by the National Health Interview Survey (NHIS). In 2002, nearly 9 million children under 18 years of age had been diagnosed with asthma. This includes children who had been told by a doctor or other health professional that they had asthma. More than 4 million of children, or 6 per 1,000 population, had suffered an asthma attack in the previous year.

NHIS data indicate important demographic and socioeconomic differences with respect to the prevalence of asthma among children. In general, asthma is more common among boys (14% vs. 10% of girls), non-Hispanic black children, and children in single-mother families and low-income households. In addition, asthma is more prevalent among older children.

ASTHMA AMONG CHILDREN 0–17 YEARS OLD BY SELECTED CHARACTERISTICS, UNITED STATES, 2002

Characteristic	Ever Diagnosed with Asthma[a]			Asthma Attack in Past 12 Months[b]		
	Number (000)	Percent	Rate[c]	Number (000)	Percent	Rate[c]
Total	**8,894**	**100.0%**	**121.9**	**4,197**	**100.0%**	**57.5**
Sex						
Male	5,190	58.4	139.1	2,518	60.0	67.5
Female	3,704	41.6	103.9	1,679	40.0	47.1
Age[d]						
Under 5	1,452	16.3	73.2	958	22.8	48.3
5–11	3,801	42.7	132.1	1,801	42.9	62.6
12–17	3,641	40.9	149.4	1,438	34.3	59.0
Race						
White, single race	6,041	67.9	111.1	2,824	67.3	51.9
Black, single race	1,873	21.1	177.1	910	21.7	86.0
American Indian or Alaska Native	74[e]	0.8[e]	147.1[e]	42[e]	1.0[e]	83.5[e]
Asian	272	3.1	106.5	111	2.6	43.5
Other, single race[f]	344	3.9	121.4	150	3.6	52.9
2 or more races[g]	285	3.2	141.3	156	3.7	77.3
Hispanic Origin						
Hispanic or Latino	1,273	14.3	101.3	558	13.3	44.4
Not Hispanic or Latino	7,621	85.7	126.2	3,639	86.7	60.2
Family Income[h]						
Less than $20,000	1,956	22.0	159.0	996	23.7	81.0
$20,000–$34,999	1,231	13.8	121.0	556	13.2	54.6
$35,000–$54,999	1,274	14.3	109.2	601	14.3	51.5
$55,000–$74,999	1,155	13.0	120.8	565	13.5	59.1
$75,000 or more	1,868	21.0	115.1	829	19.8	51.1
Health Insurance Coverage[h]						
Private	5,308	59.7	113.1	2,416	57.6	51.5
Medicaid	2,683	30.2	155.6	1,422	33.9	82.5
Other	191	2.1	130.5	79	1.9	54.0
Uninsured[i]	679	7.6	95.6	279	6.6	39.3
Region						
Northeast	2,040	22.9	151.1	889	21.2	65.9
Midwest	2,003	22.5	115.0	983	23.4	56.4
South	3,164	35.6	118.9	1,501	35.8	56.4
West	1,688	19.0	109.4	824	19.6	53.4

Source: National Center for Health Statistics. (2004). Summary Health Statistics for U.S. Children: National Health Interview Survey, 2002. At http://www.cdc.gov/nchs/data/series/sr_10/sr10_221.pdf accessed May 14, 2004.

Note: Estimates are age-adjusted to the 2000 U.S. standard population using age groups 0–4 years, 5–11 years, and 12–17 years. Some characteristics may not add to the Totals due to unknowns.

[a] Based on the NHIS question, "Has a doctor or other health professional ever told you that [child's name] had asthma?"

[b] Based on the NHIS question, "During the past 12 months, has [child's name] had an episode of asthma or an asthma attack?"

[c] Per 1,000 population.

[d] Estimates for age groups are not adjusted.

[e] Does not meet the standard of reliability or precision.

[f] Includes persons who indicated a single race other than the specific groups shown separately.

[g] Includes persons who indicated more than one racial group (e.g., "Black or African American and White").

[h] Persons with unknown family income or health insurance status are not shown, but they are included in the Totals.

[i] Includes persons without health insurance and those who had only Indian Health Service coverage or had only a private plan that paid for one type of service (e.g., accidents, dental care).

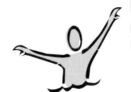

DROWNING DEATHS AND DEATH RATES IN THE UNITED STATES, 2001

In 2001, more than 3,200 people drowned in the United States, thus making drowning one of the leading causes of unintentional-injury death.

The rates of drowning deaths vary between U.S. states. Typically, the rates (per 100,000 population) are higher in Alaska and Hawaii as well as the South Atlantic, East South Central, and West South Central regions.

DROWNING DEATHS PER 100,000 POPULATION BY STATE, 2001

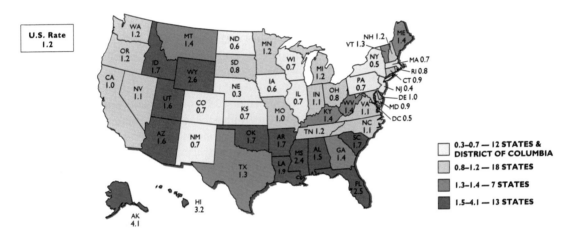

U.S. Rate 1.2

0.3–0.7 — 12 STATES & DISTRICT OF COLUMBIA	
0.8–1.2 — 18 STATES	
1.3–1.4 — 7 STATES	
1.5–4.1 — 13 STATES	

The charts below show the distribution of unintentional drowning deaths and death rates by sex and race[a]. White non-Hispanic males made up nearly one-half of the total number of fatal drowning cases. Overall and in each individual racial category, males accounted for more deaths than females. Among Hispanic and Black non-Hispanic persons, the number of drowning deaths for males was nearly five times greater than for females. Black non-Hispanic males had the highest drowning death rate, while Hispanic females had the lowest compared to other sex-race categories.

Source: National Safety Council tabulations of National Center for Health Statistics data.
[a]Does not include 28 "race unknown" cases (24 males, 4 females).

DROWNING DEATHS BY SEX AND RACE, 2001

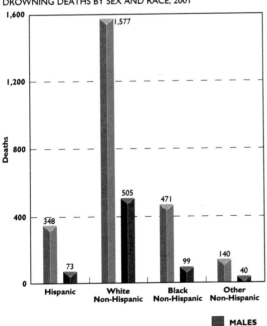

DROWNING DEATH RATES BY SEX AND RACE, 2001

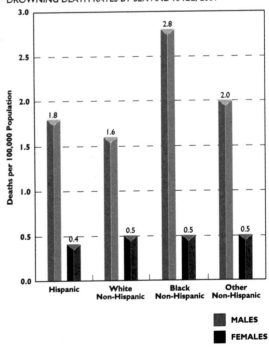

ELECTROCUTIONS ASSOCIATED WITH CONSUMER PRODUCTS

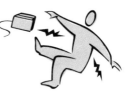

In 2000, about 400 deaths occurred as a result of electrocution. Consumer products–related electrocutions caused about 150 deaths, or more than one-third of the total.

Overall, electrocutions in the United States have decreased by 36% from 630 deaths in 1991 to 400 in 2000, according to data collected by the National Center for Health Statistics (NCHS). At the same time, the estimated number of electrocutions related to consumer products decreased from 250 to 150, a reduction of 40%. Both of these downward trends were significant, as was the 46% decline in the age-adjusted death rate from consumer product–related electrocutions (from 0.99 per million population in 1991 to 0.53 per million population in 2000).

Large appliances, including air conditioners, pumps, water heaters, furnaces, clothes dryers, refrigerators, and range hoods, accounted for the largest proportion (19%) of the electrocutions in 2000. Ladders coming in contact with power lines were the second most frequent cause of death (15%), followed by small appliances (e.g., extension cords, fans, microwaves, televisions), which contributed an additional 11%. Drills, grinding machines, saws, welding equipment, and other power tools accounted for 10% of the electrocutions. Lighting equipment such as lamps, fixtures, and work lights were responsible for 8% of the total. Installed household wiring and sports/recreational equipment represented 7% and 6% of the electrocutions deaths, respectively. The remaining 24% of the electrocutions were associated with gardening and farming equipment, miscellaneous products (e.g., pipes, poles, fences), antennas, and unspecified products.

Source: Chowdhury, R.T. (July, 2003). 2000 Electrocutions associated with consumer products. Washington, DC: U.S. Consumer Product Safety Commission.

ELECTROCUTIONS RELATED TO CONSUMER PRODUCTS, UNITED STATES, 1991–2000

Year	Total Electrocutions[a]	Consumer Product–Related Electrocutions		
		Deaths	Percent of Total	Rate[b]
1991	630	250	39.7	0.99
1992	530	200	37.7	0.78
1993	550	210	38.2	0.82
1994	560	230	41.1	0.89
1995	560	230	41.1	0.88
1996	480	190	39.6	0.72
1997	490	190	38.8	0.71
1998	550	200	36.4	0.74
1999	440	170	38.6	0.62
2000	400	150	37.5	0.53

[a] Deaths for 1991–1998 are based on the International Classification of Diseases, 9th Revision (ICD–9). Deaths for 1999–2000 are based on the International Classification of Diseases, 10th Revision (ICD–10).
[b] Deaths per 1 million population.

ELECTROCUTIONS RELATED TO CONSUMER PRODUCTS BY LOCATION, 2000

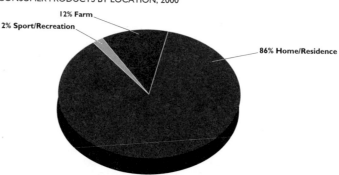

12% Farm
2% Sport/Recreation
86% Home/Residence

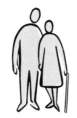

FALL-RELATED DEATHS AND HIP FRACTURES AMONG THE ELDERLY

Falls are the leading cause of injury-related mortality among the elderly. In 2001, there were 32,624 injury-related deaths among persons aged 65 and older, of which 11,623 (36%) were attributed to falls. In this age group, the death rate for fall-related injuries was 32.9 per 100,000 population.

Overall, about 54% of fatal falls among elderly persons occurred in the home. The second most common place

of occurrence for fall-related deaths were residential institutions (e.g., nursing homes), which accounted for 20% of the total. Industrial/construction areas and farms as well as athletic areas were the least likely places of occurrence for fall-related deaths, reflecting to some extent older adults' low participation in the workforce and sporting activities.

NUMBER AND PERCENT OF FALL-RELATED DEATHS BY PLACE OF OCCURRENCE AND SEX, AGES 65 AND OLDER, UNITED STATES, 2001

Place of Occurrence	Both Sexes		Male		Female	
	Deaths	Percent	Deaths	Percent	Deaths	Percent
Total deaths	11,623	100.0%	5,390	100.0%	6,233	100.0%
Home	6,258	53.8	3,027	56.2	3,231	51.8
Residential institution	2,330	20.0	812	15.1	1,518	24.4
School/public building	437	3.8	234	4.3	203	3.3
Street/highway	342	2.9	205	3.8	137	2.2
Trade/service area	181	1.6	107	2.0	74	1.2
Industrial/construction/farm	41	0.4	33	0.6	8	0.1
Sports/athletics area	16	0.1	13	0.2	3	0.0
Other specified	521	4.5	288	5.3	233	3.7
Unspecified	1,497	12.9	671	12.4	826	13.3

Source: National Safety Council tabulations of National Center for Health Statistics mortality data.

Among the elderly, falls often result in hip fracture. Hospital discharges for hip fractures among persons aged 65 and older totaled 279,771 in 2001 and averaged 290,730 cases annually between 1997 and 2001. During this 5-year period, the hip fracture hospital discharge rate for both elderly men and women

combined averaged 839.9 per 100,000 population. As the graph below indicates, women are at a much greater risk of hip fracture than men. In 2001, the hip fracture discharge rate for women (1,024.4 per 100,000 population) was more than twice the rate for men (462.4 per 100,000 population).

HIP FRACTURE[a] HOSPITAL DISCHARGE RATES, AGES 65 AND OLDER, UNITED STATES, 1997–2001

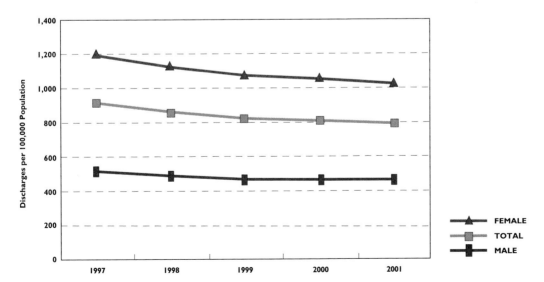

Source: HCUPnet, Healthcare Cost and Utilization Project. Agency for Healthcare Research and Quality, Rockville, MD. Available at http://www.ahrq.gov/data/hcup/hcupnet.htm.
[a]Hospital discharges for single-level Clinical Classifications Software (CCS) diagnosis category 226, "Fracture of neck of femur (hip)."

INJURY FACTS®

NATIONAL SAFETY COUNCIL

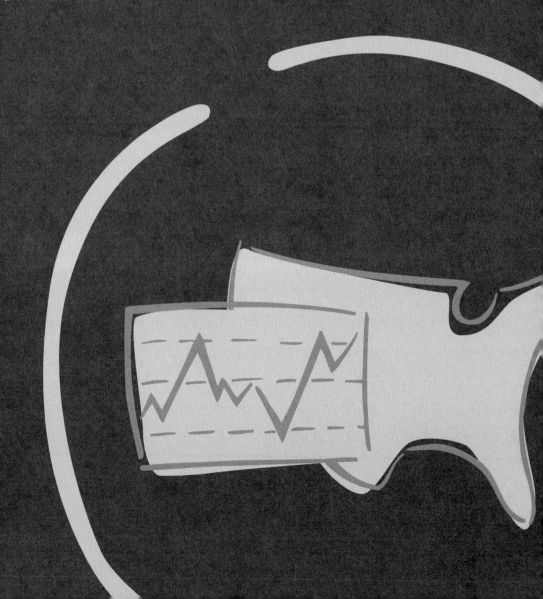

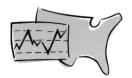

Motor-vehicle crashes are the leading cause of U-I deaths in every state.

This section on state-level data includes data for occupational and motor-vehicle injuries as well as general injury mortality.

Death rates for unintentional injuries (U-I) can vary greatly from one type of injury to the next and from state to state. The graph on the next page shows for each state the death rates (per 100,000 population) for total unintentional-injury deaths and the four leading types of unintentional-injury deaths nationally — motor-vehicle crashes, falls, poisonings, and choking (inhalation or ingestion of food or other object that obstructs breathing).

The map on page 152 shows graphically the overall unintentional-injury death rates by state.

The charts on pages 153 through 155 show (a) total unintentional-injury deaths and where U-I rank as a cause of death in each state, and (b) the five leading causes of U-I deaths in each state.

Unintentional injuries as a whole are the fifth leading cause of death in the United States and in 30 states. U-I are the third leading cause of death in Alaska, the District of Columbia, New Mexico, and Wyoming, and the fourth leading cause in ten states. U-I rank sixth in six states (California, Maryland, New Jersey, New York, Rhode Island, and Washington), and seventh in Massachusetts.

Motor-vehicle crashes were the leading cause of U-I deaths in every state. Poisoning was the leading cause in the District of Columbia. The second leading cause of U-I deaths was falls in 27 states and poisoning in 23 states. Motor-vehicle crashes was second in the District of Columbia. The most common third leading causes of U-I deaths were falls in 21 states and the District of Columbia, and poisoning in 21 states. Choking ranked third in four states (Massachusetts, Nebraska, Rhode Island, and South Dakota), fires in three states (Alabama, Arkansas, and Maryland), and

drowning in Alaska. Choking was the fourth leading cause of U-I deaths in 25 states (tied with fires in North Dakota), while the fourth ranking cause was drowning in 11 states, and fires and flames in seven states and the District of Columbia. Poisoning ranked fourth in Nebraska and Rhode Island, air transport in Alaska and New York, natural heat or cold in Montana and New Mexico, and falls in Alabama.

The table on pages 156 and 157 shows the number of U-I deaths by state for the 15 most common types of injury events. State populations are also shown to facilitate computation of detailed death rates.

The table on page 158 consists of a 4-year state-by-state comparison of unintentional-injury deaths and death rates for 1998 through 2001. Because of the change in mortality classification schemes from ICD-9 to ICD-10 in 1999, caution must be exercised in making comparisons of 1999 and later data with earlier years. A comparability study conducted by the National Center for Health Statistics indicates that if the 1998 mortality data had been coded according to ICD-10, then the U-I death total would have been about 3% greater. See the Technical Appendix for more information.

Page 159 shows fatal occupational injuries by state and counts of deaths for some of the principal types of events — transportation accidents, assaults and violent acts, contacts with objects and equipment, falls, exposure to harmful substances or environments, and fires and explosions.

Nonfatal occupational injury and illness incidence rates for most states are shown in the table on page 160 and graphically in the map on page 161. States not shown do not have state occupational safety and health plans.

Pages 162 and 163 show motor-vehicle–related deaths and death rates by state both in tables and maps. The maps show death rates based on population, vehicle miles traveled, and registered vehicles.

UNINTENTIONAL-INJURY DEATH RATES BY STATE, UNITED STATES, 2000

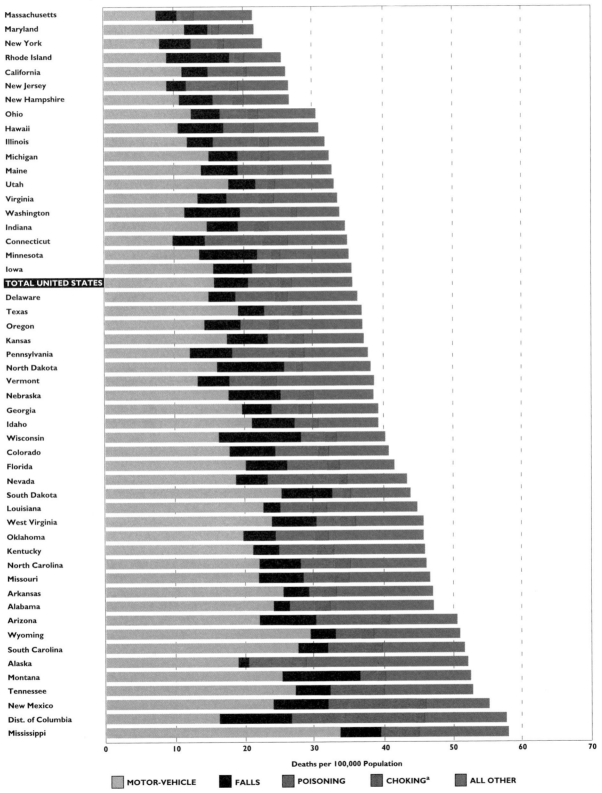

Massachusetts
Maryland
New York
Rhode Island
California
New Jersey
New Hampshire
Ohio
Hawaii
Illinois
Michigan
Maine
Utah
Virginia
Washington
Indiana
Connecticut
Minnesota
Iowa
TOTAL UNITED STATES
Delaware
Texas
Oregon
Kansas
Pennsylvania
North Dakota
Vermont
Nebraska
Georgia
Idaho
Wisconsin
Colorado
Florida
Nevada
South Dakota
Louisiana
West Virginia
Oklahoma
Kentucky
North Carolina
Missouri
Arkansas
Alabama
Arizona
Wyoming
South Carolina
Alaska
Montana
Tennessee
New Mexico
Dist. of Columbia
Mississippi

0   10   20   30   40   50   60   70

Deaths per 100,000 Population

■ MOTOR-VEHICLE   ■ FALLS   ■ POISONING   ■ CHOKINGª   ■ ALL OTHER

ªIngestion or inhalation of food or other object.

UNINTENTIONAL-INJURY DEATH RATES BY STATE

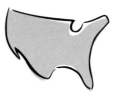

UNINTENTIONAL-INJURY DEATHS PER 100,000 POPULATION BY STATE, 2001

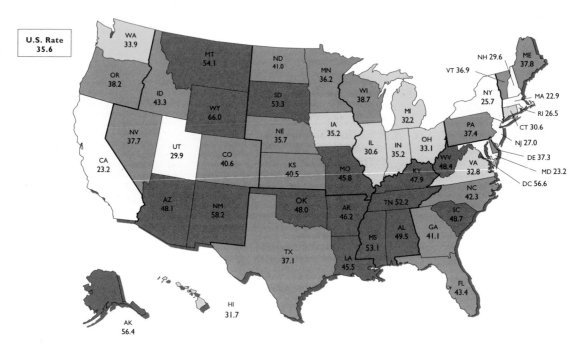

U.S. Rate
35.6

WA 33.9
MT 54.1
ND 41.0
MN 36.2
NH 29.6
ME 37.8
VT 36.9
OR 38.2
ID 43.3
SD 53.3
WI 38.7
NY 25.7
MA 22.9
WY 66.0
MI 32.2
RI 26.5
CT 30.6
NV 37.7
NE 35.7
IA 35.2
PA 37.4
NJ 27.0
CA 23.2
UT 29.9
CO 40.6
IL 30.6
IN 35.2
OH 33.1
DE 37.3
KS 40.5
MO 45.8
WV 48.4
VA 32.8
MD 23.2
DC 56.6
AZ 48.1
NM 58.2
OK 48.0
KY 47.9
NC 42.3
AR 46.2
TN 52.2
SC 48.7
TX 37.1
MS 53.1
AL 49.5
GA 41.1
LA 45.5
FL 43.4
HI 31.7
AK 56.4

REGIONAL RATES

NEW ENGLAND (CT, ME, MA, NH, RI, VT)	27.6
MIDDLE ATLANTIC (NJ, NY, PA)	29.6
EAST NORTH CENTRAL (IL, IN, MI, OH, WI)	33.2
WEST NORTH CENTRAL (IA, KS, MN, MO, NE, ND, SD)	40.3
SOUTH ATLANTIC (DE, DC, FL, GA, MD, NC, SC, VA, WV)	40.0
EAST SOUTH CENTRAL (AL, KY, MS, TN)	50.6
WEST SOUTH CENTRAL (AR, LA, OK, TX)	40.2
MOUNTAIN (AZ, CO, ID, MT, NV, NM, UT, WY)	44.3
PACIFIC (AK, CA, HI, OR, WA)	26.4

Source: National Center for Health Statistics, and U.S. Census Bureau.

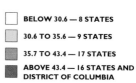

BELOW 30.6 — 8 STATES

30.6 TO 35.6 — 9 STATES

35.7 TO 43.4 — 17 STATES

ABOVE 43.4 — 16 STATES AND
DISTRICT OF COLUMBIA

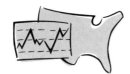
The following series of charts is a state-by-state ranking of the five leading causes of deaths due to unintentional injuries (U-I) based on 2001 data. The first line of each section gives the rank of unintentional-injury deaths among all causes of death, the total number of U-I deaths, and the rate of U-I deaths per 100,000 population. The following lines list the five leading types of unintentional-injury deaths along with the number and rate for each type.

TOTAL UNITED STATES

Rank	Cause	Deaths	Rate
5	All U-I	101,537	35.6
1	Motor-vehicle	43,788	15.4
2	Falls	15,019	5.3
3	Poisoning[a]	14,078	4.9
4	Choking[c]	4,185	1.5
5	Fires, flames, smoke	3,309	1.2

ALABAMA

Rank	Cause	Deaths	Rate
4	All U-I	2,210	49.5
1	Motor-vehicle	1,056	23.6
2	Poisoning[a]	188	4.2
3	Fires, flames, smoke	121	2.7
4	Falls	114	2.6
5	Choking[c]	110	2.5

ALASKA

Rank	Cause	Deaths	Rate
3	All U-I	357	56.4
1	Motor-vehicle	106	16.8
2	Poisoning[a]	77	12.2
3	Drowning[b]	26	4.1
4	Air transport	23	3.6
5	Falls	22	3.5

ARIZONA

Rank	Cause	Deaths	Rate
4	All U-I	2,549	48.1
1	Motor-vehicle	1,041	19.7
2	Poisoning[a]	476	9.0
3	Falls	473	8.9
4	Drowning[b]	85	1.6
5	Choking[c]	55	1.0

ARKANSAS

Rank	Cause	Deaths	Rate
5	All U-I	1,243	46.2
1	Motor-vehicle	648	24.1
2	Falls	137	5.1
3	Fires, flames, smoke	90	3.3
4	Choking[c]	63	2.3
5	Poisoning[a]	46	1.7

CALIFORNIA

Rank	Cause	Deaths	Rate
6	All U-I	8,010	23.2
1	Motor-vehicle	3,864	11.2
2	Falls	1,179	3.4
3	Poisoning[a]	1,038	3.0
4	Drowning[b]	356	1.0
5	Fires, flames, smoke	183	0.5

COLORADO

Rank	Cause	Deaths	Rate
5	All U-I	1,798	40.6
1	Motor-vehicle	761	17.2
2	Falls	288	6.5
3	Poisoning[a]	276	6.2
4	Choking[c]	59	1.3
5	Air transportation	53	1.2

CONNECTICUT

Rank	Cause	Deaths	Rate
5	All U-I	1,049	30.6
1	Motor-vehicle	306	8.9
2	Poisoning[a]	241	7.0
3	Falls	187	5.4
4	Choking[c]	92	2.7
5	Drowning[b]	31	0.9

DELAWARE

Rank	Cause	Deaths	Rate
5	All U-I	297	37.3
1	Motor-vehicle	135	17.0
2	Poisoning[a]	41	5.2
3	Falls	36	4.5
4	Fires, flames, smoke	19	2.4
5	Drowning[b]	8	1.0
5	Choking[c]	8	1.0

DISTRICT OF COLUMBIA

Rank	Cause	Deaths	Rate
3	All U-I	324	56.6
1	Poisoning[a]	104	18.2
2	Motor-vehicle	98	17.1
3	Falls	67	11.7
4	Fires, flames, smoke	12	2.1
5	Firearms	6	1.0

FLORIDA

Rank	Cause	Deaths	Rate
5	All U-I	7,093	43.4
1	Motor-vehicle	3,161	19.3
2	Poisoning[a]	1,363	8.3
3	Falls	1,084	6.6
4	Drowning[b]	406	2.5
5	Choking[c]	249	1.5

GEORGIA

Rank	Cause	Deaths	Rate
4	All U-I	3,449	41.1
1	Motor-vehicle	1,649	19.6
2	Falls	437	5.2
3	Poisoning[a]	435	5.2
4	Choking[c]	151	1.8
5	Fires, flames, smoke	140	1.7

HAWAII

Rank	Cause	Deaths	Rate
4	All U-I	388	31.7
1	Motor-vehicle	131	10.7
2	Falls	76	6.2
3	Poisoning[a]	45	3.7
4	Drowning[b]	39	3.2
5	Choking[c]	15	1.2

IDAHO

Rank	Cause	Deaths	Rate
5	All U-I	572	43.3
1	Motor-vehicle	273	20.7
2	Falls	117	8.9
3	Poisoning[a]	59	4.5
4	Drowning[b]	22	1.7
5	Struck by or against	13	1.0

ILLINOIS

Rank	Cause	Deaths	Rate
5	All U-I	3,825	30.6
1	Motor-vehicle	1,418	11.3
2	Poisoning[a]	784	6.3
3	Falls	496	4.0
4	Choking[c]	179	1.4
5	Fires, flames, smoke	161	1.3

INDIANA

Rank	Cause	Deaths	Rate
5	All U-I	2,154	35.2
1	Motor-vehicle	937	15.3
2	Falls	275	4.5
3	Poisoning[a]	154	2.5
4	Fires, flames, smoke	105	1.7
5	Choking[c]	104	1.7

IOWA

Rank	Cause	Deaths	Rate
5	All U-I	1,033	35.2
1	Motor-vehicle	441	15.0
2	Falls	225	7.7
3	Poisoning[a]	53	1.8
4	Choking[c]	45	1.5
5	Fires, flames, smoke	27	0.9

KANSAS

Rank	Cause	Deaths	Rate
5	All U-I	1,095	40.5
1	Motor-vehicle	515	19.1
2	Falls	177	6.6
3	Poisoning[a]	104	3.9
4	Choking[c]	58	2.1
5	Fires, flames, smoke	46	1.7

See footnotes on page 155.

UNINTENTIONAL-INJURY DEATHS
BY STATE (CONT.)

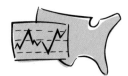

KENTUCKY

Rank	Cause	Deaths	Rate
5	All U-I	1,948	47.9
I	Motor-vehicle	862	21.2
2	Poisoning[a]	295	7.3
3	Falls	159	3.9
4	Choking[c]	80	2.0
5	Fires and flames	66	1.6

MARYLAND

Rank	Cause	Deaths	Rate
6	All U-I	1,248	23.2
I	Motor-vehicle	665	12.4
2	Falls	200	3.7
3	Fires, flames, smoke	59	1.1
4	Drowning[b]	51	0.9
5	Choking[c]	40	0.7

MINNESOTA

Rank	Cause	Deaths	Rate
5	All U-I	1,805	36.2
I	Motor-vehicle	626	12.6
2	Falls	476	9.5
3	Poisoning[a]	138	2.8
4	Drowning[b]	60	1.2
5	Mechanical suffocation	45	0.9

MONTANA

Rank	Cause	Deaths	Rate
5	All U-I	490	54.1
I	Motor-vehicle	233	25.7
2	Falls	111	12.3
3	Poisoning[a]	34	3.8
4	Natural heat, cold	14	1.5
5	Drowning[b]	13	1.4

NEW HAMPSHIRE

Rank	Cause	Deaths	Rate
5	All U-I	373	29.6
I	Motor-vehicle	142	11.3
2	Falls	72	5.7
3	Poisoning[a]	45	3.6
4	Drowning[b]	15	1.2
5	Fires, flames, smoke	14	1.1
5	Choking[c]	14	1.1

NEW YORK

Rank	Cause	Deaths	Rate
6	All U-I	4,896	25.7
I	Motor-vehicle	1,580	8.3
2	Poisoning[a]	952	5.0
3	Falls	950	5.0
4	Air transportation	257	1.3
5	Fires, flames, smoke	188	1.0

LOUISIANA

Rank	Cause	Deaths	Rate
4	All U-I	2,033	45.5
I	Motor-vehicle	994	22.3
2	Poisoning[a]	219	4.9
3	Falls	154	3.4
4	Fires, flames, smoke	100	2.2
5	Drowning[b]	84	1.9

MASSACHUSETTS

Rank	Cause	Deaths	Rate
7	All U-I	1,465	22.9
I	Motor-vehicle	534	8.3
2	Falls	237	3.7
3	Choking[c]	114	1.8
4	Fires, flames, smoke	55	0.9
5	Poisoning[a]	48	0.8

MISSISSIPPI

Rank	Cause	Deaths	Rate
4	All U-I	1,518	53.1
I	Motor-vehicle	804	28.1
2	Falls	177	6.2
3	Poisoning[a]	109	3.8
4	Choking[c]	90	3.1
5	Fires, flames, smoke	79	2.8

NEBRASKA

Rank	Cause	Deaths	Rate
5	All U-I	614	35.7
I	Motor-vehicle	265	15.4
2	Falls	140	8.1
3	Choking[c]	41	2.4
4	Poisoning[a]	38	2.2
5	Fires, flames, smoke	21	1.2

NEW JERSEY

Rank	Cause	Deaths	Rate
6	All U-I	2,296	27.0
I	Motor-vehicle	725	8.5
2	Poisoning[a]	575	6.8
3	Falls	243	2.9
4	Choking[c]	115	1.4
5	Fires, flames, smoke	71	0.8

NORTH CAROLINA

Rank	Cause	Deaths	Rate
5	All U-I	3,469	42.3
I	Motor-vehicle	1,661	20.3
2	Poisoning[a]	440	5.4
3	Falls	434	5.3
4	Choking[c]	140	1.7
5	Fires, flames, smoke	120	1.5

MAINE

Rank	Cause	Deaths	Rate
5	All U-I	486	37.8
I	Motor-vehicle	200	15.6
2	Falls	93	7.2
3	Poisoning[a]	60	4.7
4	Choking[c]	34	2.6
5	Drowning[b]	18	1.4

MICHIGAN

Rank	Cause	Deaths	Rate
5	All U-I	3,218	32.2
I	Motor-vehicle	1,394	13.9
2	Falls	507	5.1
3	Poisoning[a]	333	3.3
4	Fires and flames	130	1.3
5	Choking[c]	117	1.2
5	Drowning[b]	117	1.2

MISSOURI

Rank	Cause	Deaths	Rate
5	All U-I	2,584	45.8
I	Motor-vehicle	1,182	21.0
2	Falls	478	8.5
3	Poisoning[a]	243	4.3
4	Choking[c]	115	2.0
5	Fires, flames, smoke	93	1.7

NEVADA

Rank	Cause	Deaths	Rate
5	All U-I	790	37.7
I	Motor-vehicle	350	16.7
2	Poisoning[a]	192	9.2
3	Falls	87	4.2
4	Choking[c]	31	1.5
5	Drowning[b]	22	1.1

NEW MEXICO

Rank	Cause	Deaths	Rate
3	All U-I	1,065	58.2
I	Motor-vehicle	486	26.6
2	Poisoning[a]	227	12.4
3	Falls	156	8.5
4	Natural heat, cold	20	1.1
5	Choking[c]	19	1.0

NORTH DAKOTA

Rank	Cause	Deaths	Rate
5	All U-I	261	41.0
I	Motor-vehicle	126	19.8
2	Falls	69	10.8
3	Poisoning[a]	10	1.6
4	Fires, flames, smoke	6	0.9
4	Choking[c]	6	0.9

See footnotes on page 155.

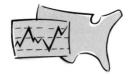
OHIO

Rank	Cause	Deaths	Rate
5	All U-I	3,774	33.1
I	Motor-vehicle	1,419	12.5
2	Poisoning[a]	607	5.3
3	Falls	587	5.2
4	Choking[c]	191	1.7
5	Fires, flames, smoke	144	1.3

OKLAHOMA

Rank	Cause	Deaths	Rate
5	All U-I	1,663	48.0
I	Motor-vehicle	711	20.5
2	Poisoning[a]	220	6.3
3	Falls	183	5.3
4	Choking[c]	93	2.7
5	Drowning[b]	59	1.7
5	Fires, flames, smoke	59	1.7

OREGON

Rank	Cause	Deaths	Rate
5	All U-I	1,328	38.2
I	Motor-vehicle	520	15.0
2	Falls	195	5.6
3	Poisoning[a]	152	4.4
4	Choking[c]	59	1.7
5	Drowning[b]	40	1.2

PENNSYLVANIA

Rank	Cause	Deaths	Rate
5	All U-I	4,595	37.4
I	Motor-vehicle	1,564	12.7
2	Poisoning[a]	825	6.7
3	Falls	714	5.8
4	Choking[c]	322	2.6
5	Fires, flames, smoke	164	1.3

RHODE ISLAND

Rank	Cause	Deaths	Rate
6	All U-I	281	26.5
I	Motor-vehicle	98	9.3
2	Falls	76	7.2
3	Choking[c]	15	1.4
4	Poisoning[a]	11	1.0
5	Fires, flames, smoke	9	0.8

SOUTH CAROLINA

Rank	Cause	Deaths	Rate
4	All U-I	1,978	48.7
I	Motor-vehicle	1,040	25.6
2	Poisoning[a]	210	5.2
3	Falls	182	4.5
4	Choking[c]	102	2.5
5	Fires, flames, smoke	68	1.7
5	Drowning[b]	68	1.7

SOUTH DAKOTA

Rank	Cause	Deaths	Rate
4	All U-I	404	53.3
I	Motor-vehicle	196	25.9
2	Falls	109	14.4
3	Choking[c]	11	1.5
4	Fires, flames, smoke	10	1.3
5	Poisoning[a]	9	1.2
5	Mechanical suffocation	9	1.2

TENNESSEE

Rank	Cause	Deaths	Rate
5	All U-I	2,999	52.2
I	Motor-vehicle	1,465	25.5
2	Poisoning[a]	350	6.1
3	Falls	349	6.1
4	Choking[c]	134	2.3
5	Fires, flames, smoke	123	2.1

TEXAS

Rank	Cause	Deaths	Rate
4	All U-I	7,920	37.1
I	Motor-vehicle	3,952	18.5
2	Poisoning[a]	1,088	5.1
3	Falls	786	3.7
4	Choking[c]	303	1.4
5	Drowning[b]	288	1.3

UTAH

Rank	Cause	Deaths	Rate
4	All U-I	681	29.9
I	Motor-vehicle	309	13.6
2	Falls	94	4.1
3	Poisoning[a]	42	1.8
4	Drowning[b]	37	1.6
5	Choking[c]	27	1.2

VERMONT

Rank	Cause	Deaths	Rate
5	All U-I	226	36.9
I	Motor-vehicle	86	14.0
2	Falls	26	4.2
2	Poisoning[a]	26	4.2
4	Choking[c]	13	2.1
5	Drowning[b]	8	1.3

VIRGINIA

Rank	Cause	Deaths	Rate
5	All U-I	2,360	32.8
I	Motor-vehicle	956	13.3
2	Poisoning[a]	339	4.7
3	Falls	309	4.3
4	Choking[c]	123	1.7
5	Drowning[b]	81	1.1

WASHINGTON

Rank	Cause	Deaths	Rate
6	All U-I	2,031	33.9
I	Motor-vehicle	703	11.7
2	Falls	467	7.8
3	Poisoning[a]	386	6.4
4	Drowning[b]	74	1.2
5	Fires, flames, smoke	67	1.1

WEST VIRGINIA

Rank	Cause	Deaths	Rate
5	All U-I	872	48.4
I	Motor-vehicle	402	22.3
2	Poisoning[a]	126	7.0
3	Falls	113	6.3
4	Choking[c]	43	2.4
5	Fires, flames, smoke	26	1.4

WISCONSIN

Rank	Cause	Deaths	Rate
5	All U-I	2,094	38.7
I	Motor-vehicle	814	15.1
2	Falls	674	12.5
3	Poisoning[a]	184	3.4
4	Choking[c]	54	1.0
5	Fires, flames, smoke	41	0.8

WYOMING

Rank	Cause	Deaths	Rate
3	All U-I	326	66.0
I	Motor-vehicle	184	37.3
2	Poisoning[a]	23	4.7
3	Falls	22	4.5
4	Drowning[b]	13	2.6
5	Choking[c]	12	2.4

Source: National Safety Council tabulations of National Center for Health Statistics mortality data for 2001.
[a] Solid, liquid, gas, and vapor poisoning.
[b] Excludes transport drownings.
[c] Inhalation or ingestion of food or other object.

UNINTENTIONAL-INJURY DEATHS BY STATE AND EVENT

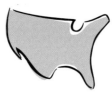

UNINTENTIONAL-INJURY DEATHS BY STATE AND TYPE OF EVENT, UNITED STATES, 2001

State	Population (000)	Total[a]	Motor-vehicle[b]	Falls	Poisoning	Choking[c]	Fires, Flames, and Smoke	Drowning[d]	Mechanical Suffocation
Total U.S.	285,094	101,537	43,788	15,019	14,078	4,185	3,309	3,281	1,370
Alabama	4,466	2,210	1,056	114	188	110	121	65	22
Alaska	633	357	106	22	77	7	14	26	16
Arizona	5,298	2,549	1,041	473	476	55	51	85	30
Arkansas	2,692	1,243	648	137	46	63	90	45	15
California	34,533	8,010	3,864	1,179	1,038	176	183	356	73
Colorado	4,429	1,798	761	288	276	59	21	29	24
Connecticut	3,433	1,049	306	187	241	92	27	31	5
Delaware	796	297	135	36	41	8	19	8	1
Dist. of Columbia	573	324	98	67	104	5	12	3	0
Florida	16,355	7,093	3,161	1,084	1,363	249	139	406	90
Georgia	8,395	3,449	1,649	437	435	151	140	116	42
Hawaii	1,225	388	131	76	45	15	4	39	6
Idaho	1,321	572	273	117	59	7	8	22	7
Illinois	12,517	3,825	1,418	496	784	179	161	83	52
Indiana	6,126	2,154	937	275	154	104	105	66	50
Iowa	2,932	1,033	441	225	53	45	27	17	11
Kansas	2,700	1,095	515	177	104	58	46	19	24
Kentucky	4,067	1,948	862	159	295	80	66	57	38
Louisiana	4,466	2,033	994	154	219	74	100	84	34
Maine	1,285	486	200	93	60	34	13	18	4
Maryland	5,383	1,248	665	200	38	40	59	51	18
Massachusetts	6,400	1,465	534	237	48	114	55	46	17
Michigan	10,005	3,218	1,394	507	333	117	130	117	76
Minnesota	4,985	1,805	626	476	138	44	42	60	45
Mississippi	2,858	1,518	804	177	109	90	79	70	14
Missouri	5,636	2,584	1,182	478	243	115	93	58	37
Montana	906	490	233	111	34	10	5	13	4
Nebraska	1,719	614	265	140	38	41	21	6	8
Nevada	2,095	790	350	87	192	31	15	22	10
New Hampshire	1,259	373	142	72	45	14	14	15	12
New Jersey	8,504	2,296	725	243	575	115	71	38	33
New Mexico	1,829	1,065	486	156	227	19	11	12	12
New York	19,075	4,896	1,580	950	952	164	188	104	68
North Carolina	8,195	3,469	1,661	434	440	140	120	94	32
North Dakota	636	261	126	69	10	6	6	4	2
Ohio	11,386	3,774	1,419	587	607	191	144	95	57
Oklahoma	3,467	1,663	711	183	220	93	59	59	12
Oregon	3,473	1,328	520	195	152	59	30	40	18
Pennsylvania	12,298	4,595	1,564	714	825	322	164	86	59
Rhode Island	1,059	281	98	76	11	15	9	8	6
South Carolina	4,060	1,978	1,040	182	210	102	68	68	33
South Dakota	758	404	196	109	9	11	10	6	9
Tennessee	5,746	2,999	1,465	349	350	134	123	71	32
Texas	21,341	7,920	3,952	786	1,088	303	217	288	94
Utah	2,280	681	309	94	42	27	11	37	11
Vermont	613	226	86	26	26	13	4	8	1
Virginia	7,193	2,360	956	309	339	123	77	81	22
Washington	5,993	2,031	703	467	386	52	67	74	28
West Virginia	1,802	872	402	113	126	43	26	25	10
Wisconsin	5,405	2,094	814	674	184	54	41	37	39
Wyoming	494	326	184	22	23	12	3	13	7

See source and footnotes on page 157.

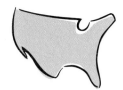
UNINTENTIONAL-INJURY DEATHS BY STATE AND TYPE OF EVENT, UNITED STATES, 2001, Cont.

State	Natural Heat or Cold	Struck By/Against Object	Firearms	Machinery	Electric Current	Water Transport	Air Transport	Rail Transport	All Other Accidents
Total U.S.	899	853	802	648	409	591	918	491	10,896
Alabama	18	16	41	14	9	8	20	14	394
Alaska	9	5	0	2	0	21	23	0	29
Arizona	44	19	17	9	5	12	21	7	204
Arkansas	9	15	18	7	5	8	10	7	120
California	53	58	94	46	35	38	67	66	684
Colorado	18	16	10	9	6	12	53	6	210
Connecticut	8	3	4	5	1	1	4	3	131
Delaware	3	0	3	4	0	1	2	0	36
Dist. of Columbia	1	2	6	2	1	0	0	1	22
Florida	27	36	23	27	37	63	35	20	333
Georgia	18	34	20	17	11	12	42	11	314
Hawaii	1	3	1	4	1	3	8	0	51
Idaho	4	13	8	8	1	9	7	0	29
Illinois	42	28	20	21	19	8	20	46	448
Indiana	19	15	23	20	12	5	12	10	347
Iowa	14	7	7	14	1	5	6	2	158
Kansas	8	14	13	12	8	3	10	1	83
Kentucky	18	21	44	17	10	8	4	6	263
Louisiana	23	21	23	7	12	39	9	12	228
Maine	3	3	2	3	2	9	2	0	40
Maryland	15	6	6	6	6	4	8	6	120
Massachusetts	23	13	4	2	2	7	7	8	348
Michigan	38	20	12	33	11	15	10	11	394
Minnesota	33	14	3	14	4	9	4	8	285
Mississippi	15	15	20	5	13	20	10	10	67
Missouri	37	24	27	28	10	8	22	11	211
Montana	14	8	3	7	1	5	6	1	35
Nebraska	5	6	5	5	2	0	2	2	68
Nevada	14	6	2	0	0	4	9	2	46
New Hampshire	2	1	3	3	2	2	1	0	45
New Jersey	21	13	10	8	7	9	4	18	406
New Mexico	20	7	8	3	4	3	10	8	79
New York	36	30	23	14	13	22	257	32	463
North Carolina	17	37	33	19	12	16	24	18	372
North Dakota	1	4	1	4	1	0	2	3	22
Ohio	23	31	24	19	15	8	6	16	532
Oklahoma	21	13	11	18	15	4	5	9	230
Oregon	12	13	20	14	1	13	6	5	230
Pennsylvania	37	38	27	20	10	4	12	22	691
Rhode Island	6	5	1	0	2	2	0	2	40
South Carolina	10	15	18	10	4	13	7	8	190
South Dakota	5	4	3	6	1	3	4	0	28
Tennessee	18	34	61	21	7	8	18	11	297
Texas	46	69	58	45	61	49	47	36	781
Utah	5	11	3	9	5	10	20	3	84
Vermont	4	3	0	1	0	2	4	1	47
Virginia	24	26	10	32	11	13	8	3	326
Washington	19	20	3	17	6	42	22	13	112
West Virginia	6	11	12	9	5	3	3	5	73
Wisconsin	27	21	14	22	1	19	20	5	122
Wyoming	5	6	0	6	1	9	5	2	28

Source: National Safety Council tabulations of National Center for Health Statistics mortality data.
[a]Deaths are by place of occurrence and exclude nonresident aliens. See also page 152.
[b]See page 162 for motor-vehicle deaths by place of residence.
[c]Suffocation by inhalation or ingestion of food or other object.
[d]Excludes water transport drownings.

UNINTENTIONAL-INJURY TRENDS BY STATE

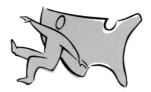

From 1998 to 2001, the greatest decrease in unintentional-injury (U-I) deaths occurred in North Dakota (-14%) and the greatest increase occurred in Alaska (+34%). The death rate decreased the most in California (-16%) and increased the most in Alaska (+31%). Nationwide, U-I deaths increased 4% over the four years and the death rate decreased 1%.

The table below shows the trend in unintentional-injury deaths and death rates by state over the most recent four years for which data are available.

UNINTENTIONAL-INJURY DEATHS BY STATE, UNITED STATES, 1998–2001

State	Deaths[a]				Deaths per 100,000 Population			
	2001[b]	2000[b]	1999	1998	2001[b]	2000	1999	1998
Total U.S.	101,537	97,900	97,860	97,835	35.6	35.6	35.9	35.9
Alabama	2,210	2,099	2,313	2,181	49.5	47.0	52.9	49.9
Alaska	357	342	294	267	56.4	52.2	47.5	43.1
Arizona	2,549	2,432	2,214	2,314	48.1	50.6	46.3	48.4
Arkansas	1,243	1,237	1,287	1,197	46.2	46.9	50.4	46.9
California	8,010	8,510	9,198	9,132	23.2	26.1	27.8	27.6
Colorado	1,798	1,702	1,519	1,542	40.6	40.7	37.4	38.0
Connecticut	1,049	1,150	1,034	1,063	30.6	34.9	31.5	32.4
Delaware	297	279	267	292	37.3	36.2	35.4	38.8
Dist. of Columbia	324	303	161	309	56.6	57.8	31.0	59.5
Florida	7,093	6,337	5,961	5,976	43.4	41.5	39.4	39.5
Georgia	3,449	3,099	3,078	3,140	41.1	39.3	39.5	40.3
Hawaii	388	387	293	319	31.7	30.7	24.7	26.9
Idaho	572	531	597	585	43.3	39.3	47.7	46.7
Illinois	3,825	3,815	4,125	3,668	30.6	31.6	34.0	30.2
Indiana	2,154	2,086	2,309	2,165	35.2	34.4	38.9	36.4
Iowa	1,033	1,031	1,123	1,068	35.2	35.5	39.1	37.2
Kansas	1,095	993	1,126	1,086	40.5	37.1	42.4	40.9
Kentucky	1,948	1,841	1,730	1,728	47.9	46.0	43.7	43.6
Louisiana	2,033	1,988	1,940	1,955	45.5	44.8	44.4	44.7
Maine	486	410	458	452	37.8	32.5	36.6	36.1
Maryland	1,248	1,135	1,296	1,334	23.2	21.5	25.1	25.8
Massachusetts	1,465	1,322	1,303	1,311	22.9	21.3	21.1	21.2
Michigan	3,218	3,127	3,188	3,059	32.2	32.2	32.3	31.0
Minnesota	1,805	1,695	1,772	1,747	36.2	35.0	37.1	36.6
Mississippi	1,518	1,637	1,642	1,697	53.1	58.0	59.3	61.3
Missouri	2,584	2,584	2,465	2,645	45.8	46.5	45.1	48.4
Montana	490	500	461	495	54.1	52.5	52.2	56.1
Nebraska	614	658	668	679	35.7	38.5	40.1	40.8
Nevada	790	811	710	777	37.7	43.2	39.2	42.9
New Hampshire	373	326	329	349	29.6	26.6	27.4	29.1
New Jersey	2,296	2,165	2,227	2,133	27.0	26.4	27.3	26.2
New Mexico	1,065	1,029	969	1,065	58.2	55.2	55.7	61.2
New York	4,896	4,118	4,797	4,520	25.7	22.6	26.4	24.8
North Carolina	3,469	3,596	3,290	3,332	42.3	46.1	43.0	43.6
North Dakota	261	253	267	303	41.0	38.1	42.1	47.8
Ohio	3,774	3,427	3,630	3,463	33.1	30.2	32.2	30.8
Oklahoma	1,663	1,546	1,609	1,565	48.0	45.7	47.9	46.6
Oregon	1,328	1,255	1,199	1,411	38.2	36.9	36.2	42.5
Pennsylvania	4,595	4,615	4,614	4,563	37.4	37.7	38.5	38.0
Rhode Island	281	254	243	252	26.5	25.4	24.5	25.4
South Carolina	1,978	1,998	1,901	1,841	48.7	51.7	48.9	47.4
South Dakota	404	341	351	369	53.3	43.8	47.9	50.3
Tennessee	2,999	2,993	2,677	2,914	52.2	52.8	48.8	53.1
Texas	7,920	7,418	7,227	7,426	37.1	36.8	36.1	37.0
Utah	681	727	650	720	29.9	32.9	30.5	33.8
Vermont	226	238	209	223	36.9	38.5	35.2	37.6
Virginia	2,360	2,337	2,214	2,295	32.8	33.3	32.2	33.4
Washington	2,031	1,971	1,914	1,893	33.9	33.6	33.3	32.9
West Virginia	872	843	798	842	48.4	45.7	44.2	46.6
Wisconsin	2,094	2,141	1,955	1,914	38.7	40.1	37.2	36.5
Wyoming	326	268	258	259	66.0	50.9	53.8	54.0

Source: National Safety Council estimates based on data from National Center for Health Statistics and U.S. Bureau of the Census. See Technical Appendix for comparability.
[a] Deaths for each state are by place of occurrence. All death totals exclude nonresident aliens.
[b] Latest official figures.

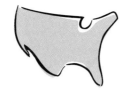

FATAL OCCUPATIONAL INJURIES BY STATE

In general, the states with the largest number of persons employed have the largest number of work-related fatalities. The four largest states — California, Florida, New York, and Texas — accounted for more than one fourth of the total fatalities in the United States. Each state's industry mix, geographical features, age of population, and other characteristics of the workforce must be considered when evaluating state fatality profiles.

FATAL OCCUPATIONAL INJURIES BY STATE AND EVENT OR EXPOSURE, UNITED STATES, 2002

State	Deaths per 100,000 Workers[a]	Total	Transportation[b]	Contact with Objects & Equipment	Assaults & Violent Acts[c]	Falls	Exposure to Harmful Substances or Environments	Fires & Explosions	All Other
Total	**4.0**	**5,524**	**2,381**	**873**	**840**	**714**	**538**	**165**	**13**
Alabama	5.1	102	36	23	19	11	13	—	—
Alaska	12.8	42	30	6	—	—	—	—	—
Arizona	3.9	101	52	8	21	10	8	—	—
Arkansas	6.4	80	37	9	7	15	10	—	—
California	2.8	478	202	62	96	58	50	9	—
Colorado	5.3	123	61	14	27	15	6	—	—
Connecticut	2.3	39	18	5	7	—	—	—	—
Delaware	2.7	11	5	—	—	—	—	—	—
Dist. of Columbia	2.5	8	—	—	—	—	—	—	—
Florida	4.5	354	167	29	52	49	52	—	—
Georgia	4.8	197	83	22	34	30	23	5	—
Hawaii	3.6	24	13	—	—	—	—	—	—
Idaho	6.1	39	29	—	—	—	—	—	—
Illinois	3.2	190	58	33	44	29	19	7	—
Indiana	4.5	136	54	30	23	9	16	—	—
Iowa	3.5	56	21	16	—	10	6	—	—
Kansas	6.7	89	38	20	9	10	9	—	—
Kentucky	7.8	146	70	20	17	20	15	—	—
Louisiana	5.5	103	49	12	—	16	15	7	—
Maine	4.6	30	25	—	—	—	—	—	—
Maryland	3.6	102	37	15	23	15	9	—	—
Massachusetts	1.4	46	14	11	9	9	—	—	—
Michigan	3.2	151	47	29	35	18	17	5	—
Minnesota	2.9	81	44	17	—	8	8	—	—
Mississippi	7.7	94	46	10	15	10	7	6	—
Missouri	6.2	175	83	22	25	24	14	5	—
Montana	11.6	51	29	8	—	6	—	—	—
Nebraska	9.0	83	43	17	8	6	6	—	—
Nevada	4.3	45	20	—	7	8	6	—	—
New Hampshire	2.8	19	9	5	—	—	—	—	—
New Jersey	3.1	129	46	13	28	21	14	7	—
New Mexico	7.3	63	37	12	5	—	—	—	—
New York	2.8	238	72	40	56	45	16	9	—
North Carolina	4.3	169	76	31	15	28	15	—	—
North Dakota	7.6	25	16	—	—	—	—	—	—
Ohio	3.6	202	79	40	30	30	19	—	—
Oklahoma	5.6	92	50	11	8	—	9	9	—
Oregon	3.7	63	23	18	5	6	—	8	—
Pennsylvania	3.1	188	77	34	23	25	21	8	—
Rhode Island	1.5	8	—	—	5	—	—	—	—
South Carolina	5.8	107	39	24	22	13	9	—	—
South Dakota	8.1	36	20	9	—	—	—	—	—
Tennessee	5.0	140	68	24	27	8	10	—	—
Texas	4.1	417	157	66	63	69	42	19	—
Utah	4.4	52	35	5	—	—	—	—	—
Vermont	3.3	11	—	—	—	—	—	—	—
Virginia	3.9	142	50	22	22	24	17	6	—
Washington	2.9	83	38	21	6	11	7	—	—
West Virginia	5.3	40	18	13	—	—	—	—	—
Wisconsin	3.1	91	36	20	13	9	10	—	—
Wyoming	12.0	32	17	6	—	—	—	—	—

Source: U.S. Department of Labor, Bureau of Labor Statistics.
Note: Dashes (—) indicate no data or data that do not meet publication criteria.
[a]Rates exclude military personnel and workers under age 16 and include the self-employed, family workers, and private household workers.
[b]Includes highway, nonhighway, air, water, and rail fatalities, and fatalities resulting from being struck by a vehicle or mobile equipment.
[c]Includes violence by persons, self-inflicted injury, and attacks by animals.

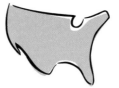

NONFATAL OCCUPATIONAL INJURY AND ILLNESS INCIDENCE RATES[a] BY STATE, PRIVATE INDUSTRY, 2002

State	Total Recordable Cases	Cases with Days away from Work[b]	Cases with Job Transfer or Restriction	Other Recordable Cases
Private Industry[c]	**5.3**	**1.6**	**1.2**	**2.5**
Alabama	5.2	1.2	1.4	2.6
Alaska	7.4	3.0	0.8	3.7
Arizona	5.0	1.4	1.1	2.5
Arkansas	5.7	1.5	1.3	2.0
California	5.6	1.8	1.5	2.2
Colorado	—	—	—	—
Connecticut	5.4	1.7	1.1	2.5
Delaware	4.3	1.6	0.7	2.0
Dist. of Columbia	—	—	—	—
Florida	5.1	1.5	1.3	2.3
Georgia	4.7	1.2	1.2	2.4
Hawaii	5.8	3.0	0.4	2.3
Idaho	—	—	—	—
Illinois	5.0	1.5	1.1	2.3
Indiana	6.9	1.7	1.8	3.4
Iowa	7.5	1.6	2.0	3.9
Kansas	6.2	1.4	1.6	3.2
Kentucky	7.2	2.2	1.8	3.2
Louisiana	3.8	1.2	0.7	1.9
Maine	8.1	2.2	2.8	3.1
Maryland	4.3	1.7	0.7	1.9
Massachusetts	4.6	1.9	0.8	1.9
Michigan	6.8	1.6	2.1	3.1
Minnesota	6.2	1.7	1.5	3.0
Mississippi	—	—	—	—
Missouri	6.0	1.4	1.6	3.0
Montana	6.8	2.3	0.8	3.7
Nebraska	5.7	1.8	1.1	2.9
Nevada	6.0	1.6	1.5	2.9
New Hampshire	—	—	—	—
New Jersey	4.3	1.6	0.7	2.0
New Mexico	5.2	1.6	1.1	2.4
New York	3.5	1.8	0.2	1.5
North Carolina	4.0	1.1	1.1	1.9
North Dakota	—	—	—	—
Ohio	—	—	—	—
Oklahoma	6.1	1.7	1.3	3.1
Oregon	6.0	1.9	1.2	2.8
Pennsylvania	—	—	—	—
Rhode Island	5.3	2.4	0.9	2.1
South Carolina	4.5	1.3	1.1	2.1
South Dakota	—	—	—	—
Tennessee	5.7	1.4	1.6	2.6
Texas	4.3	1.3	1.1	1.9
Utah	6.0	1.3	1.2	3.4
Vermont	6.7	2.1	1.3	3.3
Virginia	4.3	1.3	0.9	2.1
Washington	7.3	2.4	1.1	3.8
West Virginia	6.3	3.1	0.5	2.7
Wisconsin	7.1	2.1	1.5	3.5
Wyoming	5.6	2.2	0.6	2.8

Source: Bureau of Labor Statistics, U.S. Department of Labor.
Note: Because of rounding, components may not add to totals. Dashes (—) indicate data not available.
[a] Incidence rates represent the number of injuries and illnesses per 100 full-time workers using 200,000 hours as the equivalent.
[b] Days-away-from-work cases include those that result in days away from work with or without job transfer or restriction.
[c] Data cover all 50 states.

NONFATAL OCCUPATIONAL AND ILLNESS INCIDENCE RATES BY STATE, PRIVATE INDUSTRY, 2002

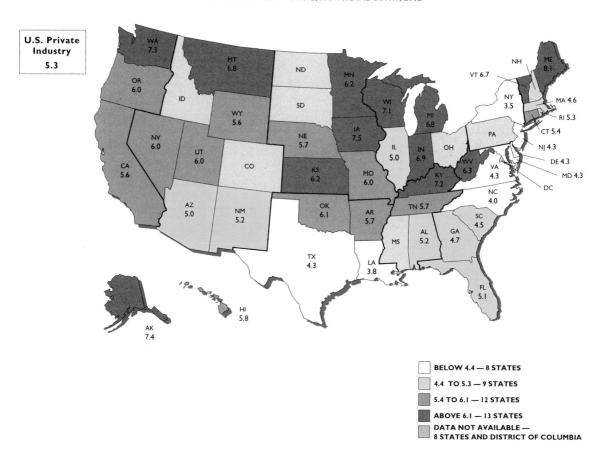

U.S. Private
Industry
5.3

WA 7.3	
MT 6.8	
ND	
MN 6.2	
NH	
ME 8.1	
VT 6.7	
OR 6.0	
ID	
SD	
WI 7.1	
NY 3.5	
MA 4.6	
WY 5.6	
MI 6.8	
RI 5.3	
NV 6.0	
NE 5.7	
IA 7.5	
PA	
CT 5.4	
UT 6.0	
CO	
IL 5.0	
IN 6.9	
OH	
NJ 4.3	
CA 5.6	
KS 6.2	
MO 6.0	
WV 6.3	
VA 4.3	
DE 4.3	
MD 4.3	
KY 7.2	
DC	
AZ 5.0	
NM 5.2	
OK 6.1	
AR 5.7	
TN 5.7	
NC 4.0	
SC 4.5	
TX 4.3	
LA 3.8	
MS	
AL 5.2	
GA 4.7	
FL 5.1	
AK 7.4	
HI 5.8	

BELOW 4.4 — 8 STATES

4.4 TO 5.3 — 9 STATES

5.4 TO 6.1 — 12 STATES

ABOVE 6.1 — 13 STATES

DATA NOT AVAILABLE —
8 STATES AND DISTRICT OF COLUMBIA

MOTOR-VEHICLE DEATHS BY STATE

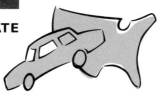

MOTOR-VEHICLE DEATHS BY STATE, UNITED STATES, 2000–2003

| State | Motor-Vehicle Traffic Deaths (Place of Accident) | | | | Total Motor-Vehicle Deaths[a] (Place of Residence) | | | |
| | Number | | Mileage Rate[b] | | Number | | Population Rate[b] | |
	2003	2002	2003	2002	2001[c]	2000	2001	2000
Total U.S.[a]	44,800	44,100	1.6	1.5	43,788	43,354	15.4	15.7
Alabama	983	1,004	1.7	1.7	1,056	1,064	23.6	23.8
Alaska	95	85	1.9	1.8	106	132	16.8	20.2
Arizona	1,120	1,104	2.2	2.1	1,041	999	19.7	20.8
Arkansas	627	641	2.1	2.1	648	680	24.1	25.8
California	4,227	4,104	1.3	1.3	3,864	3,743	11.2	11.5
Colorado	629	732	1.4	1.7	761	751	17.2	18.0
Connecticut	305	325	1.0	1.0	306	340	8.9	10.3
Delaware	145	126	1.6	1.4	135	126	17.0	16.4
Dist. of Columbia	70	50	2.0	1.3	98	56	17.1	10.7
Florida	3,179	3,137	1.8	2.0	3,161	3,057	19.3	20.0
Georgia	1,610	1,522	1.5	1.4	1,649	1,536	19.6	19.5
Hawaii	139	115	1.6	1.3	131	129	10.7	10.2
Idaho	293	265	2.1	1.9	273	271	20.7	20.1
Illinois	1,455	1,411	1.4	1.3	1,418	1,568	11.3	13.0
Indiana	787	792	1.1	1.1	937	918	15.3	15.1
Iowa	445	409	1.4	1.3	441	474	15.0	16.3
Kansas	472	510	1.6	1.8	515	495	19.1	18.5
Kentucky	931	917	2.0	1.9	862	832	21.2	20.8
Louisiana	896	865	2.1	2.1	994	1,014	22.3	22.9
Maine	205	191	1.4	1.3	200	175	15.6	13.9
Maryland	648	650	1.2	1.2	665	612	12.4	11.6
Massachusetts	462	459	0.9	0.9	534	493	8.3	7.9
Michigan	1,283	1,279	1.3	1.3	1,394	1,507	13.9	15.5
Minnesota	628	653	1.1	1.2	626	689	12.6	14.2
Mississippi	873	885	2.4	2.4	804	935	28.1	33.1
Missouri	1,232	1,203	1.8	1.7	1,182	1,097	21.0	19.8
Montana	262	268	2.5	2.6	233	234	25.7	24.6
Nebraska	293	307	1.6	1.7	265	285	15.4	16.7
Nevada	368	380	2.0	2.0	350	303	16.7	16.2
New Hampshire	126	127	1.0	1.0	142	134	11.3	10.9
New Jersey	733	786	1.0	1.1	725	772	8.5	9.4
New Mexico	437	458	1.9	1.9	486	418	26.6	22.4
New York	—	1,523	—	1.1	1,580	1,541	8.3	8.5
North Carolina	1,528	1,564	1.6	1.7	1,661	1,693	20.3	21.7
North Dakota	105	97	1.4	1.3	126	105	19.8	15.8
Ohio	1,278	1,301	1.2	1.2	1,419	1,456	12.5	12.8
Oklahoma	642	725	1.4	1.6	711	679	20.5	20.1
Oregon	511	436	1.5	1.2	520	478	15.0	14.0
Pennsylvania	—	1,618	—	1.5	1,564	1,522	12.7	12.4
Rhode Island	104	84	1.3	1.0	98	81	9.3	8.1
South Carolina	968	1,053	2.0	2.2	1,040	1,025	25.6	26.5
South Dakota	203	175	2.4	2.0	196	178	25.9	22.9
Tennessee	1,198	1,159	1.7	1.7	1,465	1,395	25.5	24.6
Texas	3,826	3,722	1.7	1.7	3,952	3,824	18.5	19.0
Utah	309	330	1.2	1.4	309	364	13.6	16.5
Vermont	69	78	0.7	0.8	86	76	14.0	12.3
Virginia	942	913	1.2	1.2	956	981	13.3	14.0
Washington	601	660	1.1	1.2	703	711	11.7	12.1
West Virginia	377	437	1.9	2.2	402	394	22.3	21.3
Wisconsin	836	805	1.4	1.4	814	890	15.1	16.7
Wyoming	165	176	1.8	2.0	184	122	37.3	23.2

Source: Motor-Vehicle Traffic Deaths are provisional counts from state traffic authorities; Total Motor-Vehicle Deaths are from the National Center for Health Statistics (see also page 156).
Note: Dashes (—) indicate data not reported.
[a] Includes both traffic and nontraffic motor-vehicle deaths. See definitions of motor-vehicle traffic and nontraffic accidents on page 175.
[b] The mileage death rate is deaths per 100,000,000 vehicle miles; the population death rate is deaths per 100,000 population. Death rates are National Safety Council estimates.
[c] Latest year available. See Technical Appendix for comparability.

MILEAGE DEATH RATES, 2003
MOTOR-VEHICLE TRAFFIC DEATHS PER 100,000,000 VEHICLE MILES

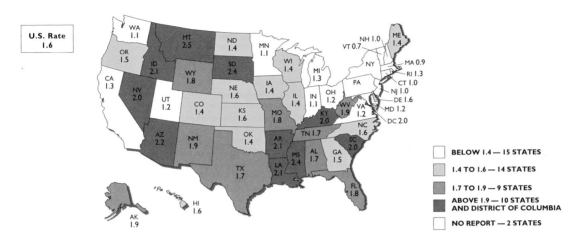

REGISTRATION DEATH RATES, 2003
MOTOR-VEHICLE TRAFFIC DEATHS PER 10,000 MOTOR VEHICLES

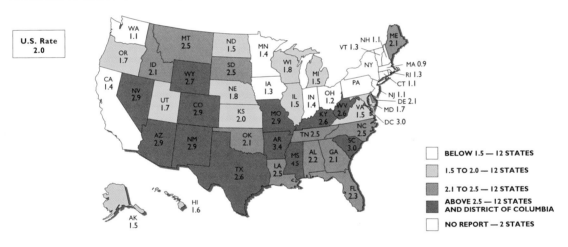

POPULATION DEATH RATES, 2003
MOTOR-VEHICLE TRAFFIC DEATHS PER 100,000 POPULATION

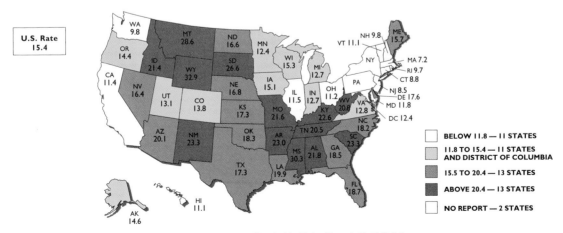

Source: Rates estimated by National Safety Council based on data from state traffic authorities, National Center for Health Statistics, Federal Highway Administration, and the U.S. Census Bureau.

INJURY FACTS®

NATIONAL SAFETY COUNCIL

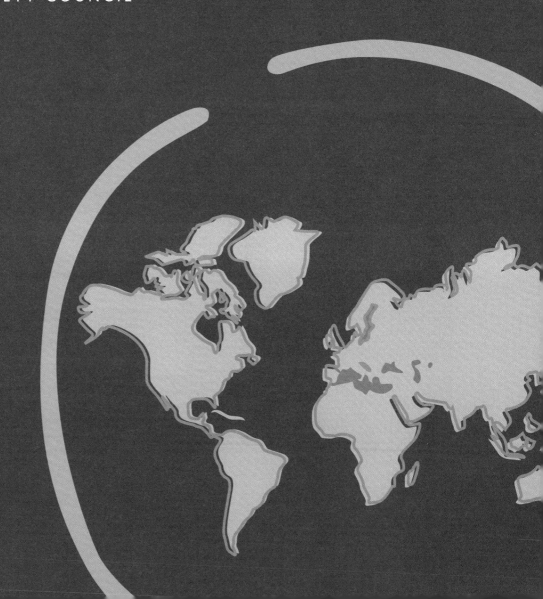

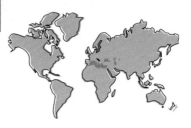
The term "Accidents and Adverse Effects" used in the International Classification of Diseases system (ICD) refers to all causes of unintentional-injury deaths, including transportation accidents, unintentional poisonings, falls, fires, burns, natural and environmental factors, drowning, suffocation, medical and surgical complications and misadventures, and other causes such as those involving machinery, firearms, or electric current. The data presented in the graph below are identified by codes E800–E949 of the ninth revision of the ICD and categories V01–X59, Y40–Y86, and Y88 of the tenth revision.

The number of unintentional-injury deaths and the death rate per 100,000 population (not adjusted for differences among countries on the age distribution of the population) are presented for 40 countries for which information was obtained. Countries are shown in ascending order of death rate for the latest year for which data were available. About half of the countries reported data for 2000. More than one-third reported data for 1999. The rest reported for 1996–1998.

The number of injury deaths ranged from 158 in Belize to more than 100,000 in the United States. The death rates per 100,000 population ranged from 9.8 in Singapore to 83.5 in Ukraine.

The mean death rate for these 40 countries was 37.8 per 100,000 population. This is not much greater than the median death rate (35.0). Half of the countries had death rates between 29.0 and 43.6 (the first and third quartile rates).

The United States, Japan, Mexico, Ukraine, and France each reported more than 30,000 injury deaths in the most recent year. The death rates for United States, Japan, and Mexico were below the mean, but the rates for Ukraine and France were above it.

A number of factors may contribute to differences in death rates among countries. Elements such as demographics, geography and climate, economic structure and development, social and religious traditions, educational and health care systems, and governmental and regulatory systems may help determine rates by influencing the overall priority of injury prevention within each society, and by influencing the kinds of prevention and control programs implemented, the intensiveness of the programs, and speed with which they are adopted.

Source: National Safety Council tabulations of World Health Organization data.

UNINTENTIONAL INJURY DEATHS AND DEATH RATES, 40 COUNTRIES, LATEST YEAR AVAILABLE

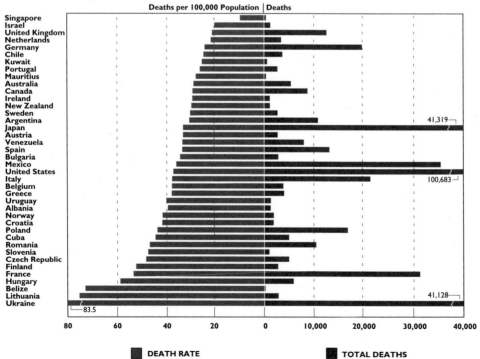

UNINTENTIONAL INJURY DEATH RATES PER 100,000 POPULATION, LATEST YEAR AVAILABLE (1998–2000)

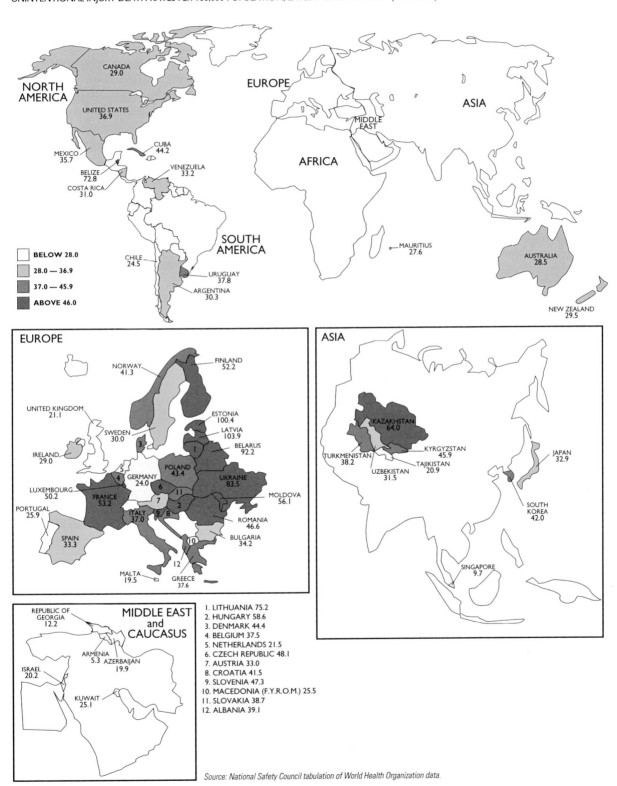

BELOW 28.0
28.0 — 36.9
37.0 — 45.9
ABOVE 46.0

NORTH AMERICA
CANADA 29.0
UNITED STATES 36.9
MEXICO 35.7
BELIZE 72.8
COSTA RICA 31.0
CUBA 44.2
VENEZUELA 33.2

SOUTH AMERICA
CHILE 24.5
URUGUAY 37.8
ARGENTINA 30.3

EUROPE
MIDDLE EAST
AFRICA
MAURITIUS 27.6

ASIA
AUSTRALIA 28.5
NEW ZEALAND 29.5

EUROPE
NORWAY 41.3
FINLAND 52.2
UNITED KINGDOM 21.1
ESTONIA 100.4
LATVIA 103.9
BELARUS 92.2
SWEDEN 30.0
IRELAND 29.0
POLAND 43.4
UKRAINE 83.5
LUXEMBOURG 50.2
GERMANY 24.0
MOLDOVA 56.1
FRANCE 53.2
PORTUGAL 25.9
ITALY 37.0
ROMANIA 46.6
SPAIN 33.3
BULGARIA 34.2
MALTA 19.5
GREECE 37.6

ASIA
KAZAKHSTAN 64.0
TURKMENISTAN 38.2
KYRGYZSTAN 45.9
TAJIKISTAN 20.9
UZBEKISTAN 31.5
JAPAN 32.9
SOUTH KOREA 42.0
SINGAPORE 9.7

MIDDLE EAST and CAUCASUS
REPUBLIC OF GEORGIA 12.2
ARMENIA 5.3
AZERBAIJAN 19.9
ISRAEL 20.2
KUWAIT 25.1

1. LITHUANIA 75.2
2. HUNGARY 58.6
3. DENMARK 44.4
4. BELGIUM 37.5
5. NETHERLANDS 21.5
6. CZECH REPUBLIC 48.1
7. AUSTRIA 33.0
8. CROATIA 41.5
9. SLOVENIA 47.3
10. MACEDONIA (F.Y.R.O.M.) 25.5
11. SLOVAKIA 38.7
12. ALBANIA 39.1

Source: National Safety Council tabulation of World Health Organization data.

INTERNATIONAL MOTOR-VEHICLE DEATHS AND DEATH RATES

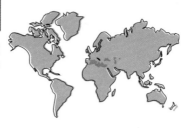

The International Classification of Diseases system (ICD) identifies motor-vehicle traffic accidents by codes E810–E819 in the ninth ICD revision and more than 280 individual four-character codes in the range from V01 to V89 of the tenth revision. A motor vehicle is a mechanically or electrically powered device used in the transportation of persons or property on a land highway. A motor-vehicle traffic accident involves a motor vehicle in transport (i.e., in motion or on a roadway) on a public highway.

The graph below shows both the number of motor-vehicle deaths and the death rate per 100,000 population for 40 countries analyzed. Countries are shown in ascending order of death rate for the most recent year for which data were available. The data range from 1996 to 2000, with 34 of the 40 countries reporting for 1999 or 2000.

Of the countries reporting, the United States has the highest number of motor-vehicle deaths—41,091

(1999), followed by Japan—11,670 (1999), Mexico—8,871 (2000), and France—7,852 (1999).

Among the 40 countries, Belize has the highest motor-vehicle death rate with 44.2 deaths per 100,000 population in 1998, followed by Greece at 21.1 (1999), Lithuania at 18.4 (2000), Venezuela at 17.4 (2000), and Kuwait at 16.6 (2000). Albania (1.7 per 100,000 population in 2000) reported the lowest rate, while Singapore (5.4 per 100,000 population in 2000) and Sweden (5.5 per 100,000 in 1999) reported the second and third lowest rate of motor-vehicle deaths, respectively.

The mean death rate for these 40 countries was 11.8 per 100,000 population. This is about the same as the median death rate, which was 10.4. Half of the countries had death rates between 7.7 and 14.7 (the first and third quartile rates).

Source: National Safety Council tabulations of World Health Organization data.

DEATHS AND DEATH RATES DUE TO MOTOR-VEHICLE TRAFFIC ACCIDENTS, 40 COUNTRIES, LATEST YEAR AVAILABLE

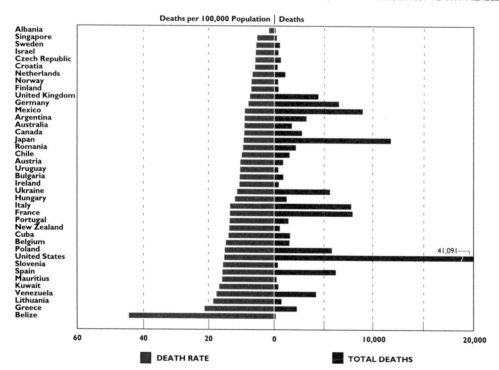

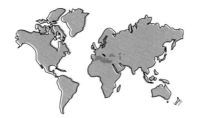

INJURIES DUE TO MOTOR-VEHICLE TRAFFIC ACCIDENTS, 2000

The table below presents data on nonfatal motor-vehicle injuries in European countries, Israel, and the United States. These statistics are compiled by the secretariat of the United Nations Economic Commission for Europe (UNECE) based on data reported by UNECE member countries and other official national and international organizations.

Nonfatal traffic accidents included are those in which at least one moving vehicle was directly or indirectly involved and that (a) occurred or originated on a road open to public traffic and (b) resulted in one or more persons being injured.

NONFATAL MOTOR-VEHICLE INJURIES AND INJURY RATES BY AGE, 2000

Country	Injuries		Injuries per 100,000 Population							
	Total	Change from 1999	All Ages	0–9	10–14	15–17	18–20	21–24	25-64	65 & Over
Albania[a]	336	−12%	9.88	(b)	(b)	(b)	(b)	(b)	(b)	(b)
Tajikistan	1,465	−15%	23.44	7.60	32.25	(b)	(b)	(b)	(b)	(b)
Azerbaijan	2,199	−5%	27.21	10.31	11.47	14.92	17.79	29.69	40.89	23.73
Romania	6,315	−4%	28.15	18.63	22.60	23.19	30.18	32.95	30.96	26.15
Armenia	1,163	−9%	30.59	16.00	12.68	9.52	(b)	(b)	(b)	(b)
Georgia	2,079	−4%	42.04	6.99	28.80	(b)	240.17	(b)	47.80	26.05
Belarus	6,494	−3%	65.00	31.40	40.29	86.23	125.99	130.37	68.15	30.80
Kyrgyzstan	3,292	0%	67.08	32.37	36.99	29.56	110.81	99.43	62.24	228.16
Ukraine	36,636	−4%	74.71	39.02	46.33	84.59	150.89	139.41	80.80	36.67
Republic of Moldova	3,147	2%	86.36	54.13	48.12	84.04	170.03	149.81	93.02	48.58
Kazakhstan	13,254	−3%	89.30	47.02	61.01	(c)	(c)	(c)	92.21	59.95
Bulgaria	8,030	−12%	98.53	52.81	72.96	114.74	201.87	168.13	100.77	67.16
Macedonia[d]	2,340	−22%	115.21	61.04	81.99	132.40	237.62	192.22	120.49	73.10
Russia	179,401	−1%	123.88	63.15	85.37	159.82	225.47	231.35	128.87	65.09
Estonia	1,843	9%	134.90	91.18	111.01	211.27	331.67	278.00	129.31	61.66
Finland	8,508	−6%	164.21	52.94	126.80	431.16	468.59	276.85	154.45	119.53
Denmark	9,092	−3%	169.97	45.36	117.84	425.23	611.79	378.10	162.10	105.96
Poland	71,638	5%	185.38	(b)	(b)	(b)	(b)	(b)	(b)	(b)
Slovakia	10,094	−12%	186.84	(b)	(b)	(b)	(b)	(b)	(b)	(b)
Lithuania	6,960	−10%	188.49	141.76	151.13	247.65	452.25	340.92	180.55	104.63
Turkey[a]	136,751	9%	212.55	82.60	119.72	167.93	274.34	262.48	266.90	206.29
Hungary[a]	22,698	−8%	226.00	104.19	176.77	295.52	400.05	401.46	237.64	136.67
Latvia	5,449	4%	230.29	132.71	154.14	288.39	482.83	514.44	227.85	101.50
Sweden	22,032	0%	248.03	74.35	155.54	426.38	633.75	520.00	268.77	144.23
Norway	11,662	2%	259.67	82.92	156.03	577.38	890.54	539.98	256.61	144.66
France	162,117	−3%	274.59	90.78	180.27	587.17	753.49	633.16	269.79	132.77
Greece[a]	30,803	−6%	292.76	(b)	(b)	(b)	(b)	(b)	(b)	(b)
Malta[a]	1,169	3%	307.47	315.26	1,353.79	1,821.84	1,289.02	419.91	(b)	(b)
Czech Republic	32,439	−7%	315.97	179.33	241.87	430.91	740.83	648.24	304.79	165.07
Ireland	12,043	−2%	318.01	97.64	134.01	244.53	581.28	461.90	304.47	128.57
Switzerland	30,058	2%	416.95	154.29	304.41	730.63	1,124.95	911.90	428.26	230.96
Croatia	20,501	13%	467.91	214.76	252.52	(c)	(c)	(c)	443.96	220.58
Italy	301,559	−5%	521.33	90.23	213.17	881.76	1,289.82	1,264.12	541.85	217.70
Cyprus	3,586	−3%	535.94	(b)	(b)	(b)	(b)	(b)	(b)	(b)
United Kingdom[e]	316,874	0%	545.79	241.71	492.59	838.44	1,379.26	1,061.90	564.99	236.09
Slovenia	11,574	29%	581.58	219.39	343.21	1,012.59	1,673.14	1,457.68	548.16	222.81
Germany[a]	504,074	−3%	613.50	263.96	500.19	1,223.24	2,088.40	1,459.00	592.45	272.09
Israel	39,817	−12%	625.16	222.65	222.12	501.64	1,524.56	1,366.78	749.08	299.45
Portugal[a,f]	59,924	−8%	631.44	293.71	358.57	824.75	1,446.41	1,258.22	633.16	381.87
Belgium	67,961	−4%	662.17	227.19	434.13	1,386.64	1,928.72	1,543.74	645.07	268.43
Austria	54,929	0%	676.36	249.57	416.20	1,662.33	2,142.95	1,511.24	649.42	347.83
United States	3,189,000	−1%	1,161.18	444.66	583.34	2,233.82	2,790.95	2,285.56	1,204.47	723.14

Source: United Nations. (2002). Statistics of Road Traffic Accidents in Europe and North America. Vol. XLVII. Geneva: UN Commission for Europe.
[a] Population estimates and age distribution for 1999.
[b] Injury data not available.
[c] Comparable population and injury data not available.
[d] The former Yugoslav Republic of Macedonia.
[e] Great Britain.
[f] Continental territory only.

FATAL OCCUPATIONAL INJURIES BY COUNTRY

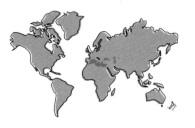

Counts and rates of work-related deaths are shown on this page and the next. Comparisons between countries should be made with caution and take into account the differences in sources, coverage, and kinds of cases included.

OCCUPATIONAL DEATHS BY COUNTRY, 1998–2002

Country	Deaths					Source of Data	Maximum Period[a]	Coverage		
	1998	1999	2000	2001	2002			Worker Types[b]	% of Total Employment[c]	Economic Activities Excluded
Occupational Injuries Only — Compensated Cases										
France	683	717	730	—	—	I	varies	E	75	P
Tunisia	114	129	158	159	—	I	—	E	39	P
Occupational Injuries Only — Reported Cases										
Argentina	1,092	1,069	915	—	—	I	—	E, SE	60	none
Austria	140	131	142	122	130	I	none	E, SE	71	none
Azerbaijan	44	34	37	27	59	N	—	E	—	—
Belarus	294	298	258	234	228	N	same year	E	—	none
Chile	339	261	362	302	345	—	—	IE	47	none
Czech Republic	208	191	223	231	206	N	none	E, SE	95	AF, Pol
Denmark	80	69	68	50	—	N	1 year	E, SE	100	ASO
Hungary	158	154	151	124	163	N	90 days	E, SE	98	none
Japan	1,844	1,992	1,889	1,790	1,658	N	—	E	—	none
Poland	651	523	594	554	515	N	6 months	E, SE	76	Agr
Portugal	—	236	368	—	—	N	1 year	E, SE	67	PA, AF
Slovakia	138	115	88	100	87	N	none	IE	98	none
Spain	1,075	1,104	1,136	1,030	1,104	N	none	I	85	PA, AF
Sweden	68	67	59	56	—	I	none	E, SE	97	none
Taiwan, China	631	650	602	543	—	—	—	—	—	—
Ukraine	1,504	1,321	1,239	1,325	1,227	N	4 months	E	71	AF
United Kingdom	200	173	219	210	—	N	1 year	E, SE	92	SF, AT
United States	5,117	5,184	5,022	5,042	4,716	C	none	E, SE	100	none
Occupational Injuries and Commuting Accidents — Compensated Cases										
Belgium	66	64	78	69	—	I	none	IE	48	P, AF
Brazil	—	—	2,053	—	—	I	none	E	27	none
Germany	1,287	1,293	1,153	1,107	—	I	none	E, SE	100	none
Greece	78	120	80	—	—	I	none	E	48	none
Italy	1,232	1,188	1,115	1,241	—	I	none	I	76	none
Occupational Injuries and Commuting Accidents — Reported Cases										
Burkina Faso	12	17	8	—	—	I	none	I	—	none
Egypt[d]	149	143	113	130	121	N	6 months	E	11	none
Hong Kong, China	240	235	199	176	—	N	none	E	77	none
Romania	531	454	489	440	415	N	same year	E, SE	61	AF, P
Russian Federation	4,300	4,260	4,400	4,370	—	N	none	E	5	Low
Occupational injuries and Occupational Diseases — Compensated Cases										
Australia[e]	265	242	231	210	198	I	3 years	E	83	AF
Canada	798	833	882	919	934	I	none	E, SE	85	AF
Switzerland	105	83	82	72	—	I	same year	IE	88	none
Occupational injuries and Occupational Diseases — Reported Cases										
Sri Lanka	—	37	41	27	36	N	1 year	E	35	M,E,TSC,C
Turkey	1,252	1,333	1,291	1,008	—	I	—	IE	25	none
Zimbabwe	174	169	96	101	—	I	1 year	IE	—	PA, D, Inf
Occupational injuries, Occupational Diseases, and Commuting Accidents — Compensated cases										
Israel	300	114	120	100	—	I	same year	E, SE	100	none
Malaysia	1,273	912	1,004	958	858	I	—	I	—	—
Thailand	790	610	616	597	—	I	—	I	16	none
Occupational injuries, Occupational Diseases, and Commuting Accidents — Reported cases										
Bulgaria	104	89	138	138	—	N	—	E, SE	35	none
Mexico	1,141	1,128	1,740	1,502	—	I	none	IE	32	none
Togo	10	9	7	10	—	I	—	E	—	Agr, PA, F

Source: National Safety Council tabulation of International Labour Organization data.
Note: Dash (—) means data not available.
[a]Maximum period between accident and death for death to be counted.
[b]Types of workers included in the data.
[c]Workers covered by the statistics as a percentage of total employment; latest year available.
[d]Establishments with 50 or more workers.
[e]Excluding Victoria and Australian Capital Territory.

Source of Data	Worker Types	Economic Activities		
C = Census	E = Employees	AF = Armed forces	D = Domestic services	PA = Public administration
I = Insurance system	I = Insured persons	Agr = Agriculture	E = Electricity, gas, and water	Pol = Police
N = Notification system	IE = Insured employees	ASO = Air, sea, offshore accidents	Inf = Informal sector	SF = Sea fishing
S = Survey	SE = Self-employed	AT = Air transport	Low = Activities with low rates of injuries	TSC = Transport, storage, and communications
		C = Construction	M = Manufacturing	
			P = Public sector	

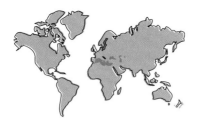

About 350,000 workers died in occupational accidents in 2002 according to estimates made by the International Labour Organization (ILO). The ILO also estimates that universal use of best prevention practices could prevent about 300,000 of those deaths.

Source: "Global Estimates of Fatalities Caused by Work Related Diseases and Occupational Accidents, 2002" [www.ilo.org/public/English/protection/safework/accidis/globest_2002/dis_world.htm accessed 4/19/04]. Takala, J. (2002). Introductory Report: Decent Work—Safe Work. *Geneva: International Labour Organization.*

OCCUPATIONAL DEATH RATES BY COUNTRY, 1998–2002

Country	1998	1999	2000	2001	2002
Deaths per 100,000 employed persons					
Occupational injuries only — Compensated cases					
France	4.5	4.5	4.4	—	—
Occupational injuries only — Reported cases					
Azerbaijan	4	4	4	3	6
Belarus	7.4	7.4	6.4	5.8	5.9
Denmark	3	3	2	2	—
Hungary	4.31	4.06	3.98	3.21	4.21
Poland	5.5	—	5.2	5.1	4.9
Sweden	1.7	1.7	1.5	1.4	—
Ukraine	10.2	9.2	9.5	10.5	10.0
United Kingdom	0.8	0.7	0.9	0.8	—
Occupational injuries and commuting accidents — Compensated cases					
Brazil	—	—	11.5	—	—
Germany	3.42	3.42	3.05	2.95	—
Occupational injuries and commuting accidents — Reported cases					
Egypt	9	8	7	7	7
Hong Kong, China	10.1	9.7	8.0	7.1	—
Romania	8	7	7	7	7
Russian Federation	14.2	14.4	14.9	15.0	—
Occupational injuries and occupational diseases — Compensated cases					
Australia	4	3	3	3	2
Canada	6.7	6.7	7.1	7.2	7.2
Occupational injuries and occupational diseases — Reported cases					
United States	3.9	3.9	3.8	3.7	3.6
Occupational injuries, occupational diseases, and commuting accidents — Compensated cases					
Israel	—	4.1	4.3	4.2	—
Occupational injuries, occupational diseases, and commuting accidents — Reported cases					
Bulgaria	8.6	8.3	7.3	7.3	—
Togo	17.4	15.1	11.7	16.8	—
Deaths per 100,000 insured persons					
Occupational injuries only — Compensated cases					
Tunisia	11.7	13.0	15.1	14.6	—
Occupational injuries only — Reported cases					
Argentina	23.7	21.6	18.6	—	—
Austria	5.3	4.9	5.3	4.5	—
Chile	13	10	14	12	13
Czech Republic	4.4	4.2	4.9	5.2	4.6
Portugal	—	7.4	8.7	—	—
Slovakia	6.27	5.47	4.27	4.91	4.29
Spain	9.8	9.5	9.2	8.0	8.3
Taiwan, China	8.4	8.5	7.7	6.9	—
Occupational injuries and commuting accidents — Compensated cases					
Greece	4.1	6.2	4.1	—	—
Italy	8	7	7	—	—
Occupational injuries and commuting accidents — Reported cases					
Burkina Faso	7.5	9.9	4.4	—	—
Occupational injuries and occupational diseases — Compensated cases					
Switzerland	3.2	2.4	2.3	2.0	—
Occupational injuries and occupational diseases — Reported cases					
Turkey	22.5	22.9	24.6	20.6	—
Zimbabwe	13.5	13.5	8.4	10.1	—
Occupational injuries, occupational diseases, and commuting accidents — Compensated cases					
Malaysia	15.1	10.6	11.3	10.9	10.8
Thailand	15.4	11.5	11.3	—	—
Occupational injuries, occupational diseases, and commuting accidents — Reported cases					
Mexico	10	9	14	12	—
Deaths per 1,000,000 hours worked					
Occupational injuries only — Reported cases					
Japan	0.01	0.01	0.01	0.01	0.01
Occupational injuries and occupational diseases — Reported cases					
Sri Lanka	—	0.072	0.009	0.007	0.008
Occupational injuries and commuting accidents — Compensated cases					
Belgium	0.02	0.02	0.03	0.02	—

Source: National Safety Council tabulation of International Labour Organization data.
Note: Dash (—) means data not available.
See limitations of data on page 170.

TECHNICAL APPENDIX
OTHER SOURCES
GLOSSARY
INDEX

INJURY FACTS®

NATIONAL SAFETY COUNCIL

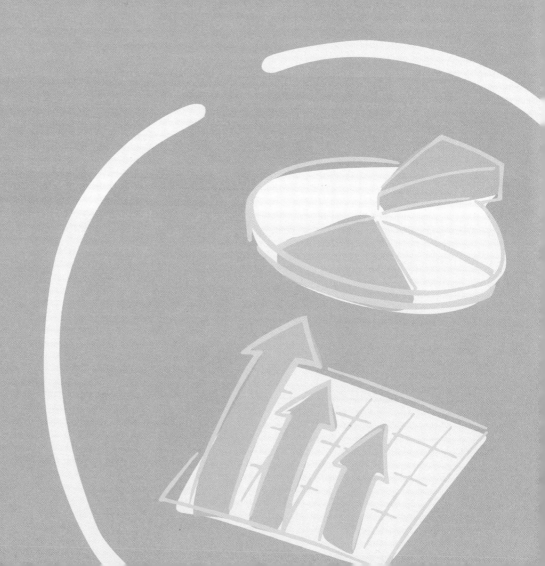

This appendix gives a brief explanation of some of the sources and methods used by the National Safety Council (NSC) Statistics Department in preparing the estimates of deaths, injuries, and costs presented in this book. Because many of the estimates depend on death certificate data provided by the states or the National Center for Health Statistics (NCHS), it begins with a brief introduction to the certification and classification of deaths.

Certification and classification. The medical certification of death involves entering information on the death certificate about the disease or condition directly leading to death, antecedent causes, and other significant conditions. The death certificate is then registered with the appropriate authority and a code is assigned for the underlying cause of death. The underlying cause is defined as "(a) the disease or injury which initiated the train of morbid events leading directly to death, or (b) the circumstances of the accident or violence which produced the fatal injury" (World Health Organization [WHO], 1992). Deaths are classified and coded on the basis of a WHO standard, the *International Statistical Classification of Diseases and Related Health Problems*, commonly known as the International Classification of Diseases, or ICD (WHO, 1992). For deaths due to injury and poisoning, the ICD provides a system of "external cause" codes to which the underlying cause of death is assigned. (See pages 18–19 of *Injury Facts®* for a condensed list of external cause codes.)

Comparability across ICD revisions. The ICD is revised periodically and these revisions can affect comparability from year to year. The sixth revision (1948) substantially expanded the list of external causes and provided for classifying the place of occurrence. Changes in the classification procedures for the sixth revision as well as the seventh (1958) and eighth (1968) revisions classified as diseases some deaths previously classified as injuries. The eighth revision also expanded and reorganized some external cause sections. The ninth revision (1979), provided more detail on the agency involved, the victim's activity, and the place of occurrence. The tenth revision, which was adopted in the United States effective with 1999 data, completely revised the transportation-related categories. Specific external cause categories affected by the revisions are noted in the historical tables.

The table at the end of this appendix (page 179) shows the ICD-9 codes, the ICD-10 codes, and a comparability ratio for each of the principal causes of unintentional-injury death. The comparability ratio represents the net effect of the new revision on statistics for the cause of death. The comparability ratio was obtained by classifying a sample of death certificates under both ICD-9 and ICD-10 and then dividing the number of deaths for a selected cause classified under ICD-10 by the number classified to the most nearly comparable ICD-9 cause. A comparability ratio of 1.00 indicates no net change due to the new classification scheme. A ratio less than 1.00 indicates fewer deaths assigned to a cause under ICD-10 than under ICD-9. A ratio greater than 1.00 indicates an increase in assignment of deaths to a cause under ICD-10 compared to ICD-9.

The broad category of "accidents" or "unintentional injuries" under ICD-9 included complications and misadventures of surgical and medical care (E870–E879) and adverse effects of drugs in therapeutic use (E930–E949). These categories are not included in "accidents" or "unintentional injuries" under ICD-10. In 1998, deaths in these two categories numbered 3,228 and 276, respectively.

Under ICD-9, the code range for falls (E880–E888) included a code for "fracture, cause unspecified" (E887). A similar code does not appear in ICD-10 (W00–W19), which probably accounts for the low comparability ratio (0.8409). In 1998, deaths in code E887 numbered 3,679.

Beginning with 1970 data, tabulations published by NCHS no longer include deaths of nonresident aliens. In 2001, there were 688 such deaths, of which 303 were motor-vehicle related.

Fatality estimates. The Council uses four classes to categorize unintentional injuries: Motor Vehicle, Work, Home, and Public. Each class represents an environment and an intervention route for injury prevention through a responsible authority such as a police department, an employer, a home owner, or public health department.

Motor vehicle. The Motor-Vehicle class can be identified by the underlying cause of death (see the table on page 179).

Work. The National Safety Council adopted the Bureau of Labor Statistics' Census of Fatal Occupational Injuries (CFOI) figure, beginning with the 1992 data year, as the authoritative count of unintentional work-related deaths. The CFOI system is described in detail in Toscano and Windau (1994).

The 2-Way Split. After subtracting the Motor-Vehicle and Work figures from the unintentional-injury total (ICD-10 codes V01–X59, Y85–Y86), the remainder belong to the Home and Public classes. The Home class can be identified by the "place of occurrence" subclassification (code .0) used with most nontransport deaths; the Public class is the remainder. Missing "place of occurrence" information, however, prevents the direct determination of the Home and Public class totals. Because of this, the Council allocates nonmotor-vehicle, nonwork deaths into the Home and Public classes based on the external cause, age group, and cases with specified "place of occurrence." This procedure, known as the 2-Way Split, uses the most recent death certificate data available from the NCHS and the CFOI data for the same calendar year. For each cause-code group and age group combination, the Motor-Vehicle and Work deaths are subtracted, and the remainder, including those with "place of occurrence" unspecified, are allocated to Home and Public in the same proportion as those with "place of occurrence" specified.

The table on page 179 shows the ICD-10 cause-codes and CFOI event codes for the most common causes of unintentional-injury death. The CFOI event codes (BLS, 1992) do not match exactly with ICD cause codes, so there is some error in the allocation of deaths among the classes.

State reporting system. The Council operates a reporting system through which participating states send tabulations of unintentional-injury death data by age group, class, and type of event or industry. This is known as the Injury Mortality Tabulation reporting system. These data are used to make current year estimates based on the most recent 2-Way Split and CFOI data.

Linking up to current year. The benchmark data published by NCHS are usually two years old and the CFOI data are usually one year old. The link-relative technique is used to make current year estimates from

these data using the state vital statistics data. This method assumes that the change in deaths from one year to the next in states reporting for both years reflects the change in deaths for the entire nation. The ratio is calculated and multiplied times the benchmark figure resulting in an estimate for the next year. It may be necessary to repeat the process, depending on the reference year of the benchmark. For example, the 2001 NCHS and CFOI data were used this year for a 2-Way Split, and state data were used to make estimates for 2002 and 2003 Home and Public classes using the link-relative technique. CFOI data for 2002 were also available so it was necessary only to make 2003 Work estimates.

Revisions of prior years. When the figures for a given year are published by NCHS, the 2-Way Split based on those figures and the CFOI become the final estimate of unintentional-injury deaths by class, age group, and type of event or industry. Subsequent years are revised by repeating the link-relative process described above. For example, in the 2004 edition of *Injury Facts*®, the 2001 NCHS and CFOI data were used to produce final estimates using the 2-Way Split, the 2002 estimates were revised using more complete state data and 2002 CFOI figures, and the new 2003 estimates were made with the state data available in the spring of 2004.

Nonfatal injury estimates. The Council uses the concept of "disabling injury" to define the kinds of injuries included in its estimates. See page 23 for the definition of disabling injury and the National Health Interview Survey (NHIS) injury definitions.

Injury-to-death ratios. There is no national injury surveillance system that provides disabling injury estimates on a current basis. The National Health Interview Survey, a household survey conducted by the NCHS (see page 23), produces national estimates using its own definition of injury (Schiller & Bernadel, 2004). For this reason, the Council uses injury-to-death ratios to estimate nonfatal disabling injuries for the current year. Complete documentation of the procedure, effective with the 1993 edition, may be found in Landes, Ginsburg, Hoskin, and Miller (1990). The resulting estimates are not direct measures of nonfatal injuries and should not be compared with prior years.

Population sources. All population figures used in computing rates are taken from various reports published by the Bureau of the Census, U.S. Department of Commerce, on their Internet web site (www.census.gov). *Resident* population is used for computing rates.

Costs (pp. 4–7). The procedures for estimating the economic losses due to fatal and nonfatal unintentional injuries were extensively revised for the 1993 edition of *Accident Facts*®. New components were added, new benchmarks adopted, and a new discount rate assumed. All of these changes resulted in significantly higher cost estimates. For this reason, it must be reemphasized that the cost estimates should not be compared to those in earlier editions of the book.

The Council's general philosophy underlying its cost estimates is that the figures represent income not received or expenses incurred because of fatal and nonfatal unintentional injuries. Stated this way, the Council's cost estimates are a measure of the economic impact of unintentional injuries and may be compared to other economic measures such as gross domestic product, per capita income, or personal consumption expenditures. (See page 91 and "lost quality of life" [p. 177] for a discussion of injury costs for cost-benefit analysis.)

The general approach followed was to identify a benchmark unit cost for each component, adjust the benchmark to the current year using an appropriate inflator, estimate the number of cases to which the component applied, and compute the product. Where possible, benchmarks were obtained for each class: Motor Vehicle, Work, Home, and Public.

Wage and productivity losses include the value of wages, fringe benefits, and household production for all classes, and travel delay for the Motor Vehicle class.

For fatalities, the present value of after-tax wages, fringe benefits, and household production was computed using the human capital method. The procedure incorporates data on life expectancy from the NCHS life tables, employment likelihood from the Bureau of Labor Statistics household survey, and mean earnings from the Bureau of the Census money income survey. The discount rate used was 4%, reduced from 6% used

in earlier years. The present value obtained is highly sensitive to the discount rate; the lower the rate, the greater the present value.

For permanent partial disabilities, an average of 17% of earning power is lost (Berkowitz & Burton, 1987). The incidence of permanent disabilities, adjusted to remove intentional injuries, was computed from data on hospitalized cases from the National Hospital Discharge Survey (NHDS) and nonhospitalized cases from the National Health Interview Survey and National Council on Compensation Insurance data on probabilities of disability by nature of injury and part of body injured.

For temporary disabilities, an average daily wage, fringe benefit, and household production loss was calculated and this was multiplied by the number of days of restricted activity from the NHIS.

Travel delay costs were obtained from the Council's estimates of the number of fatal, injury, and property damage crashes and an average delay cost per crash from Miller et al. (1991).

Medical expenses, including ambulance and helicopter transport costs, were estimated for fatalities, hospitalized cases, and nonhospitalized cases in each class.

The incidence of hospitalized cases was derived from the NHDS data adjusted to eliminate intentional injuries. Average length of stay was benchmarked from Miller, Pindus, Douglass, and Rossman (1993b) and adjusted to estimate lifetime length of stay. The cost per hospital day was benchmarked to the National Medical Expenditure Survey (NMES).

Nonhospitalized cases were estimated by taking the difference between total NHIS injuries and hospitalized cases. Average cost per case was based on NMES data adjusted for inflation and lifetime costs.

Medical cost of fatalities was benchmarked to data from the National Council on Compensation Insurance (1989) to which was added the cost of a premature funeral and coroner costs (Miller et al., 1991).

Cost per ambulance transport was benchmarked to NMES data, and cost per helicopter transport was benchmarked to data in Miller et al. (1993a). The number of cases transported was based on data from Rice and MacKenzie (1989) and the National Electronic Injury Surveillance System.

Administrative expenses include the administrative cost of private and public insurance, which represents the cost of having insurance, and police and legal costs.

The administrative cost of motor-vehicle insurance was the difference between premiums earned (adjusted to remove fire, theft, and casualty premiums) and pure losses incurred, based on data from A. M. Best. Workers' compensation insurance administration was based on A. M. Best data for private carriers and regression estimates using Social Security Administration data for state funds and the self-insured. Administrative costs of public insurance (mainly Medicaid and Medicare) amount to about 4% of the medical expenses paid by public insurance, which were determined from Rice and MacKenzie (1989) and Hensler et al. (1991).

Average police costs for motor-vehicle crashes were taken from Miller et al. (1991) and multiplied by the Council's estimates of the number of fatal, injury, and property damage crashes.

Legal expenses include court costs, and plaintiffs' and defendants' time and expenses. Hensler et al. (1991) provided data on the proportion of injured persons who hire a lawyer, file a claim, and get compensation. Kakalik and Pace (1986) provided data on costs per case.

Fire losses were based on data published by the National Fire Protection Association in the *NFPA Journal*. The allocation into the classes was based on the property use for structure fires and other NFPA data for nonstructure fires.

Motor-vehicle damage costs were benchmarked to Blincoe and Faigin (1992) and multiplied by the Council's estimates of crash incidence.

Employer costs for work injuries is an estimate of the productivity costs incurred by employers. It assumes each fatality or permanent injury resulted in 4 person-months of disruption, serious injuries 1 person-month, and minor to moderate injuries 2 person-days. All injuries to nonworkers were assumed to involve 2 days

of worker productivity loss. Average hourly earnings for supervisors and nonsupervisory workers were computed and then multiplied by the incidence and hours lost per case. Property damage and production delays (except motor-vehicle related) are not included in the estimates but can be substantial.

Lost quality of life is the difference between the value of a statistical fatality or statistical injury and the value of after-tax wages, fringe benefits, and household production. Because this does not represent real income not received or expenses incurred, it is not included in the total economic cost figure. If included, the resulting *comprehensive costs* can be used in cost-benefit analysis because the total costs then represent the maximum amount society should spend to prevent a statistical death or injury.

Work deaths and injuries (p. 48). The method for estimating total work-related deaths and injuries is discussed above. The breakdown of deaths by industry division for the current year is obtained from the CFOI and state Injury Mortality Tabulation figures using the link-relative technique (also discussed above).

The estimate of nonfatal disabling injuries by industry division is made by multiplying the estimate of employment for each industry division by the BLS estimate of the incidence rate of cases involving days away from work for each division (e.g., BLS, 2003) and then adjusting the results so that they add to the work-injury total previously established. The "private sector" average incidence rate is used for the government division, which is not covered in the BLS survey.

Employment. The employment estimates for 1992 to the present were changed for the 1998 edition. Estimates for these years in prior editions are not comparable. The total employment figure used by the Council represents the number of persons in the civilian labor force, aged 16 and older, who were wage or salary workers, self-employed, or unpaid family workers, plus active-duty military personnel resident in the U.S. The total employment estimate is a combination of three figures — total civilian employment from the Current Population Survey (CPS) as published in *Employment and Earnings*, plus the difference between total resident population and total civilian population, which represents active duty military personnel.

Employment by industry is obtained from an unpublished Bureau of Labor Statistics table titled "Employed and experience unemployed persons by detailed industry and class of worker, Annual Average [year] (based on CPS)."

Time lost (p. 51) is the product of the number of cases and the average time lost per case. Deaths average 150 workdays lost in the current year and 5,850 in future years; permanent disabilities involve 75 and 565 days lost in current and future years, respectively; temporary disabilities involve 17 days lost in the current year only. Off-the-job injuries to workers are assumed to result in similar lost time.

Off-the-job (p. 52) deaths and injuries are estimated by assuming that employed persons incur injuries at the same rate as the entire population.

Motor-Vehicle section (pp. 86–117). Estimates of miles traveled, registered vehicles, and licensed drivers are published by the Federal Highway Administration in *Highway Statistics* and *Traffic Volume Trends*.

In addition to the death certificate data from NCHS and state registrars, the Council receives annual summary reports of traffic crash characteristics from about 15 states. Most national estimates are made using various ratios and percent distributions from the state crash data.

Beginning with the 1998 edition of *Accident Facts®*, national estimates of crashes by manner of collision (p. 90) and motor-vehicles involved in crashes by type of vehicle (p. 100) are made using the percent changes from the previous year to the current year as reported by the states. This percent change is then applied to benchmark figures obtained from the National Highway Traffic Safety Administration (NHTSA), Fatality Analysis Reporting System (FARS), and General Estimates System (GES) data for the previous year, which yields the current year estimates. These current year estimates are then adjusted to add to the Councils overall number of deaths, injuries, and fatal, injury, and property damage–only crashes that are listed on page 86. Because of these changes, comparisons to previous years should not be made.

Berkowitz, M., & Burton, J.F., Jr. (1987). *Permanent Disability Benefits in Workers' Compensation.* Kalamazoo, MI: W.E. Upjohn Institute for Employment Research.

Blincoe, L.J., & Faigin, B.M. (1992). *Economic Cost of Motor Vehicle Crashes,* 1990. Springfield, VA: National Technical Information Service.

Bureau of Labor Statistics [BLS]. (1992). *Occupational Injury & Illness Classification Manual.* Itasca, IL: National Safety Council.

Bureau of Labor Statistics [BLS]. (2003, December 18). *Workplace Injuries and Illnesses in 2002.* Press release USDL-03-913.

Hensler, D.R., Marquis, M.S., Abrahamse, A.F., Berry, S.H., Ebener, P.A., Lewis, E.D., Lind, E.A., MacCoun, R.J., Manning, W.G., Rogowski, J.A., & Vaiana, M.E. (1991). *Compensation for Accidental Injuries in the United States.* Santa Monica, CA: The RAND Corporation.

Hoyert, D.L., Arias, E., Smith, B.L., Murphy, S.L., & Kochanek, K.D. (2001). Deaths: final data for 1999. *National Vital Statistics Reports, 49*(8).

Kakalik, J.S., & Pace, N. (1986). *Costs and Compensation Paid in Tort Litigation.* R-3391-ICJ. Santa Monica, CA: The RAND Corporation.

Landes, S.R., Ginsburg, K.M., Hoskin, A.F., & Miller, T.A. (1990). *Estimating Nonfatal Injuries.* Itasca, IL: Statistics Department, National Safety Council.

Miller, T., Viner, J., Rossman, S., Pindus, N., Gellert, W., Douglass, J., Dillingham, A., & Blomquist, G. (1991). *The Costs of Highway Crashes.* Springfield, VA: National Technical Information Service.

Miller, T.R., Brigham, P.A., Cohen, M.A., Douglass, J.B., Galbraith, M.S., Lestina, D.C., Nelkin, V.S., Pindus, N.M., & Smith-Regojo, P. (1993a). Estimating the costs to society of cigarette fire injuries. *Report to Congress in Response to the Fire Safe Cigarette Act of 1990.* Washington, DC: U.S. Consumer Product Safety Commission.

Miller, T.R., Pindus, N.M., Douglass, J.B., & Rossman, S.B. (1993b). *Nonfatal Injury Incidence, Costs, and Consequences: A Data Book.* Washington, DC: The Urban Institute Press.

Rice, D.P., & MacKenzie, E.J. (1989). *Cost of Injury in the United States: A Report to Congress.* Atlanta, GA: Centers for Disease Control and Prevention.

Schiller, J.S., & Bernadel, L. (2004). Summary health statistics for the U.S. population: National health interview survey, 2002. *Vital and Health Statistics, Series 10,* No. 220. Hyattsville, MD: National Center for Health Statistics.

Toscano, G., & Windau, J. (1994). The changing character of fatal work injuries. *Monthly Labor Review, 117*(10), 17-28.

World Health Organization. (1977). *Manual of the International Statistical Classification of Diseases, Injuries, and Causes of Death.* Geneva, Switzerland: Author.

World Health Organization. (1992). *International Statistical Classification of Diseases and Related Health Problems* — Tenth Revision. Geneva, Switzerland: Author.

SELECTED UNINTENTIONAL-INJURY CODE GROUPINGS

Manner of Injury	ICD-9 Codes[a]	ICD-10 Codes[b]	Comparability Ratio[c]	OI & ICM[d] Event Codes
Unintentional Injuries	E800–E869, E880–E929[e]	V01–X59, Y85–Y86	1.0305 (1.0278–1.0333)[f]	00–60, 63–9999
Railway accident	E800–E807	V05, V15, V80.6, V81(.2–.9)	n/a	44
Motor-vehicle accident	E810–E825	V02–V04, V09.0, V09.2, V12–V14, V19.0–V19.2, V19.4–V19.6, V20–V79, V80.3–V80.5, V81.0–V81.1, V82.0–V82.1, V83–V86, V87.0–V87.8, V88.0–V88.8, V89.0, V89.2	0.9754 (0.9742–0.9766)	41, 42, 43
Water transport accident	E830–E838	V90–V94	n/a	45
Air transport accident	E840–E845	V95–V97	n/a	46
Poisoning by solids & liquids	E850–58, E860–66	X40–X49	n/a	344
Poisoning by gases and vapors	E867–E869			341
Falls	E880–E888	W00–W19	0.8409 (0.8313–0.8505)	1
Fires and burns	E890–E899	X00–X09	0.9743 (0.9568–0.9918)	51
Drowning	E910	W65–W74	0.9965 (0.9716–1.0213)	381
Suffocation by ingestion or inhalation	E911–E912	W78–W80	n/a	382
Mechanical suffocation	E913	W75–W77, W81–W84	n/a	383, 384, 389
Firearms	E922	W32–W34	1.0579 (1.0331–1.0828)	0220, 0222, 0229 with source = 911[g]

Source: National Safety Council.
Note: n/a means comparability ratio not calculated or does not meet standards of reliability or precision.
[a]WHO (1977).
[b]WHO (1992).
[c]Hoyert, Arias, Smith, et al. (2001). Table III.

[d]BLS (1992).
[e]The National Safety Council has used E800–E949 for unintentional injuries. The code group in the table omits complications and misadventures of surgical and medical care (E870–E879) and adverse effects of drugs in therapeutic use (E930–E949).
[f]Figures in parentheses are the 95% confidence interval for the comparability ratio.
[g]Struck by flying object where the source of injury was a bullet.

OTHER SOURCES

The following organizations may be useful for obtaining more current data or more detailed information on various subjects in *Injury Facts®*.

American Association of Poison Control Centers
3201 New Mexico Avenue, Suite 310
Washington, DC 20016
(202) 362-7217
www.aapcc.org
aapcc@poison.org

Bureau of Labor Statistics
U.S. Department of Labor
2 Massachusetts Avenue, NE
Washington, DC 20212
(202) 691-7828
www.bls.gov
blsdata_staff@bls.gov

Bureau of the Census
U.S. Department of Commerce
Public Information Office
Washington, DC 20233-8200
(301) 457-2794
www.census.gov

Bureau of Justice Statistics
810 7th Street, NW
Washington, DC 20531
(202) 307-5933
www.ojp.usdoj.gov

Bureau of Transportation Statistics
U.S. Department of Transportation
400 7th Street, SW, Room 3103
Washington, DC 20590
(800) 853-1352
www.bts.gov
answers@bts.gov

Centers for Disease Control and Prevention
1600 Clifton Road
Atlanta, GA 30333
(404) 639-3534 or (800) 311-3435
www.cdc.gov

Chemical Safety Board
2175 K Street, NW, Suite 400
Washington, DC 20037
(202) 261-7600
www.chemsafety.gov
info@csb.gov

Eno Transportation Foundation
1634 I Street, NW, Suite 500
Washington, DC 20006
(202) 879-4700
www.enotrans.com

Environmental Protection Agency, U.S.
1200 Pennsylvania Avenue, NW
Washington, DC 20460
(202) 260-2090
www.epa.gov
public-access@epa.gov

European Agency for Safety and Health at Work
Gran Via, 33
E-48009 Bilbao, Spain
Phone: +34 944-794-360
Fax: +34 944-794-383
http://europe.osha.eu.int
information@osha.eu.int

Federal Aviation Administration
U.S. Department of Transportation
National Aviation Safety Data Analysis Center
800 Independence Avenue, SW
Washington, DC 20591
(202) 366-4000
www.faa.gov

Federal Bureau of Investigation
935 Pennsylvania Avenue, NW
Washington, DC 20535-0001
(202) 324-3000
www.fbi.gov

Federal Highway Administration
U.S. Department of Transportation
400 7th Street, SW
Washington, DC 20590
(202) 366-0660
www.fhwa.dot.gov
execsecretariat.fhwa@fhwa.dot.gov

Federal Motor Carrier Safety Administration
U.S. Department of Transportation
400 7th Street, SW
Washington, DC 20590
(800) 832-5660
www.fmcsa.dot.gov

Federal Railroad Administration
U.S. Department of Transportation
1120 Vermont Avenue, NW
Washington, DC 20590
(202) 366-2760
www.fra.dot.gov

Federal Transit Administration
400 7th Street, SW
Washington, DC 20590
www.fta.dot.gov

FedStats
Gateway to official statistical information available to the
public from more than 100 federal agencies.
www.fedstats.gov

FirstGov
Gateway to federal, state, local, tribal, and international
government websites.
www.firstgov.gov

Insurance Information Institute
110 William Street
New York, NY 10038
(212) 346-5500
www.iii.org

Insurance Institute for Highway Safety
1005 N. Glebe Road, Suite 800
Arlington, VA 22201
(703) 247-1500
www.highwaysafety.org

International Hunter Education Association
P.O. Box 490
Wellington, CO 80549-0490
(970) 568-7954
www.ihea.com
ihea@frii.com

International Labour Office
4, rue des Morillons
CH-1211 Geneva 22
Switzerland
Phone: +41-22-799-6111
Fax: +41-22-798-8685
www.ilo.org
ilo@ilo.org

Mine Safety and Health Administration
1100 Wilson Boulevard, 21st Floor
Arlington, VA 22209-3939
(202) 693-9400
www.msha.gov

Motorcycle Safety Foundation
2 Jenner Street, Suite 150
Irvine, CA 92718-3812
(714) 727-3227
www.msf-usa.org

National Academy of Social Insurance
1776 Massachusetts Avenue, NW, Suite 615
Washington, DC 20036-1904
(202) 452-8097
www.nasi.org
nasi@nasi.org

National Center for Education Statistics
U.S. Department of Education
1990 K Street, NW
Washington, DC 20006
(202) 502-7300
http://nces.ed.gov

National Center for Health Statistics
3311 Toledo Road, Room 2217
Hyattsville, MD 20782
(301) 458-4636
www.cdc.gov/nchs

National Center for Injury Prevention and Control
Office Of Communication Resources, Mail Stop K65
4770 Buford Highway, NE
Atlanta, GA 30341-3724
(770) 488-1506
www.cdc.gov/ncipc
ohcinfo@cdc.gov

National Clearinghouse for Alcohol and Drug Information
P.O. Box 2345
Rockville, MD 20847-2345
(301) 468-2600 or (800) 729-6686
www.health.org

National Climatic Data Center
151 Patton Avenue
Asheville, NC 28801-5001
(828) 271-4800
http://lwf.ncdc.noaa.gov/oa/ncdc.html
ncdc.info@noaa.gov

National Collegiate Athletic Association
700 W. Washington Street
P.O. Box 6222
Indianapolis, IN 46206-6222
(317) 917-6222
www.ncaa.org

National Council on Compensation Insurance
901 Peninsula Corporate Circle
Boca Raton, FL 33487
(800) NCCI-123 (800-622-4123)
www.ncci.com

National Fire Protection Association
P.O. Box 9101
Batterymarch Park
Quincy, MA 02269-0910
(617) 770-3000 or (800) 344-3555
www.nfpa.org
osds@nfpa.org

National Highway Traffic Safety Administration
U.S. Department of Transportation
400 7th Street, SW
Washington, DC 20590
(202) 366-0123 or (800) 424-9393
www.nhtsa.dot.gov
    National Center for Statistics and Analysis (NRD-30)
    (202) 366-4198 or (800) 934-8517
    NCSAweb@nhtsa.dot.gov

National Institute for Occupational Safety and Health
Clearinghouse for Occupational Safety and Health
    Information
4676 Columbia Parkway
Cincinnati, OH 45226
(800) 356-4674
www.cdc.gov/niosh
eidtechinfo@cdc.gov

National Spinal Cord Injury Association
6701 Democracy Boulevard, Suite 300-9
Bethesda, MD 20817
(301) 588-6959
www.spinalcord.org
nscia2@aol.com

National Sporting Goods Association
1601 Feehanville Drive, Suite 300
Mt. Prospect, IL 60056
(847) 296-6742
www.nsga.org
info@nsga.org

National Transportation Safety Board
490 L'Enfant Plaza East, SW
Washington, DC 20594
(202) 314-6000
www.ntsb.gov

Occupational Safety and Health Administration
U.S. Department of Labor
Office of Statistics
200 Constitution Avenue, NW
Washington, DC 20210
(800) 321-OSHA (6742)
www.osha.gov

Prevent Blindness America
500 E. Remington Road
Schaumburg, IL 60173
(800) 331-2020
www.preventblindness.org
info@preventblindness.org

Transportation Research Board
500 5th Street, NW
Washington, DC 20001
(202) 334-2934
www.nas.edu/trb

U.S. Coast Guard
2100 2nd Street, SW
Washington, DC 20593-0001
(800) 368-5647
www.uscgboating.org
uscginfoline@gcrm.com

U.S. Consumer Product Safety Commission
National Injury Information Clearinghouse
Washington, DC 20207-0001
(301) 504-0424
www.cpsc.gov
clearinghouse@cpsc.gov

World Health Organization
20, avenue Appia
CH-1211 Geneva 27
Switzerland
Phone: +41-22-791-2111
Fax: +41-22-791-0746
www.who.int
info@who.int

Accident is that occurrence in a sequence of events that produces unintended injury, death, or property damage. *Accident* refers to the event, not the result of the event (see *unintentional injury*).

Death from accident is a death that occurs within one year of the accident.

Disabling injury is an injury causing death, permanent disability, or any degree of temporary total disability beyond the day of the injury.

Fatal accident is an accident that results in one or more deaths within one year.

Home is a dwelling and its premises within the property lines including single-family dwellings and apartment houses, duplex dwellings, boarding and rooming houses, and seasonal cottages. Excluded from *home* are barracks, dormitories, and resident institutions.

Incidence rate, as defined by OSHA, is the number of occupational injuries and/or illnesses or lost workdays per 100 full-time employees (see formula on page 61).

Injury is physical harm or damage to the body resulting from an exchange, usually acute, of mechanical, chemical, thermal, or other environmental energy that exceeds the body's tolerance.

Motor vehicle is any mechanically or electrically powered device not operated on rails, upon which or by which any person or property may be transported upon a land highway. The load on a motor vehicle or trailer attached to it is considered part of the vehicle. Tractors and motorized machinery are included while self-propelled in transit or used for transportation. *Nonmotor vehicle* is any road vehicle other than a motor vehicle, such as a bicycle or animal-drawn vehicle, except a coaster wagon, child's sled, child's tricycle, child's carriage, and similar means of transportation; persons using these latter means of transportation are considered pedestrians.

Motor-vehicle accident is an unstabilized situation that includes at least one harmful event (injury or property damage) involving a motor vehicle in transport (in motion, in readiness for motion, or on a roadway but not parked in a designated parking area) that does not result from discharge of a firearm or explosive device and does not directly result from a cataclysm. [See Committee on Motor Vehicle Traffic Accident Classification (1997), *Manual on Classification of Motor Vehicle Traffic Accidents*, ANSI D16.1-1996, Itasca, IL: National Safety Council.]

Motor-vehicle traffic accident is a motor-vehicle accident that occurs on a trafficway — a way or place, any part of which is open to the use of the public for the purposes of vehicular traffic. *Motor-vehicle nontraffic accident* is any motor-vehicle accident that occurs entirely in any place other than a trafficway.

Nonfatal injury accident is an accident in which at least one person is injured and no injury results in death.

Occupational illness is any abnormal condition or disorder other than one resulting from an occupational injury caused by exposure to environmental factors associated with employment. It includes acute and chronic illnesses or diseases that may be caused by inhalation, absorption, ingestion, or direct contact (see also page 61).

Occupational injury is any injury such as a cut, fracture, sprain, amputation, etc., which results from a work accident or from a single instantaneous exposure in the work environment (see also page 61).

Pedalcycle is a vehicle propelled by human power and operated solely by pedals; excludes mopeds.

Pedestrian is any person involved in a motor-vehicle accident who is not in or upon a motor vehicle or nonmotor vehicle. Includes persons injured while using a coaster wagon, child's tricycle, roller skates, etc. Excludes persons boarding, alighting, jumping, or falling from a motor vehicle in transport who are considered occupants of the vehicle.

Permanent disability (or permanent impairment) includes any degree of permanent nonfatal injury. It includes any injury that results in the loss or complete loss of use of any part of the body or in any permanent impairment of functions of the body or a part thereof.

Property damage accident is an accident that results in property damage but in which no person is injured.

Public accident is any accident other than motor-vehicle that occurs in the public use of any premises. Includes deaths in recreation (swimming, hunting, etc.), in transportation except motor-vehicle, public buildings, etc., and from widespread natural disasters even though some may have happened on home premises. Excludes accidents to persons in the course of gainful employment.

Source of injury is the principal object such as tool, machine, or equipment involved in the accident and is usually the object inflicting injury or property damage. Also called *agency* or *agent*.

Temporary total disability is an injury that does not result in death or permanent disability but that renders the injured person unable to perform regular duties or activities on one or more full calendar days after the day of the injury.

Total cases include all work-related deaths and illnesses and those work-related injuries that result in loss of consciousness, restriction of work or motion, or transfer to another job, or require medical treatment other than first aid.

Unintentional injury is the preferred term for accidental injury in the public health community. It refers to the *result* of an accident.

Work hours are the total number of hours worked by all employees. They are usually compiled for various levels, such as an establishment, a company, or an industry. A work hour is the equivalent of one employee working one hour.

Work injuries (including occupational illnesses) are those that arise out of and in the course of gainful employment regardless of where the accident or exposure occurs. Excluded are work injuries to private household workers and injuries occurring in connection with farm chores that are classified as home injuries.

Workers are all persons gainfully employed, including owners, managers, other paid employees, the self-employed, and unpaid family workers but excluding private household workers.

Work/Motor-vehicle duplication includes *work injuries* that occur in *motor-vehicle accidents* (see definitions for work injuries and motor-vehicle accident on this page).

INDEX